# RHETORIC AND MEDICINE IN EARLY MODERN EUROPE

# Literary and Scientific Cultures of Early Modernity

***Series editors*:**



For more than a decade now, *Literary and Scientific Cultures of Early Modernity* has provided a forum for groundbreaking work on the relations between literary and scientific discourses in Europe, during a period when both fields were in a crucial moment of historical formation. We welcome proposals that address the many overlaps between modes of imaginative writing typical of the sixteenth and seventeenth centuries—poetics, rhetoric, prose narrative, dramatic production, utopia—and the vocabularies, conceptual models, and intellectual methods of newly emergent 'scientific' fields such as medicine, astronomy, astrology, alchemy, psychology, mapping, mathematics, or natural history. In order to reflect the nature of intellectual inquiry during the period, the series is interdisciplinary in orientation and publishes monographs, edited collections, and selected critical editions of primary texts relevant to an understanding of the mutual implication of literary and scientific epistemologies.

# Rhetoric and Medicine in Early Modern Europe

Edited by
STEPHEN PENDER
*University of Windsor, Canada*

and

NANCY S. STRUEVER
*The Johns Hopkins University, USA*

Routledge
Taylor & Francis Group
LONDON AND NEW YORK

First Published 2012 by Ashgate Publisher

2 Park Square, Milton Park, Abingdon, Oxon OX14 4RN
711 Third Avenue, New York, NY 10017, USA

*Routledge is an imprint of the Taylor & Francis Group, an informa business*

First issued in paperback 2016



**British Library Cataloguing in Publication Data**
Rhetoric and medicine in early modern Europe. – (Literary and scientific cultures of early modernity)
1. Rhetoric – Europe – History – 16th century. 2. Rhetoric – Europe – History – 17th century. 3. Rhetoric – Europe – History – 18th century. 4. Medicine – Language – History – 16th century. 5. Medicine – Language – History – 17th century. 6. Medicine – Language – History – 18th century.
I. Series II. Pender, Stephen, 1967– III. Struever, Nancy S.
808'.0094-dc23

**Library of Congress Cataloging-in-Publication Data**
Rhetoric and medicine in early modern Europe / edited by Stephen Pender and Nancy S. Struever.
p. cm. — (Literary and scientific cultures of early modernity)
Includes bibliographical references and index.
ISBN 978-1-4094-3022-3 (hardcover: alk. paper)
1. Rhetoric—Europe—History. 2. Medicine—Language—History. 3. Rhetoric—Early works to 1800. 4. Literature and science—Europe—History. 5. Europe—History—1492–1648. 6. Europe—History—1648–1715. I. Pender, Stephen, 1967– II. Struever, Nancy S.
P301.3.E85R48 2012
808.0094—dc23

2012011241

ISBN 978-1-4094-3022-3 (hbk)
ISBN 978-1-138-24622-5 (pbk)

# Contents

# List of Contributors

**Andrea Carlino** teaches history of medicine at the University of Geneva. In the field of the history of anatomy and of scientific visual culture, he has published *Books of the Body: Anatomical Ritual and Renaissance Learning* (Chicago and London 1999), *Paper Bodies: A Catalogue of Anatomical Fugitive Sheets (1538–1687)* (London 1999) and, in collaboration with Deanna Petherbridge and Claude Ritschard, the catalogue of the exhibition *Corps à vif: Art et Anatomie* (Geneva 1998). His current research is focused on the relationship of literature, medicine, and natural philosophy, on the humanist foundations of scientific culture, as well as on literary practices and techniques in early modern science and medicine. He has recently co-edited *Littérature et médecine: approches et perspectives* (XVI$^{e}$-XIXe siècles) (Geneva 2007) and, with Michel Jeanneret, *Vulgariser la médecine: A la recherche d'un style médical en France et en Italie (XVI et XVII siècles)* (Geneva 2008).

**Guido Giglioni** is the Cassamarca Lecturer in Neo-Latin Cultural and Intellectual History 1400 to1700 at the Warburg Institute, University of London. He is the author of *Immaginazione e malattia. Saggio su Jan Baptiste van Helmont* (Angeli, 2000) and *Latin Manuscripts of Francis Glisson (1): Philosophical Papers* (Cambridge Wellcome Unit, 1996) as well as numerous articles on Cardano, women in early modern science, Boyle, Leibniz, and Tommaso Campanella.

**Daniel M. Gross** is associate professor of English and director of composition at the University of California, Irvine. Currently at work on a monograph entitled *The Art of Listening*, he has published *The Secret History of Emotion: From Aristotle's* Rhetoric *to Modern Brain Science* (Chicago, 2006) and, with Ansgar Kemman, edited *Heidegger and Rhetoric* (SUNY, 2005) and numerous articles in, for example, *History of the Human Sciences*, *Rhetorica*, and *Philosophy and Rhetoric*.

**Jean Dietz Moss** is professor emerita of English at The Catholic University of America. She is the author of numerous books and articles including, as editor, *Rhetoric and Praxis: The Contribution of Classical Rhetoric to Practical Reasoning* (Catholic University of America, 1986), *Novelties in the Heavens: Rhetoric and Science in the Copernican Controversy* (Chicago, 1993) and, with William Wallace, *Rhetoric and Dialectic in the Time of Galileo* (Catholic University of America, 2003).

**Stephen Pender** is associate professor, English, at the University of Windsor, Canada and is a specialist in the poetry and prose of early modern Britain, intellectual history, the history of medicine, and the history of rhetoric. He has published articles in *Philosophy and Rhetoric*, *Rhetorica*, *Early Science and*

*Medicine*, the *British Journal for the History of Science*, and the *Dalhousie Review*, as well as a number of chapters in collections of essays. He is currently at work on the relationship between rhetoric, medicine, and emotion in early modern England, medical thought in contemporary historiography, the history of the imagination, and laughter.

**Amy M. Schmitter** is associate professor and associate chair in the department of philosophy, University of Alberta, Canada. She has taught at the University of Pittsburgh and the University of New Mexico, and has held a fellowship at the Stanford Humanities Centre, Stanford University. She is a specialist in the history of the passions and in early modern philosophy, and has published numerous articles in *Philosophical Studies, Journal of the History of Ideas, Archiv für Geschichte der Philosophie*, and in several collection of essays. She is at work on a book entitled *Passions, Affects, and Sentiments: A Genealogy of Early Modern Theories of the Emotions*.

**Julie R. Solomon** is former scholar-in-residence at The American University in Washington, D.C. and is author of *Objectivity in the Making: Francis Bacon and the Politics of Inquiry* (Johns Hopkins, 1998), editor, with Catherine Gimelli Martin, of *Francis Bacon and the Refiguring of Early Modern Thought* (Ashgate, 2005), and numerous articles on Calvin, Shakespeare, and Thomas Harriot.

**Nancy Struever** is professor emerita of history at Johns Hopkins University. Among her numerous publications are *The Language of History in the Renaissance: Rhetoric and Historical Consciousness in Florentine Humanism* (Princeton, 1970), *Theory as Practice: Ethical Inquiry in the Renaissance* (Chicago, 1992), and, most recently, *The History of Rhetoric and the Rhetoric of History* (Ashgate, 2009) and *Rhetoric, Modality, Modernity* (Chicago, 2009).

**Richard Sugg** is research fellow in literature and medicine in the department of English studies at Durham University. He is the author of *John Donne* (Palgrave, 2007) and *Murder After Death: Literature and Anatomy in Early Modern England* (Cornell, 2007), and he is at work on books on the soul and on early modern cannibalism and medicine.

**Grant Williams** is associate professor of English at Carleton University, Ottawa, Canada and editor, with Christopher Ivic, of *Forgetting in Early Modern English Literature and Culture: Lethe's Legacy* (Routledge, 2004) and, with Donald Beecher, of *Ars reminiscendi: Mind and Memory in Renaissance Culture* (Centre for Reformation and Renaissance Studies, 2009). He is currently working on a book on the ethical dimensions of the blazon in early modernity.

# Acknowledgements and Permissions

The editors would like to thank all participants in the original series of panel discussions at the Renaissance Society of America conference in Scottsdale, Arizona, 2003, as well as those who offered us papers and advice over the many years this collection was taking shape. Stephen Pender acknowledges the support of a Standard Research Grant in intellectual history from the Social Sciences and Humanities Research Council of Canada and funds from the Research Leadership Chair Programme at the University of Windsor, Canada. He also thanks librarians and staff at the Leddy Library, University of Windsor, the British Library, the Wellcome Institute, Fisher Rare Books Library, the University of Toronto, the Union Theological Seminary, the New York Public Library, and the following individuals: D.D.C. Chambers, Thomas Dilworth, Erika Gaffney, David Galbraith, Elizabeth Harvey, Dale Jacobs, C. Suzanne Matheson, Jeff Noonan, Katherine Quinsey, Jonathan Sawday, Michael Schoenfeldt, Nancy S. Stuever, Gregory Taylor, Christopher Tindale, Richard Todd, Patricia Vicari, and all our patient contributors. Elisa Durante deserves special mention, and profound thanks, as research assistant for this project.

The translation of Andrea Carlino's paper is printed with the kind permission of the author, and the revision of Stephen Pender's paper is printed with the permission of Christoph Lüthy, editor of *Early Science and Medicine*, in which it first appeared, and Brill.

# Introduction
# Reading Physicians

Stephen Pender

Among the *badinages* and missives meant for paramours and patrons, techy suitors and incorrigible sons in W. Elder's *Pearls of Eloquence, or The School of Complements* (1656) is a model exchange between a patient and a physician. The "sick loving Patient" urges his physician to his bedside, while the physician advises his patient against excessive passion: "let a merry heart be your best Physician," he writes, "for conceit is hurtfull, if it be not contentive, and it is past the reach of my Reason to cure a corrupted mind." But psychic cure is the physician's point: he gently cautions against hypochondriasis, delicately asserts his authority, and insists that his client embrace patience and "put off melancholly," lest strong feeling amplify his pain.[1] This imagined correspondence—in which the patient is importuning but deferential, the physician generous, voluble—suggests civility and concern, consolation and reciprocity of sentiment. "[I]magine that I am with you," the physician writes, and do not be "weak in spirit." As much as the physician promises freedom from both illness and treatment, he also assures: a sound imagination, moderate passions, and calm spirits are crucial to recovery, prophylaxes against relapse. Extant seventeenth century letters from physicians to patients enjoin similar caution: while explaining the cause of one distemper, John Symcotts, for example, insists that his patient forego his "author Vaughan," whose "vain and frivolous" prognostications discomfort.[2] Although some physicians were reluctant to consult patients from afar,[3] casebooks and *consilia*, diaries and

[1] W. Elder, *Pearls of Eloquence, or The School of Complements* (London, 1656), 123–24. For similar, model letters, in this case between patients, see W. P., *The Wits Academy: or, The Muses Delight* (London, 1677), 90–92.

[2] *A Seventeenth-Century Doctor and His Patients: John Symcotts, 1592? –1662*, ed. F. N. L. Poynter and W. J. Bishop, Publications of the Bedfordshire Historical Society, vol. 31 (Streatley, 1951), 25–6. Symcotts has in mind the popular text by William Vaughan, *Approved Directions for Health, Both Naturall and Artificiall: Derived from the Best Physicians as well Modern as Ancient* (London, 1612 [1600, 1602, 1607, etc.]).

[3] See, for example, the letter from Thomas Hariot to Theodor Turquet de Mayerne, in which Hariot writes, "I thought it neither necessary nor useful to confer by letter on the details in a case [cancer, it seems] so bristling with difficulties, and it was preferable to proceed from ocular examination and mutual consultation for all to be properly understood" (John W. Shirley, *Thomas Hariot: a Biography* [Oxford: Oxford University Press, 1983], 436–8). For examples of letters between physicians, see Josiah C. Trent, "Five Letters

collections of *historiae* evidence rich, varied forms of correspondence between sufferers and physicians, including texts that detail complex medical recipes, offer counsel, and probe regimen, recovery, reputation.[4]

Yet this imagined exchange is refractive, and invites critique. Aside from a request that the physician visit the sickbed, Elder envisions an ideal interaction, untainted by the frustrations and disappointments that accompanied medical treatment, free from criticisms directed at medical practitioners, and evacuated of the power that defined patient-physician relationships. Arguments about the uncertainty of medicine, its perils and promises, the incommensurability of medical theory and practice, the character and conduct of its agents,[5] and the status

---

of Marcus Aurelius Severinus," *Bulletin of the History of Medicine* 15 (1944): 306–323. Letters to and from patients are often modelled on *consilia*; see Brian Nance, "Wondrous Experience as Text: Valleriola and the *Observationes Medicinales*," in *Textual Healing: Essays on Medieval and Early Modern Medicine*, ed. Elizabeth Lane Furdell (Leiden: Brill, 2005), 101–117, esp. 114. Jan Groeneveldt et al.'s *Oracle for the Sick* (London, 1685) is expressly devoted to treating patients by letter. On the emergent *res publica medicorum*, see Ian Maclean, "The Medical Republic of Letters before the Thirty Years War," *Intellectual History Review* 18.1 (2008): 15–30 and sources. Maclean notes that the first book with the title 'medical letters' (1521) included "humanist discussion of ancient sources ...; consilia; polemic with colleagues over remedies ...; engagement with the latest publications and latest ideas; accounts of rare and marvellous happenings; acts of eye-witnessing" (19).

4 See Michael MacDonald, *Mystical Bedlam: Madness, Anxiety, and Healing in Seventeenth-Century England* (Cambridge: Cambridge University Press, 1981), Roy Porter, "The Patient's View: Doing Medical History from Below," *Theory and Society* 14.2 (1985): 175–98, Lucinda McCray Beier, *Sufferers and Healers: The Experience of Illness in Seventeenth-Century England* (London: Routledge and Kegan Paul, 1997), Margaret Pelling, *Medical Conflicts in Early Modern London: Patronage, Physicians, and Irregular Practitioners, 1550–1640* (Oxford: Clarendon Press, 2003), esp. 225–74, and *Historia: Empiricism and Erudition in Early Modern Europe*, ed. Gianna Pomata and Nancy G. Siraisi (Cambridge, MA.: MIT Press, 2005). See also Ronald C. Sawyer, "Patients, Healers, and Disease in the Southeast Midlands, 1597–1634" (Ph.D. Dissertation, University of Wisconsin-Madison, 1986). For a later period, see Dora B. Wiener, *The Citizen-Patient in Revolutionary and Imperial Paris* (Baltimore: Johns Hopkins, 1993). On early modern English letter writing, see Gary Schneider, *The Culture of Epistolarity: Vernacular Letters and Letter Writing in Early Modern England, 1500–1700* (Cranbury, NJ: Associated University Presses, 2005), and on medical letters, see E. Foster, "From a Patient's Point of View: Illness and Heath in the Letters of Lisolette von der Pfalz (1652–1722)," *Bulletin of the History of Medicine* 60 (1986): 297–320,M. Louis-Courvoisier and A. Mauron, "'He Found Me Very Well; for Me, I Was Still Feeling Sick': the Strange Worlds of Physicians and Patients in the 18th and 21st Centuries," *Journal of Medical Ethics: Medical Humanities* 28 (2002): 9–13, and especially Wayne Wild, *Medicine-By-Post: The Changing Voice of Illness in Eighteenth-Century British Consultation Letters and Literature* (Amsterdam: Rodopi, 2006).

5 These are numerous but see, for example, John Oberndorff, *The Anatomyes of the True Physician, and Counterfeit Mounte-Bank*, trans. F. H. (London, 1602), John Cotta, *A Short Discoverie of the Unobserved Dangers of Severall Sorts of Ignorant and*

of the profession—one that trafficked in urine and blood, faeces and decay—flourished in medical and non-medical texts and contexts in the sixteenth and seventeenth centuries.[6] Although medicine was frequently lauded in encomia and *paragoni*, usually in university settings, physicians and surgeons were impugned in both learned and popular fora for breaking sabbath or atheism, indifference, incompetence, or lucre. Central to learned criticism is the notion that healing is "oftentymes done more by chaunce, then by any certayne Methode or Reason."[7] To Robert Underwood in 1605, for example, the "chiefest rules of this Art, / yea and his greatest ground, / Stand but on observations, / and on conjectures fraile."[8] In 1616, Geoffrey Goodman offers the derisive suggestion that the fullness of the *materia medica* is related to the deficiency of medical knowledge: the multiplication of remedies preserves the "mysteries and secrets" of the physician's art and "raises the price of their physicke," while physicians "doe but guesse at their physicke."[9] In the preface to *The Passions of the Soul* (1649), Descartes writes that "nowhere is our need to acquire new learning more apparent than in things that concern Medicine." Practitioners are unsure about common illnesses, "which all the most learned Physicians cannot understand, and only aggravate by their remedies when they undertake to dispel them." To Descartes, medicine ignored physics, was poor in theory, and even the most "prudent" physicians were content with maxims and

*Unconsiderate Practisers of Physicke in England* (London, 1612) and Jonathan Goddard, *A Discourse Setting Forth the Unhappy Condition of the Practice of Physick in London* (London, 1670).

6 See Christopher Hill, "The Medical Profession and its Radical Critics," *Change and Continuity in Seventeenth-Century England* (New Haven: Yale University Press, 1991), 157–78 and Harold J. Cook, *The Decline of the Old Medical Regime in Stuart London* (Ithaca and London, 1986). Lucinda Beier usefully summarizes the issues in her *Sufferers and Healers*, 151–81, 242–59, and Winfried Schleiner, *Medical Ethics in the Renaissance* (Washington, D.C.: Georgetown University Press, 1995), esp. 20–29. See also Stephen Pender, "Examples and Experience: the Uncertainty of Medicine," *British Journal for the History of Science* 39.1 (2006): 1–28 and, for similar criticism of the new science, Peter Harrison, "'The Fashioned Image of Poetry or the Regular Instruction of Philosophy?': Truth, Utility, and the Natural Sciences in Early Modern England," in *Science, Literature, and Rhetoric in Early Modern England*, ed. Juliet Cummins and David Burchill (Aldershot: Ashgate, 2007), 15–35. The latter collection does not treat medicine.

7 John Securis, *A Detection and Querimonie of the Daily Enormities and Abuses Committed in Physick* (np, 1566), sig. Biiii$^r$.

8 Underwood, *A New Anatomie. Wherein the Body of Man is Fit and Aptly (Two Wayes) Compared: 1 To a Household, 2 To a Cittie* (London, 1605), 22.

9 *The Fall of Man, or the Corruption of Nature, Proved by the Light of our Naturall Reason* (London, 1616), 97.

rules gleaned from experience alone.[10] Perhaps least susceptible to improvement, to the virtuoso Robert Boyle, was the "semeiotical part" of medicine.[11]

By 1684, in a book dedicated to Boyle, Lionardo di Capoa could declare that physic is "a Profession, so doubtful and uncertain in it self, [that] has neither Learning nor Principles, upon which others may lay any firm Foundation . [it is] an Art, of its own nature in the highest degree uncertain, dubious, and unconstant."[12] Although it was still gentlemanly to have some knowledge of medicine, "especially the Diagonostick part … as also the prognostick part," no "discipline is more subject to deception with regard to cause, than is medicine."[13] In a period that witnessed physicians' and surgeons' uneven arrogation of authority, various attempts to discipline unorthodox practitioners, and an accelerated investment in 'scientific medicine' (in the form of anatomical studies or iatrochemistry, animadversions on the methodus medendi or the classification of fevers), medicine continued to be disparaged as poor philosophy, worse practice, "the lowest of Professions."[14] This ongoing debate was expressly political, as Nancy Struever argues in this volume: uncertainty may inspire dependence on ostensible expertise, and thus enhance physicians' authority, even in the absence of adequate theoretical explanation or suitable etiologies of technique. Still, contractual 'cure agreements,' often specifying exclusivity between patient and practitioner, were broken or contested, for reasons ranging from failure to cure to length of treatment.[15] As Elder's letters show, patients were actively engaged in treatment: some were ready to change

---

10 *The Passions of the Soul*, trans. Stephen H. Voss (Indianapolis and Cambridge: Hackett, 1989), 6–7; on writing as a physician, see 17.

11 Robert Boyle, *The Works of the Honourable Robert Boyle*, ed. Thomas Birch, second edition, 6 vols. (London, 1772), 2.89–90.

12 Lionardo Di Capoa, *The Uncertainty of the Art of Physic*, trans. John Lancaster ( London, 1684), 17, preface sig. B2r, 4.

13 *The Life of Edward, First Lord Herbert of Cherbury, Written by Himself*, ed. J. M. Shuttleworth (London: Oxford University Press, 1976), 21; Friedrich Hoffmann, *Fundamenta Medicinae ex Principiis Naturae Mechanicis in Usum Philiatrorum Succinte Proposita* [1695], trans. Lester S. King ( London: MacDonald, 1971), 115.

14 John Stuteville to Sir Justinian Isham, 12 January 1656, in Frances Parthenope Verney, *Memoirs of the Verney family*, 3 vols. (London: Longman, 1892–1899), 3.200. Pliny, *Naturalis Historiae*, trans. W. H. S. Jones, 10 vols. (Cambridge, MA.: Harvard University Press, 1938), 29.1–8 is the *locus classicus* for discussions of the uncertainty of medicine. See Philemon Holland's translation of Pliny's *History of the World, Commonly Called, The Natural History of C. Plinius Secundus* (London, 1601), book 2, 343–9. As Roger French notes, "Pliny's criticism of doctors may well have shaped later attacks" on medicine (*Medicine Before Science: the Rational and Learned Doctor from the Middle Ages to the Enlightenment* [Cambridge: Cambridge University Press, 2003], 65ff. and citations).

15 Pelling, *Medical Conflicts*, 249–74.

doctors or refuse payment, and many who were able consulted various practitioners during a single illness, to some physicians' consternation.[16]

The pressures of medical uncertainty affected the ways in which physicians and patients imagined not only the negotiation of authority but therapy itself, especially treatment for emotional or psychological distemper. While medical theory and practice was historically contested, eclectic, for distempers caused or exacerbated by passion, early modern physicians embraced a broad, variegated ensemble of remedies, perhaps because physical therapies—bleeding, emetics, laxatives—were frequently ineffective, sometimes perilous. The problem was grave: as the physician Edward Jorden writes, the "perturbations of the minde" are often to blame for disease, and we are like "battered Citties without walles, or shippes tossed in the Sea, exposed to all manner of assaults and daungers, even to the overthrow of our owne bodies." His remedies for hysteria include religious instruction, inspiring contrary passions in sufferers, "divers sorts of fallacies," and "good counsell and perswasions."[17] As Francis Bacon avers in *De dignitate et augmentis scientiarum*, "there is no physician of any skill [*paulo prudentior*] who does not attend to the accidents of the mind [*accidentia animi*]" as essential to both remedy and recovery.[18] Indeed, in Elder's terms, physicians remedy 'hurtful conceits,' assuage the imagination, urge a 'merry heart' as tonic; the 'lowest of professions' confects medical, philosophical, and rhetorical intervention, and has done so since antiquity. And it must: its theoretical and methodological resources are frequently poor, its practice rough and invasive, its results fragile. Perhaps that is why one early modern commonplace insists: *illa medicum informat ubi namque desinit Philosophus ibi incipit Medicus* (that physician informs [us] that where philosophy ends, medicine begins).[19]

---

16 See Pelling, *Medical Conflicts*, esp. 225–32, including sources and, for example, *A Seventeenth-Century Doctor and His Patients*, 28. 'Misomedon,' Mandeville's fictional patient, visits several physicians during his lengthy illness; see *A Treatise*, esp. 19, 28–9. The patient was sometimes figured as both active and passive, as the physician David Abercromby suggests in 1686: the chief "Secret of Physick" consists in the physician's timely application of remedies, but half the work is the patient's, who "must contribute towards his own cure by an exact submission, and scrupulous performance of what he is order'd to do, take, or observe" (*The Discourse of Wit*, 220).

17 *A Briefe Discourse of a Disease Called the Suffocation of the Mother* (London, 1603), 15, 23–5. On Jorden, see the introduction to *Witchcraft and Hysteria in Elizabethan London: Edward Jorden and the Mary Glover Case*, ed. Michael Macdonald (London: Tavistock / Routledge, 1991), vii-lxiv.

18 *The Works of Francis Bacon*, ed. James Spedding et al., 12 vols. (London: Longman, 1857–74), 1.585, 4.378.

19 Everard Digby, *Theoria Analytica* (London, 1579), 374. On Digby, see W. S. Howell, *Logic and Rhetoric in England 1500–1700* (Princeton: Princeton University Press, 1956), 194–96, J. W. Binns, *Intellectual Culture in Elizabethan and Jacobean England: the Latin Writings of the Age* (Leeds: Francis Cairns, 1990), 389 and references (Binns' claims that Digby "still awaits detailed study by professional historians of philosophy") and Nancy

This apothegm rests on ancient authority. Greek and Roman orators, philosophers, and physicians retail broad comparisons between medicine, moral philosophy, and their interventionist programmes; medicine and philosophy shared forms of inference, interest in psychology and physiology, and commitment to theoretical inquiry and empirical practice, one often at odds with the other.[20] From the Hippocratean *On Regimen* through Aristotle's views about the fundamental intrication of *dianoia* and somatic states (especially in the *Physiognomica* [805a1ff.]) to Hellenistic conceptions of hygiene, ancients were certain that bodies affected minds, that the psyche disposed the soma, that medicine and philosophy were consanguine. Habits and sensibilities, temperaments and passions occasioned as well as remedied illness; dietetics might provide "a physiologically founded doctrine of 'the good life.'"[21] Physicians should be skilled philosophers, and the "most accomplished investigators into nature generally push their studies so far

Struever, *Theory as Practice: Ethical Inquiry in the Renaissance* (Chicago: University of Chicago Press, 1992), 135ff. This collocation of healing and philosophical knowledge, medicine and discursive therapy, was explored thoroughly in early modernity. In William Bullein's rangy *A Dialogue against the Fever Pestilence* (1578 [1564]), for example, the characters Antonius and 'Medicus' discuss the virtues of astrological and natural philosophical knowledge for a physician. "What do the knowledge of these thynges profite to Phisike, I praie you tel me?" Antonius asks. Medicus' answer is telling: physicians must have "knowledge of tymes and seasons, and bee acquainted with complexions of men," with the climate, air, and diet. For "where the Philosopher doth leave, there the Phisition doth begin" (*A Dialogue against the Fever Pestilence* [1578 (1564)], ed. Mark W. Bullen and A. H. Bullen [London: Early English Text Society, 1931 (1888)], 32. See also R. Bostocke, *The Difference betwene the Auncient Phisicke ... and the Latter Phisicke Proceeding from Idolaters, Ethnickes, and Heathen* [London, 1585], sig. A5v). The sentiment appears on stage—in his straights, Christopher Marlowe's Doctor Faustus bids philosophy and *oeconomy* farewell "and Galen come" (*Doctor Faustus* in *Marlowe's Doctor Faustus 1604-1616*, ed. W. W. Greg [Oxford: Clarendon Press, 1950], 165 [prologue, 1604, ll. 30–45]). This concept also appears in Paracelsus and Hippocrates; see *Die Grosse Wundarznei* in *Samtliche Werke*, ed. Karl Sudhoff, part 1, X.291 and *Ancient Medicine*, chapter 20)—and is noted with approbation by Robert Boyle: "such is the affinity between Natural Philosophy and Physick, or the dependence of this on that, that we need not wonder at the judicious Observation of *Aristotle*, where he thus writes [de sensu et sensibili, cap.1], *Naturalium fere plurimus & Medicorum, qui magis Philosophice artem prosequuntur, illi quidem finiunt ad ea, quae de Medicina, hi vero ex iis quae de Natura, incipiunt quae de Medicina*" (Boyle, *Usefulness of Natural Philosophy* [1663], part 2, section 1, in *The Works of Robert Boyle*, ed. Michael Hunter and Edward B. Davis, 14 vols. [London: Pickering & Chatto, 1999], 3.299).

20 See, for example, Gorgias, *Encomium of Helen*, Isocrates, *Busiris*, 22, in *Isocrates*, trans. Larue van Hook, 3 vols. (Cambridge, MA.: Harvard University Press, 1954), 115 and, especially, Philip J. van der Eijk, *Medicine and Philosophy in Classical Antiquity: Doctors and Philosophers on Nature, Soul, Health, and Disease* (Cambridge: Cambridge University Press, 2005), which is the finest work on ancient medical thought to date.

21 Theodor J. Tracy, *Physiological Theory and the Doctrine of the Mean in Plato and Aristotle* (The Hague: Mouton, 1969), esp. 276ff. and van der Eijk, *Medicine and Philosophy in Classical Antiquity*, esp. 206–237.

as to conclude with an account of medical principles."[22] Able physicians bolster both inquiry and practice with philosophical knowledge and, as Descartes later recognised, the finest philosophers embrace healing as a cardinal aim.[23] As one seventeenth-century physician avers, the "two grandees in the common-wealth of learning, the Philosopher and the Physician" are "happy stars" when they agree, "but opposed, they portend a deluge of Barbarisme."[24]

Not only were ancient physicians concerned with rhetorical display,[25] most doctors and philosophers agreed that healing depends, in part, on discursive therapy, on 'contentive' conceits. If medicine begins where philosophy ends — a maxim "*universally receiv'd among Physicians*" in the seventeenth century[26] — one point of intersection is the 'therapeutic word.'[27] In the recovery of ancient philosophical and rhetorical learning, speech was figured not only as an "instrument

---

22 *De sensu,* 436a18-b2; *De respiratione* 480b22–30.

23 See the preface to the French edition of *The Principles of Philosophy* (1647 [1644 in Latin]), where Descartes claims that the whole of philosophy is like a tree: the roots are metaphysics, the trunk physics, and the many branches emerging from the trunk might be reduced to three principal areas of study and intervention, medicine, mechanics, and morals. Earlier, in the *Discourse on Method* (1637), he insists that "the mind depends so much on the temperament and disposition of the bodily organs that if it is possible to find some means of making men in general wiser and more skilful .... I believe that we must look for it in medicine." In a 1645 letter to the Marquess of Newcastle, Descartes writes that the "preservation of health has always been the principal end of my studies" (*The Philosophical Writings of Descartes,* ed. John Cottingham et al., 3 vols. [Cambridge: Cambridge University Press, 1985], 1.186 87, 143, 3.275).

24 Anonymous, *Anthropologie Abstracted: or the Idea of Humane Nature Reflected in Briefe Philosophicall, and Anatomicall Collections* (London, 1655), 109. A preface by the important printer Henry Herringman states that the work was authored by a physician, "esteemed ... as one of the most hopefull of his Profession" (sig. A2v).

25 See, for example, Heinrich Von Staden, "Anatomy as Rhetoric: Galen on Dissection and Persuasion," *The Journal of the History of Medicine and Allied Sciences* 10 (1995): 47–66, Lisa Keränen, "The Hippocratic Oath as Epideictic Rhetoric: Reanimating Medicine's Past for its Future," *Journal of Medical Humanities* 21 (2001): 55–68, and Susan P. Mattern, *Galen and the Rhetoric of Healing* (Baltimore: Johns Hopkins University Press, 2008).

26 Jeremiah Wainwright, *A Mechanical Account of the Non-Naturals: Being a Brief Explication of the Changes Made in Humane Bodies by Air, Diet, &c.* (London, 1707), sig. A2v. See also Walter Harris, *Pharmacologia Anti-Empiric* (London, 1683), 36. We might see in these formulations the Cartesian programme—in which moral philosophy sits somewhat awkwardly on the shoulders of medical thought—*avant la lettre*.

27 On the 'therapeutic word,' see Pedro Lain Entralgo, *The Therapy of the Word in Classical Antiquity*, trans. L.J. Rather and John M. Sharp (New Haven and London: Yale University Press, 1970); Cicero, *Tusculan Disputations*, 3.34.81–4; George W. McClure, "Healing Eloquence: Petrarch, Salutati, and the Physicians," *Journal of Medieval and Renaissance Studies* 15 (1985): 317–46; and James S. Baumlin and Tita French Baumlin, "Psyche / Logos: Mapping the Terrains of Mind and Rhetoric," *College English* 51.3 (1989): 245–61.

for exhortation and persuasion," but for "consoling the afflicted and assuaging the fears of the terrified, for curbing passion and quenching appetite and anger …"[28] Early modern practitioners emulated ancient physicians and philosophers, orators and counsellors, who enlisted discursive therapies and embraced *to prepon* in speech and conduct. As the Hippocratean *On Decorum* specifies, physicians should be "serious, artless, … graceful in speech, gracious in disposition," and must comfort patients with "solicitude and attention."[29] Consolation is central to early Greek figurations of both philosophy and medicine, as it was to Cicero, who proposed that various salves might be found even in the speeches of the sophists, and who presented some of his own work as a compendium of remedies.[30] Again, speech is therapeutic: *oratio* could exhort, admonish, praise, and heal.[31] As Daniel Gross points out in this volume, early modern physicians recognise "the ways in which everyday language can be a site for curative, psychosomatic intervention." Robert Burton cites Galen: many "have been cured by good counsel and persuasion alone. . a gentle speech is the true cure of a wounded soul" (2.2.6.2: 475). Several early moderns follow Galen, too, insisting that confidence and trust in a physician, both secured rhetorically, are essential to healing.[32] Thus the notion that rhetoric "could claim little direct relevance for medicine" depends in part on a very narrow conception of rhetoric as trope and ornament.[33] In contrast, past practitioners recognised rhetoric as a form of inquiry, as a lissom method for reasoning about signs and symptoms in a suffering body, and as a discourse of *kairos* and *krisis* with close parallels to medical thought; both are uncertain, interventionist, and depend, for their authority, on systems and rules which claim to organise both occasion and practice. Rhetorical inquiry is interested in experience, attuned to assessing and changing varying capacities for speaking and listening, for ethical, therapeutic, and interpretative action. As Aristotle suggests, rhetoric

---

28 Cicero, *De natura deorum*, trans. H. Rackham (Cambridge: Harvard University Press, 1933), 2.148.267.

29 *Hippocrates*, trans. W. H. S. Jones, 8 vols. (Cambridge, MA: Harvard University Press, 1923), 3.281–82, 12, 295, 16–298–99.

30 Cicero, *De natura deorum*, 2.59.49.

31 McClure, "Healing Eloquence," 317.

32 As Thomas Fienus insists, Galen "says that the faith of the sick man in the physician does a great deal for the health ... the physician will therefore heal better who can persuade better" (L. J. Rather, "Thomas Fienus' (1567–1631) Dialectical Investigation of the Imagination as Cause and Cure of Bodily Disease," *Bulletin of the History of Medicine* 41 (1967): 349–67; 363). Burton agrees (1.2.3.2: 223). Both drew on Galen's *Prognostics*, in which he argues that "Hippocrates shows us here how the first benefit ... that comes from a knowledge of prognosis is that it leads the sick to trust in the physician and to put themselves in his hands" (quoted in M. R. McVaugh, "Bedside Manners in the Middle Ages," *Bulletin of the History of Medicine* 71.2 [1997]: 209–223; 208).

33 Charles Schmitt, "Aristotle among the Physicians," in *The Medical Renaissance of the Sixteenth Century*, ed. A. Wear, R. K. French, and I. M. Lonie (Cambridge: Cambridge University Press, 1985), 1–15, esp. 14.

is a counterpart of both dialectic and ethics, and has the appearance (σχῆμα or *schema*) of politics (1356a25ff.): the form of inquiry against which appear the practices noted above is hermeneutic, devoted to investigating "civil interests, tasks, performances, carried in texts, signs," that sifts, distinguishes, and reinvents means for examining and directing, describing and redescribing civil capacities.[34] Practical activity necessarily involves persuasion, and *praxis* is often figured and undertaken using rhetorical terms and concepts, methods and metaphors. If rhetoric is in part defined by the ability to discern probabilities, that 'discernment' is a prudential enterprise. Capable rhetors and the practically wise are interdependent; as Luis de Granada insists in his textbook on preaching (1576), "prudence … is the guide of all actions and so also of our speech."[35] Rhetoric as a way of perceiving probabilities and adjusting one's argument to the audience and circumstance offers a model of ethical action and interaction; rhetorical inquiry informs the practice of private and public virtue, it ensures an effective transfer of remedial efforts between philosophy and medicine, as I have argued in my contribution to this collection. The art of persuasion is central to public life. But as an ensemble of techniques that investigates the changing vicissitudes of human experience, as an art moored to action and intervention, rhetoric is also a discourse of probability and proof.[36] Medicine, too, is pragmatic and thus cannot be divorced from its contested figurations, its multiple styles, or its discursive practices in various contexts.

## Inquiry and Remediation

One context is the early modern bedside.[37] In sickbed conversations, patients told physicians "what was wrong: when and how the complaint had started, what events

34 Nancy S. Struever, *Rhetoric, Modality, Modernity* (Chicago: University of Chicago Press, 2009), 1.

35 Granada, *Ecclesiasticæ Rhetoricæ, sive de Ratione Concionandi, libri sex* (1576), quoted and translated in Winfried Schleiner, *The Imagery of John Donne's Sermons* (Providence: Brown University Press, 1970), 15–16. As Eugene Garver has argued, "any prudential use of knowledge in action must ... involve rhetoric to some degree" (*Machiavelli and the History of Prudence* [Madison: University of Wisconsin Press, 1987]11, 21). See Lois S. Self, "Rhetoric and *phronēsis*: The Aristotelian Ideal," *Philosophy and Rhetoric* 12 (1979): 130–145 and compare Charles Trinkaus, who argues orators encounter and discuss, if not resolve, genuine philosophical problems in the course of practising their art ("Truth in Rhetoric and Anthropology," in *Renaissance Eloquence: Studies in the Theory and Practice of Renaissance Rhetoric*, ed. James J. Murphy [Berkeley: University of California Press, 1983], 207–220; 209).

36 Carlo Ginzburg, *History, Rhetoric, and Proof* (London and Hanover: University Press of New England, 1999).

37 See, for example, Saul Jarcho, "Morgagni, Vicarius, and the Difficulty of Clinical Diagnosis," in *Medicine, Science, and Culture: Historical Essays in Honor of Owsei Temkin*, ed. Lloyd G. Stevenson and Robert P. Multhauf (Baltimore: Johns Hopkins University Press, 1968), 87–95, Jerome Bylebyl, "The Manifest and the Hidden in the

had precipitated it, the characteristic pains and symptoms, its periodicity." The patient would describe "key lifestyle features," like "eating and sleeping habits, his bowel motions, recent emotional traumas, and so forth."[38] External causes of disease are discovered by "the inquisition of the Physitian, and the relation of the patient."[39] That trauma is among a practitioner's concerns is telling: Sir Thomas Elyot's cure for sorrow enjoins sufferers to embrace the "holsome counsayles" in scripture and "bokes of morall doctrine."[40] Since soul and body are knit together, remedying physical suffering means "care must be taken, to sweeten and abate the troubles of the mind with pleasing words. ... *A good speech is a Physitian for a sick mind.*"[41] In order to cure "spirituall sicknesses," the 'frivolous' William Vaughan recommends that physicians "invent and devise some spirituall pageant

---

Renaissance Clinic," in *Medicine and the Five Senses*, ed. W. F. Bynum and Roy Porter (Cambridge: Cambridge University Press, 1993), 40–60, and Michael Solomon, *Fictions of Well-Being: Sickly Readers and Vernacular Medical Writing in Late Medieval and Early Modern Spain* (Philadelphia: University of Pennsylvania Press, 2010), esp. 40ff. For a division of bedside medical inquiry into naturals, non-naturals, and illnesses, see 'Alius Medicus,' *Animadversions on the Medicinal Observations, of ... Frederick Loss* (London, 1674), 4–9, and for a lengthy, fictional *historia*, see Bernard de Mandeville, *A Treatise of the Hypochondriack and Hysterick Passions* (London, 1711), 2ff.

[38] Roy Porter, "The Rise of Physical Examination," in *Medicine and the Five Senses*, ed. W. F. Bynum and Roy Porter (Cambridge: Cambridge University Press, 1993), 182; see also McVaugh, "Bedside Manners in the Middle Ages," and Solomon, *Fictions of Well-Being*, 40–70. As G. S. Rousseau observes, every time "a patient enters a practitioner's office a literary experience is about to occur: replete with characters, setting, time, place, language, and a scenario that can end in a number of predictable ways. Literature enriches the sense of this daily drama" ("The Discourses of Literature and Medicine: Theory and Practice [1]" [1981] in his *Enlightenment Borders: Pre- and Postmodern Discourses*, vol. 2: *Medical, Scientific* [Manchester and New York: Manchester University Press, 1991], 10–11; the whole article is germane). This was commonplace by Cicero's time: a rhetor should resemble a "a careful physician who, before he attempts to administer a remedy to his patient, must investigate not only the malady of the man he wishes to cure, but also his habits when in health, and his physical constitution" (*De oratore*, 2.44.186). As Giovanni Battista da Monte suggests, "first we will consider the symptoms recited by [the patient], which ought to be diligently explained" (quoted in Bylebyl, "The Manifest and the Hidden," 57).

[39] Philemond Holland, *Gutta Podagrica: A Treatise of the Gout* (London, 1633), 13.

[40] Sir Thomas Elyot, *The Castel of Helth* (1541 [1533]), sig. 64v.

[41] Levinus Lemnius, *The Secret Miracles of Nature*, no trans (London, 1658), 65. For example, William Fenner notes that the affections are motions, "so they are *sensible motions too*. For the will stirs up the inferiour faculties of the Soul, and they stirre up the humours and parts of the body .... This is the reason why the affections are called passions, for they make the soul to suffer, and the body to suffer." When "there is a great apprehension of either [good or evil], not only the soul is *deeply* affected, but also the body is mightily compatible" (*A Treatise of the Affections; or The Souls Pulse* [London, 1650], 6–7).

to fortifie and help the imaginative facultie, which is corrupted and depraved"—imprinting "another conceit, whether it be wise or foolish, in the Patients braine, thereby to put out all former phantasies."[42] Although sufferers commonly "hate good comfort in words when the cause of [their] comfort indeedis gone,"[43] the corrupt "imaginative facultie" must be healed by 'invention'—a technique Cardano recommends—strengthened in order to relieve suffering. A sick person "is to be wrought into an Imagination quite contrary" to the offending passions that accompany distemper.[44] As the melancholy physician Caspar Barlaeus writes in a letter of 1638, "perhaps I have more to suffer from the affection of my imagination than from the obstruction in the hypochondrium, even though they ... conspire against me in a less than friendly manner."[45] Those who are vigorous and cheerful seldom require medical help—or should not, at least after age thirty, according to an early modern commonplace drawn from Suetonius and Celsus.[46] Writing in the early fifteenth century, one physician notes that a state of "temperate gaiety" purifies the blood, distributes natural heat, sharpens the wit and "makes the understanding more capable" as well as promoting a "healthy complexion and a pleasing appearance."[47]

In this intimate scene of inquiry and remediation, both patients' and practitioners' activities are largely rhetorical: praying, detailing symptoms, reading self-help manuals and regimens, chatting with visitors and physicians, receiving counsel, occasioning or assuaging emotion.[48] Of course, physicians attended to a myriad of circumstances, principally organised by the categories of the non-naturals and prognostic signs, but some indications were available

---

42 William Vaughan, *Approved Directions for Health, Both Naturall and Artificiall: Derived from the Best Physicians as well Modern as Ancient,* fourth edition (London, 1612), 90.

43 Thomas Wilson, *The Art of Rhetoric* (1560), ed. Peter E. Medine (University Park: Pennsylvania University Press, 1994), 113.

44 Johannes Jonstonus, *The Idea of Practical Physick,* trans. Nicholas Culpeper (London, 1657), 8.4.21.

45 Letter to Petrus Cunaeus, 1 March 1638 in F.F. Blok, *Caspar Barlaeus: From the Correspondence of a Melancholic* (Amsterdam: Van Gorcum, 1976), 63–4.

46 In *De medicina,* Celsus writes that a healthy man, "who is both vigorous and his own master, should be under no obligatory rules, and have no need either for a physician or an ointment-healer [iatrolepta]" (trans. W. G. Spencer, 3 vols. [Cambridge, MA., 1971], 1.1); see also Suetonius, *Lives of the Caesars,* trans. Catherine Edwards (Oxford: Oxford University Press, 2000), 68.131.

47 Benedetto Reguardati, *Pulcherimum et utilissimum opus ad sanitatis conservationem* (1477), f. 124v–125r, quoted in Glending Olson, *Literature as Recreation in the Later Middle Ages* (Ithaca and London: Cornell University Press, 1982), 50.

48 John Donne's *Devotions Upon Emergent Occasions* (1624) is a fine example of the range of feeling, activity, and consultation at the sickbed; see Stephen Pender, "Essaying the Body: Donne, Affliction, and Medicine," in *John Donne's Professional Lives*, ed. David Colclough (Cambridge: D.S. Brewer, 2002), 215–48.

only in discursive form, in sufferers' narrations or in case histories. Frequently occasioned by a rote ensemble of questions, and thus somewhat restrictive of both the patient's and the physician's expression, *historiae* and *consilia* nevertheless pose questions concerning the relationship between particular cases and general remedies, evidence and narrative, discourse and practice.[49] This admixture of consolation and consultation, assurance and application suggests the organising presence of rhetoric in medical practice and, as this collection demonstrates, in medical theory, in styles of care and counsel, and in establishing medical authority. Rhetoric shapes the experience of suffering as well as clinical encounters, and rhetoric's role in propagandising shifts in medical and philosophical thought is clear: changes in theory and practice were secured rhetorically and, then as now, rhetoric was an essential component in reforming styles of investigation, scenes of inquiry, and therapeutics, as Jean Dietz Moss argues in her chapter on physicians and the waters of Bath.

## Physicians Reading

This array of concerns—the physician's discourse, demeanour, and style, the relationship between ancient and contemporary practice, medical uncertainty—was addressed in various prescriptions for reading, for both patients and physicians. With respect to patients, reading both caused and remedied illness; if excessive, it was considered disturbing, but it was also remedial, a notion moored to the recovery of ancient moral philosophy, particularly Stoicism and Epicureanism.[50] But what should physicians themselves read? This question has a curious, and under-explored, history. One thorough account of medical curricula in the late middle ages demonstrates that physicians read widely in natural philosophy and philosophy, including ethics and rhetoric, logic and method, Greek, Latin, and Arabic texts, especially Avicenna. All seven liberal arts were thought necessary to the study of medicine, and there were strong efforts to "reconcile" philosophy and medicine, the Aristotelian and the Hippocratic-Galenic traditions, in medical education.[51] Of course, what physicians read at humanist grammar schools and universities in the sixteenth and seventeenth centuries is well-established. In

---

49 See Nancy Siraisi, "Girolamo Cardano and the Art of Medical Narrative," *Journal of the History of Ideas* 52 (1991): 581–602, Jole Agrimi and Chiara Crisciani, *Les "Consilia" Médicaux*, trans. Caroline Viola (Turnhout, Belgium: Brepols, 1994), Siraisi, "Anatomizing the Past: Physicians and History in Renaissance Culture," *Renaissance Quarterly* 53 (2000): 1–30, and Brian Nance, *Turquet de Mayerne as Baroque Physician: the Art of Medical Portraiture* (Amsterdam: Rodopi, 2001), esp. 23–65.

50 See George W. McClure, *Sorrow and Consolation in Italian Humanism* (Princeton: Princeton University Press, 1991).

51 Nancy G. Siraisi, *Taddeo Alderotti and His Pupils: Two Generations of Italian Medical Learning* (Princeton: Princeton University Press, 1981), 96–202; 140, 201. See also Carole Rawcliffe, *Medicine and Society in Later Medieval England* (Stroud: Sutton, 1995), esp. 105–110.

England, for example, before studying Galen and Hippocrates, often in a second degree, like all scholars of the period students of medicine read Terence and Seneca, Virgil, Ovid, and Horace, Cicero and Quintilian, Curtius and Suetonius.[52] Should students not pursue a degree in medicine, instruction in medicine was frequently informal, and found its place alongside standard humanist curricula.[53] Even unorthodox physicians, eager to establish their own authority, confirmed that the "man which intends the practice of Physick, must be qualified with good Litterature, and lay a Philosophical foundation, that he may be able to discourse and reason with himself, the causes and effects of things, both in Nature and Art."[54]

But for the Spanish humanist Juan Luis Vives, all except the most gifted physicians should abjure poetry and grammar, history and philosophy, "Cicero or Demosthenes, Virgil or Homer," after their initial acquaintance with the *studia humanitatis*. Although physicians may write of their own experiences "for the use of posterity," they must devote time to their art, which is already "obscure"— there is enough to master in medicine alone to fill a whole lifetime.[55] Yet in the

[52] There were innovative pedagogical programmes that enjoin all pupils to be exposed to natural philosophy and medicine, but for the most part medical studies were taken after immersion in the liberal arts, increasingly dominated by the study of logic and rhetoric. See William T. Costello, *The Scholastic Curriculum of Early Seventeenth-Century Cambridge* (Cambridge, MA: Harvard University Press, 1958), 45–64, T. W. Baldwin, *Shakespere's Small Latine and Lesse Greeke*, 2 vols. (Urbana: University of Illinois Press, 1944), and, for medical education, Paul F. Grendler, *The Universities of the Italian Renaissance* (Baltimore: Johns Hopkins University Press, 2002), 314–352, Phyllis Allen, "Medical Education in 17th Century England," *Journal of the History of Medicine and Applied Sciences* 1 (1946): 115–143 and Roger K. French, *William Harvey's Natural Philosophy* (Cambridge: Cambridge University Press, 1994), ch. 1–4, and Jean Dietz Moss and William A. Wallace, *Rhetoric and Dialectic in the Time of Galileo* (Washington: The Catholic University of America, 2003), 12–21. For a sense of what sixteenth-century English physicians were reading, see Eric Sangwine, "The Private Libraries of Tudor Doctors," *Journal of the History of Medicine and Allied Sciences* 33 (1978): 167–84.

[53] See Gillian Lewis, "The Faculty of Medicine," in T. H. Aston, ed., *The History of the University of Oxford*, 8 vols. (Oxford: Clarendon Press, 1984-), vol. 3: "The Collegiate University," ed. James McConica (1986), 213–256, esp. 238–41.

[54] Everard Maynwaring, *Medicus Absolutus ... The Compleat Physician, Qualified and Dignified* (London, 1668), 46. On Maynwaring, see Stephen Pender, "Seeing, Feeling, Judging: Pain in the Early Modern Imagination," in *The Sense of Suffering: Constructions of Physical Pain in Early Modern Culture*, ed. Jan Frans van Dijkhuizen and Karl A. E. Enenkel (Leiden: Brill, 2009), 477–503.

[55] *Vives: On Education, a Translation of the De Tradendis Disciplinis of Juan Luis Vives*, trans. Foster Watson (Cambridge: Cambridge University Press, 1913), 223, 222. See also *De disiplinis*, ed. Henry Jackson (London, 1612), 343–44 and *Opera omnia*, ed. Francisco Fabian y Fuero, 8 vols. (Valencia, 1745; reprint London: Gregg Press, 1964), 6.383. On 'science' as a component of 'letters,' see F. Edward Cranz, "The *Studia Humanitatis* and *Litterae* in Cicero and Leonardo Bruni," in *Perspectives on Early Modern and Modern Intellectual History*, ed. Joseph Marino and Melinda Schlitt (Rochester: University of Rochester Press, 2000), 3–26, esp. 14.

sixteenth and seventeenth centuries physicians routinely occupied themselves, and plied their audiences, with 'good Litterature': as well translating Galen's *De sanitate tuenda* and *De temperamentis*, Thomas Linacre wrote a Latin grammar; John Caius published on the sweating disease, Latin and Greek pronunciation, and English dogs; Thomas Cogan wrote on the widsom of the old testament, edited Cicero's familiar letters, and published the popular *Haven of Health* (1584, 1588, 1589, 1605, etc.); Philemon Holland and Thomas Lodge exerted grand efforts to present Roman history and Stoic philosophy to an English readership; and John Bulwer engaged in a broad, ambitious, and lifelong project exploring rhetoric and embodiment, natural history and anthropology.[56] Niccolo Leoncino was perhaps one of the best known physician-philologues, as Andrea Carlino notes in his chapter on Vesalius. William Harvey, too, demonstrates his intimate knowledge of the history of rhetoric and philosophy by directing his listeners to Cicero for both the function of nerves and the use of the parts of the body in his early Lumleian lectures.[57] Although his modern editor insists he is "overenthusiastic" in his reference to Cicero, Harvey's point is clear: he is, in part, retracing the steps of ancient philosophers and rhetoricians, probing the body, exploring the relationships between parts and wholes, matter and spirit, as he speaks to an audience of surgeons in 1616.[58] Harvey displays remarkable rhetorical sophistication, using ancient literature, particularly Terence, to impugn accepted medical tenets. His

---

[56] See Antonia Maclean, *Humanism and the Rise of Science in Tudor England* (London: Heinemann, 1972), 186–209, R. J. Dürling, "Linacre and Medical Humanism," in *Linacre Studies: Essays on the Life and Work of Thomas Linacre, c. 1460-1524*, ed. Francis Maddison, Margaret Pelling, and Charles Webster (Oxford: Clarendon Press, 1977), 76–106, Vivian Nutton, "John Caius and the Linacre Tradition," *Medical History* 23 (1979): 373–91, *idem*, "John Caius and the Eton Galen: Medical Philology in the Renaissance," *Medizinhistorisches Journal* 20 (1985): 227–52, various works by Holland and Lodge, especially the former's Pliny and the latter's Seneca, and, for example, Bulwer's *Pathomyotomia, or A Dissection of the Significative Muscles of the Affections of the Minde* (London, 1649).

[57] In the *Tusculan Disputations*, trans. J. E. King (Cambridge, MA.: Harvard University Press, 1927), 1.20.46–48, Cicero speculates about the "passages" from the seat of the soul to the eyes, ears and nose, and at 2.9.25, 11.30, 23.59–60, 27.93-96, 47.122, and especially 54–9.133–150, Cicero discusses the relationships between parts and wholes (*De Natura Deorum*, trans. H. Rackham [Cambridge, MA.: Harvard University Press, 1933]).

[58] William Harvey, *Lectures on the Whole of Anatomy*, ed. and trans. C.D. O'Malley, F.N.L. Poynter, K.F. Russell (Berkeley and Los Angeles: University of California Press, 1961), 235. On Harvey's *Prelectiones*, see Roger K. French, "Natural Philosophy and Anatomy," *Le Corps à la Renaissance: Actes due XXX^e^ Colloque de Tours 1987*, ed. Jean Céard, Marie M. Fontaine and Jean-Claude Margolin (Paris: Aux Amateurs de Livres, 1990), 447–460, *idem*, *Harvey's Natural Philosophy*, esp. ch. 4, and Luke Wilson, "William Harvey's *Prelectiones*: The Performance of the Body in the Renaissance Theater of Anatomy," *Representations* 17 (1987): 62–95. The lectures, including annual, winter anatomies transacted over five days ("if the bodies may so last without annoie"), proved popular and prestigious (*Lectures*, 4).

"classical literary citations and allusions" are integral to his scientific inquiry; they underwrite his apologia for "an unclassical medicine."[59] While curious to us, Harvey's references to Cicero and his redaction of Terence are far from antic.

Girolamo Cardano prided himself on "his ability to read rapidly and seize the essential content of a volume." According to Nancy Siraisi, his reading might have been "wider" than most of his colleagues, including texts on mathematics, astronomy, and the new world. He wrote on a wide array of subjects, too, including music, ethics, dreams and, famously, himself, as Guido Giglioni demonstrates in this volume.[60] Though a parsimonious writer, the Hugenot physician Theodore Turquet de Mayerne read, with interest, Herbert of Cherbury's *De veritate*.[61] And, in his treatment of melancholy, Burton demonstrated the breadth and depth of reading that might be brought to bear on a psycho-physiological condition.[62] Indeed, one early seventeenth-century Sussex physician turned to the *Anatomy of Melancholy* for assistance.[63] This breadth of reading speaks to a contemporary commitment to eclecticism: medical practitioners, apothecaries included, were by far the largest group practising natural history in the period, exploring and expanding the *materia medica*, a development reflected in the increased numbers of herbals and medical books published in the later half of the sixteenth century.[64] Natural history developed out of medical humanism, and rhetoric had a central

---

[59] Marjorie O'Rourke Boyle, "William Harvey's Soliloquy to the College of Physicians: Reprising Terence's Plot," *Medical History* 52 (2008): 365–86; 369, 386. Boyle demonstrates Harvey's ties to Linacre and Caius (374).

[60] Nancy Siraisi, *The Clock and the Mirror: Girolamo Cardano and Renaissance Medicine* (Princeton: Princeton University Press, 1997), 53, passim.

[61] Hugh Trevor-Roper, *Europe's Physician: the Various Life of Sir Theodore de Mayerne* (New Haven: Yale University Press, 2006), 8; see also Nance, Turquet de Mayerne as Baroque Physician, 12–13.

[62] The latest work on Burton evidences his wide reading; see, for example, Angus Gowland, *The Worlds of Renaissance Melancholy: Robert Burton in Context* (Cambridge: Cambridge University Press, 2006) and Grant Williams, "Disfiguring the Body of Knowledge: Anatomical Discourse and Robert Burton's The *Anatomy of Melancholy*," ELH 68 (2001): 593–613.

[63] Edward Poeten of Petworth, Sussex, who was active in the 1620s and 1630s, and an assistant to Sir Thomas Bonham; see *Sloane Manuscripts 1965*, folios 122ff. and Harold Cook, "Against Common Right and Reason: the College of Physicians against Sir Thomas Bonham," *American Journal of Legal History* 29.4 (1985): 301-322; 321.

[64] See H. S. Bennett, *English Books and Readers 1558 to 1603* (Cambridge: Cambridge University Press, 1965), 179–189 and his companion volume for the seventeenth century, *English Books and Readers 1603 to 1640* (Cambridge: Cambridge University Press, 1970), 140–149, Elizabeth Lane Furdell, *Publishing and Medicine in Early Modern England* (Rochester: University of Rochester Press, 2002) and, especially, Harold J. Cook, "The Cutting Edge of a Revolution? Medicine and Natural History Near the Shores of the North Sea," in *Renaissance and Revolution: Humanists, Scholars, Craftsmen, and Natural Philosophers in Early Modern Europe*, ed. J. V. Field and Frank A. J. L. James (Cambridge: Cambridge Univ. Press, 1993), 45–61.

role in refining not only historical consciousness but 'scientific' sensibilities. Across disciplines, attention to natural and historical particulars was inspired by a revivified and broad conceptualisation of decorum that encouraged attention to the exigencies of time and place.[65] Ecumenical, then, in their attention to ancient sources of medical and philosophical knowledge, physicians were active in the new science, in natural history and natural philosophy, and central to the emergence of a republic of letters. They essayed the fragile commensurability of theory and intervention, their professional status as investigators of contingency, and the ways in which particulars might yield general knowledge.

As Giovanni Argentario notes, medical terminology — and, by implication, medical practice — cannot be immured from other disciplines, and thus it is impossible to draw a clear line between medicine and philosophy.[66] But medicine is also intimate with rhetoric. Perhaps that is why Vives ends his disquisition on physicians' reading and training with a paean to the appropriateness, decorum, and *kairos* that they would have learned from humanist curricula. Drawing on Hippocrates' *On Decorum* and the standard skills developed and refined in rhetorical study, he recommends that physicians dress neatly rather than sumptuously, that they question the patient "in an urbane and affable fashion," and that they form just judgements, eschewing emotion. But his focus is conversation: if "the kind of illness of body or weakness of mind disinclines the patient to conversation, the physician will transact his inquiries with few and specially prudent words." If a patient can endure conversation, physicians should "narrate some anecdote, wittily, pleasantly, suited to the mood of [the] patient" and enlist the patient's trust.[67] Elsewhere, Vives insists that emotional distemper is susceptible to medical treatment, including phlebotomy, but he also recommends discursive therapy: meditation and the alteration of opinion (as species of *aversione cognitatis*), driving one passion out with another, walking, wine, and music, and "the distraction of occupations" and "pleasant little stories" (*narratiumculis lepidis*).[68] Where might a physician gather *narratiumculis lepidis* but from reading?

## Finders of Occasion

In the late seventeenth century, one physician worried about not only what but how physicians read. To Giorgio Baglivi, physicians should be "industrious bees," gathering precepts and practices from various areas of inquiry, rather than spiders,

---

65 See Nancy Struever, *The Language of History in the Renaissance: Rhetoric and Historical Consciousness in Florentine Humanism* (Princeton: Princeton University Press, 1970) and Brian W. Ogilvie, *The Science of Describing: Natural History in Renaissance Europe* (Chicago and London: University of Chicago Press, 2006), 35, 85, 118–19.

66 Heikki Mikkeli, *Hygiene in the Early Modern Medical Tradition* (Helsinki: Academia Scientiarum Fennica, 1999), 36.

67 Vives, *On Education,* 225–26.

68 Carlos G. Noreña, *Juan Luis Vives and the Emotions* (Carbondale: Southern Illinois University Press, 1989), 213–18.

spinning complex, unsubstantiated webs of speculation about illness and cure.[69] This common Senecan metaphor appears in his *De praxi medica ad priscam observandi rationem revocanda* (1696), dedicated to his patron and patient, Innocent XII, at Rome. Baglivi was Croatian; he studied and taught in Italy, was a member of the Royal Society (1697), and finished his career, after three years as assistant to Marcello Malpighi, as professor of theoretical medicine at the Sapienza. *De praxi medica* was Englished twice in the early eighteenth century (1704, 1723). The "Learned *Baglive*, ... a late Author of Note," was conservative: although he supported the reigning iatromechanical model of physiology for its exactitude, he had enormous respect for the ancients, and for Galen and Hippocrates in particular.[70] His own eclecticism is reflected in his advice to novice practitioners. While knowledge of "Meteors, Astronomy, Eloquence, or the Art of Persuading," moral philosophy, and prudence is necessary for a physician, and a "considerable Ornament" (24–5), it does little for the "curative" part of medicine. Yet Baglivi frequently offers discursive and ethical strictures for his ideal practitioner: a physician must read judiciously, manage analogies and similitudes appropriately, temper his moods and dispositions, and master the art of persuading. By "the mere Force of Words," a physician "fastens . such a Vertue upon his Remedies, and raises the Faith and Hopes of the Patient to that Pitch, that sometimes he masters difficult Diseases with the silliest Remedies" (171). The greatest sagacity and industry should be devoted to assuaging a sufferer's spirits via "fair Words," agreeable medicines, "pretending" that the remedies to hand are the most effective—what one late sixteenth-century Spanish physician calls "rhetorical insinuation."[71] "I can scarce express what Influence the Physicians Words have upon the Patient's Life," Baglivi writes, "and how much they sway the Fancy" (171). Grief, sorrow, and melancholy are "easily cur'd" by rhetorical intervention and by regimen, "by agreeable Conversation ... or else by a Way of living adjusted by a prudent Physician" (162). As a contemporary English physician insists, when "a Sick Person comes to stand in need of the *Physitians* help, those surely of all others are most likely to do him good, who may be presumed to sympathize with him the most feelingly in his Afflictions."[72]

For Baglivi, prudence is determined by the physician's temperament and a course of sanctioned reading. Disposition effects treatment and cure: our "innate Temperaments do oftentimes oblige us to embrace Error, and make false Judgments of Things." A physician "naturally Timorous and Melancholick" by habit of mind avoids "Spiritous Volatile Med'cines," attempting to cure instead by remedies "less Active" (16). The "false Idols" of physicians, the "prepossession

[69] Giorgio Baglivi, *The Practice of Physick*, no. trans., second edition (London, 1723), 129–130.

[70] The quotation is from Mandeville, *A Treatise*, 38.

[71] Miguel Sabuco de Nantes, *Coloquio del Conocimiento de Sí Mismo* (1587), quoted in Maureen Flynn, "Taming Anger's Daughters," *Renaissance Quarterly* 51 (1998): 875.

[72] Richard Griffith, *A la Mode Phlebotomy No Good Fashion ...* (London, 1681), 184.

of false Opinions," gleaned by the "preposterous reading of Books," impede the improvement of medicine (15). A "great Part of Wisdom" in curing diseases is keeping the mind untainted with prejudice, theory "clear of the Errors of the Schools," and "unbypass'd by Humour and Inclination" (75). Baglivi builds his insights on Juan Huarte, whom he cites (49), and who argued that differences in capacity should organise professional calling; and those differences depend on temperament and the non-naturals.[73] Physicians who are fine theorists are poor practitioners, and vice versa; imaginative facility should organise vocation. The understanding is a power "impertinent for curing," whereas the imagination, which traffics in particulars, is condign: encountering a patient, an imaginative physician "knoweth things which seem impossible" (177, 180). Diagnostic knowledge is secured, Huarte argues, by "a grace which springeth from the fruitfulnesse of the imagination, which by another name is termed a readinesse of capacitie, which by common signes, and by uncertain conjectures, … knoweth 1000 differe[n]ces of things, wherein the force of curing and prognosticating with certaintie consisteth" (180). In addition, the imagination determines the right application of remedies, the "greatest part of practice," which is why "*Galen* said, that the proper name of a phisition, was "The finder out of occasion" (182).[74] The other 'finders of occasion' are rhetors.

Like Huarte, then, Baglivi seeks a moderate practitioner who understands theory, but practices with wit and imagination, in full awareness of the strengths and weaknesses of his own temperament. Unsurprisingly, Baglivi ardently praises experience as the ground of medical efficacy, but forms of proper reading, note-taking, and commentary assist in knowing and adjusting one's sensibilities and compensating for the limits of experience and the uncertainty of practice. Medicine is never exclusively philological, of course, but "seasonal and considerate" reading develops sagacity and prudence (39, see 46). Reading haphazardly, reading "sorry" books (39), perusing only books indulgent in novelty or discredited ancient learning (43–4), and "over-reading" (46), which constrains the exercise of reason (42), throw physicians "headlong either into Scepticism or Madness" (41). Yet keeping a commonplace book contributes to curing by firmly rivetting sentences and precepts in the mind (47). In the production of commentary on ancient medical texts, Baglivi urges physician-philologues to avoid judgement and follow texts scrupulously, word for word (57–8). Despite its necessity, in the end erudition falters: physicians will not find "a more learned Book than the

---

[73] Juan Huarte, *Examen de Ingenios*, trans. M. Camillo Camilli, Englished from the Italian by Richard Carew (London, 1594; rpt. Gainsville: Scholars' Facsimiles, 1959), 21-2, 57, 74–5. Further references are included in parenthesis in the text. On Huarte, see Malcolm K. Read, *Juan Huarte de San Juan* (Boston: Twayne, 1981).

[74] 'Occasions' are another term for the non-naturals. Writing in the 1120s, Hugh of St. Victor cites Galen's *Tegni*, from the commentary by Hunayn Ibn Ishaq al-Ibadi (d. 873): "Occasiones ... aut faciunt sanitatem aut conservant" (quoted in *The* Didascalicon *of Hugh of St. Victor*, ed. and trans. Jerome Taylor [New York: Columbia University Press, 1961], 206 n. 76).

Patient himself, whose Disease will quickly and faithfully lay open to the diligent Observer" (48, see 50). A "tumultuary and inconsiderate way of Reading" (38) might simply enforce prejudice, the "Idols of the Mind" (57), unless physicians proceed with care, and embrace the range of sensibilities and discernment that licit reading engenders.

## A Salutary Conversation

Inquiry concerning the relationship between reading and medicine, literature and science, rhetoric and natural history in the early modern period is increasingly rich. Recent scholarship has developed and refined our sense of the affinities between literature and medicine: Jonathan Sawday has explored thoroughly the "culture of dissection" in early modernity, William Kerwin has argued that early modern drama 'shapes' medical history, and Richard Sugg has deftly suggested that "literature spurred medicine."[75] Gail Kern Paster has coined the phrase "early modern habits of bodily thought and sensation" to describe the ways in which perceptions of physiology intersect with cultural and political forms.[76] Similarly, parsing "pleasures, anxieties, and interests" in early modern England, Stephen Greenblatt argues for a lineal affinity between medical discourse and theatrical practice. Medicine and theatre are not related as "cause and effect or source and literary realization," but share a code, "a set of interlocking tropes and similitudes

75 Jonathan Sawday, *The Body Emblazoned: Dissection and the Human Body in Renaissance Culture* (London and New York: Routledge, 1995), Andrew Cunningham, *The Anatomical Renassiance: the Resurrection of the Anatomical Projects of the Ancients* (Aldershot: Scolar Press, 1997), Andrea Carlino, *Books of the Body: Anatomical Ritual and Renaissance Learning,* trans. John and Anne C. Tedeschi (Chicago: University of Chicago Press, 1999), William Kerwin, *Beyond the Body: the Boundaries of Medicine and English Renaissance Drama* (Amherst and Boston: University of Massachusetts Press, 2005), 5, 131, and Richard Sugg, *Murder after Death: Literature and Anatomy in Early Modern England* (Ithaca and London: Cornell University Press, 2007), 2. On these anatomical animadversions, see Stephen Pender, "Signs of Interiority, or Epistemology in the Bodyshop," *The Dalhousie Review* 85.2 (2005): 221–37, idem, review of Sugg, *Murder After Death, The Times Literary Supplement* (2 November 2007) and, idem, review of William Kerwin, *Beyond the Body, Renaissance Quarterly* 59.2 (2006): 635–37.

76 Gail Kern Paster, "Nervous Tension: Networks of Blood and Spirit in Early Modern England," in *The Body in Parts: Fantasies of Corporeality in Early Modern Europe,* ed. David Hillman and Carla Mazzio (London: Routledge, 1997), 107. In her investigation of 'cheap print' and the representation of the womb, pregnancy, and childbirth, Mary Fissell suggests that early modern habits of thought were "enacted through the body" (*Vernacular Bodies: the Politics of Reproduction in Early Modern England* [Oxford: Oxford University Press, 2004], 10). See also Katharine A. Craik, *Reading Sensations in Early Modern England* (Basingstoke: Palgrave Macmillan 2007).

that function not only as the objects but the conditions of representation."[77] These scholars build on early attempts to trace the broad affinities between medicine and literature, a field of inquiry now emerging from adolescence.[78]

Recently, too, various scholars have argued for a gradual and decisive incursion of rhetoric into demonstrative argument in early modern scientific discourse and intellectual history.[79] Rhetoric was "employed not only to frame discussions, to

---

[77] Stephen Greenblatt, *Shakespearean Negotiations: the Circulation of Social Energy in Renaissance England* (Berkeley and Los Angeles: University of California Press, 1988), 1–20, 86.

[78] See, for example, Kester Svendson, *Milton and Science* (Cambridge, MA: Harvard University Press, 1956), Herbert Silvette, *The Doctor on Stage: Medicine and Medical Men in Seventeenth-Century England,* ed. Francelia Butler (Knoxville: University of Tennessee Press, 1967), Irving I. Edgar, *Shakespeare, Medicine, and Psychiatry: An Historical Study in Criticism and Interpretation* (New York: Philosophical Library, 1970), Barbara J. Shapiro, *Probability and Certainty in Seventeenth-Century England: A Study of the Relationships Between Natural Science, Religion, History, Law, and Literature* (Princeton: Princeton University Press, 1983), M.A. Screech, *Montaigne and Melancholy: The Wisdom of the Essays* (Selinsgrove: Susquehanna University Press, 1984), Raymond A. Anselment, *The Realms of Apollo: Literature and Healing in Seventeenth-Century England* (Newark: University of Delaware Press, 1985), John Wiltshire, *Samuel Johnson in the Medical World: The Doctor and the Patient* (Cambridge: Cambridge University Press, 1991), F. David Hoeniger, *Medicine and Shakespeare in the English Renaissance* (Newark: University of Delaware Press, 1992), Karen L. Edwards, *Milton and the Natural World: Science and Poetry in Paradise Lost* (Cambridge: Cambridge University Press, 1999), *Disease, Diagnosis, and Cure on the Early Modern Stage,* ed. Stephanie Moss and Kaara L. Peterson (Aldershot: Ashgate, 2004), *Textual Healing: Essays on Medieval and Early Modern Medicine,* ed. Elizabeth Lane Furdell (Leiden: Brill, 2005), M. A. Katritzky, *Women, Medicine, and Theatre, 1500-1750: Literary Mountebanks and Performing Quacks* (Aldershot: Ashgate, 2007), Louis M. Bishop, *Words, Stones, and Herbs: The Healing Word in Medieval and Early Modern England* (New York: Syracuse University Press, 2007), Todd H. J. Pettigrew, *Shakespeare and the Practice of Physic: Medical Narratives on the Early Modern English Stage* (Newark: University of Delaware Press, 2007), and *Rhetorics of Bodily Disease and Health in Medieval and Early Modern England,* ed. Jennifer C. Vaught (Aldershot: Ashgate, 2010). There is also some very fine work being done concerning the relationship between medicine and the visual arts; for excellent examples, see Pamela H. Smith, "Science and Taste: Painting, the Passions, and the New Philosophy in Seventeenth-century Leiden," Isis 90 (1999): 420–61 and Laurinda S. Dixon, *Perilous Chastity: Women and Illness in Pre-Enlightenment Art and Medicine* (Ithaca: Cornell University Press, 1995).

[79] See, for example, R. W. Serjeantson, "Proof and Persuasion," in *The Cambridge History of Science*, 7 vols., *Early Modern Science*, ed. Katherine Park and Lorraine Daston (Cambridge: Cambridge University Press, 2006), 3.132–175. See also Susan James, *Passion and Action: The Emotions in Seventeenth-Century Philosophy* (Oxford: Clarendon Press, 1997), 208-24 ("The Value of Persuasion"). In a more recent survey of early modern science, Pamela H. Smith does not treat rhetoric, and treats medicine hardly at all ("Science on the Move: Recent Trends in the History of Early Modern Science," *Renaissance Quarterly* 62 [2009]: 345–75).

prepare the ground, to clarify, or to underscore the importance of the positions assumed on a question, but it was … introduced into the scientific proofs of the arguments" concerning, for example, Copernican cosmology or anatomical controversy.[80] Embracing a notion of experiment predicated on its discursive accounts, Peter Dear has argued that the "creation of experimental natural philosophy must be understood through the exploitation and deformation of that framework by literary techniques and strategies."[81] As Maurice Slawinski argues in an important, but neglected, piece from 1991, there is an "intimate link between natural philosophy and rhetoric." Both seek "to analyse facts, draw inferences, and marshal evidence," and both are fundamentally concerned with persuasion: to "adopt rhetorical forms of argument so as to gain public credence invariably involves a rhetoricization of scientific logic itself."[82] The "rhetorical form" of scientific texts, even of objects of scrutiny, is "constitutive of their meaning, not separable from it."[83]

The importance of reading and rhetoric to medical theory and practice has been recognised by a number of modern scholars. As Nancy Struever argued in the 1990s, from the fourteenth century, particularly in the work of Pietro d'Abano, rhetorical figures were used to explain medical theory, and both medicine and rhetoric were pragmatic and interventionist: one devoted to the body, the other to the body politic and the soul. Struever has investigated this "rhetorical-medical mind set," the intrication of therapy and cure, in Pietro d'Abano, Petrarch, Descartes, and others; and she has proposed a dual history of rhetoric and medicine in order to account for these habits of thought.[84] Struever builds on these insights in this volume.

---

[80] Jean Dietz Moss, *Novelties in the Heavens: Rhetoric and Science in the Copernican Controversy* (Chicago: University of Chicago Press, 1993), 2. Although her work is devoted to Copernicus' reception, her point is general; see also Alan G. Gross, *The Rhetoric of Science* (Cambridge, MA: Harvard University Press, 1990), James Franklin, *The Science of Conjecture: Evidence and Probability before Pascal* (Baltimore: Johns Hopkins University Press, 2001), esp. 102–130, and spurring work by Matthew L. Jones, *The Good Life in the Scientific Revolution: Descartes, Pascal, Leibniz and the Cultivation of Virtue* (Chicago: University of Chicago Press, 2006), esp. 55–86.

[81] "Narratives, Anecdotes, and Experiments: Turning Experience into Science in the Seventeenth Century," in *The Literary Structure of Scientific Argument: Historical Studies*, ed. Peter Dear (Philadelphia: University of Pennsylvania Press, 1991), 135–163; 163.

[82] Maurice Slawinski., "Rhetoric and Science / Rhetoric of Science / Rhetoric as Science," in *Science, Culture, and Popular Belief in Renaissance Europe*, ed. Stephen Pumfrey, Paolo L. Rossi, and Maurice Slawinski (Manchester: Manchester University Press, 1991), 72, 90.

[83] Serjeantson, "Proof and Persuasion," 133.

[84] Nancy S. Struever, "Petrarch's *Invective Contra Medicum*: An Early Confrontation of Rhetoric and Medicine," *Modern Language Notes* 108 (1999), 659–79, "Rhetoric and Medicine in Descartes' *Passions de l'Āme*: The Issue of Intervention," in *Renaissance-Rhetorik / Renaissance Rhetoric,* ed. Heinrich F. Plett (Berlin, 1993), 196–212, and "The

Several years ago, in a remarkably wide-ranging essay, David Harley argued that all medical practitioners, from village wise women to members of the College of Physicians, had to provide explanations of medical theory and medical practice that satisfied their sometimes credulous, sometimes sceptical patients. All medical writing, Harley continued, can "profitably be seen as competition for the control of meaning" rather than simply advertisement.[85] Rhetoric has always been "more central to medicine than it is to the natural sciences," Harley continues, not least because "the objects of inquiry are not alert to the rhetoric" (421). Thus rhetoric "structures and constitutes the experience" of healing (421), an argument made by Hans-Georg Gadamer some time ago: "in all medical treatment … the discussion and shared dialogue between doctor and patient plays a decisive role."[86]

Harley has also explored the profusion of medical metaphors in early modern preaching,[87] as has Richard Sugg, and they are ubiquitous, frequently laudatory, and often disclose a writer's aspirations for piercing, perspicacious analysis. As one early modern writer suggests in his introduction to a selection of ancient

---

Discourse of Cure: Rhetoric and Medicine in the Late Renaissance," in *Rhetoric and Pedagogy: Its History, Philosophy, and Practice*, ed. Winifred Bryan Horner and Michael Leff (Mahwah, N.J.: Lawrence Erlbaum, 1995), 277–93. On Struever's signal contributions to intellectual history and the history of rhetoric, to the "revolution of sensibility" to which rhetoric was central in early modernity, see John O. Ward, "Rhetoric: *Disciplina* or Epistemology? Nancy Struever and Writing the History of Medieval and Renaissance Rhetoric," in *Perspectives on Early Modern and Modern Intellectual History: Essays in Honor of Nancy S. Struever*, ed. Joseph Marino and Melinda W. Schlitt (Rochester: University of Rochester Press, 2001), 348–74. Other intellectual historians have been less concerned with medicine; for example, I was surprised to find next to no reference to medical thought in Donald Kelley's *The Descent of Ideas: the History of Intellectual History* (Aldershot: Ashgate, 2002), a history of philosophical eclecticism. The importance of medical thought to the period Kelley identifies as the matrix of intellectual history—the late eighteenth and the early nineteenth centuries—deserves sustained attention, as does the intimate association between, say, history and medicine in ancient Greece. That probable reasoning, sign inference, and conjectural history matured, in part, in ancient medical thought, suggests its relevance to Kelley's 'story.' And what is more 'eclectic,' in both theory and practice, than early modern medicine? On the history of the term 'habits of thought,' see Stephen Pender, "Habits of Thought, Structures of Feeling," in *Renaissance Tropologies: The Cultural Imagination of Early Modern England*, ed. Jeanne Shami (Pittsburgh: Duquesne University Press, 2008), 281–307.

[85] David Harley, "Rhetoric and the Social Construction of Sickness and Healing," *Social History of Medicine* 12 (1999): 407–35; 414–415. Further references included in parenthesis in the text.

[86] *The Enigma of Health: The Art of Healing in a Scientific Age,* trans. John Gaiger and Nicholas Walker (Oxford: Polity Press, 1996), 77; see 41, 131–2. See also Byron J. Good, *Medicine, Rationality, and Experience: An Anthropological Perspective* (Cambridge: Cambridge University Press, 1994).

[87] "Medical Metaphors in English Moral Theology, 1560–1660," *Journal of the History of Medicine and Allied Sciences* 48 (1993): 396–435.

letters, rhetoric is not unlike medicine: so that, "as the Physician, to heale many and sundrie maladies, wherewith his weake patients are infected, vseth many and sundrie sortes of medicines: in like manner, to write formally to persons diuers in degree, thou haste here ready to serue thy turne, many presidents [*sic*] and examples …, drawne out of the most pure and cleare founteines of the finest and eloquentest Rhetoricians[.]"[88] Metaphorically occupying the position of a doctor or surgeon is a powerful rhetorical stance; but even surgery might be seen as a struggle for language, for settled terminology, for discursive authority since, as recent scholarship has argued, for physicians and surgeons, authority depends, in part, on ethos, decorum, and honour.[89] Trust and confidence, the reputation and persona of the healer, the manner and style of clinical inquiry, the conversation between patient and doctor: all depend on, are secured by, rhetoric.

## Authority, Anatomy, Style

This collection is the first to specifically address the relationship between medicine and rhetoric in early modern Europe. While recent work has explored the rhetoric of disease, the valence of drugs and remedies on and off stage, and the fragile accumulation of authority among physicians in early modernity, no work, to my knowledge, takes the intimate relationship between rhetoric and medicine as its focus. Scholars of early modern intellectual and cultural history have built on the work of researchers concerned with the rhetoric and narrative in contemporary medicine, particularly in patient-physician relationships, in order to deepen our understanding of the role of persuasion in establishing a natural philosophical foundation for medicine, in shaping an emerging and troubled profession, and in defining aspects of medical theory and practice, as I argue in the first chapter.[90]

---

[88] Abraham Flemming, *A Panoplie of Epistles or, A Looking Glass for the Unlearned London 1576,* sigs. ¶Vv-¶VIr. For numerous other examples, see Robert Cawdrey's *A Treasure or Store-House of Similies* (London, 1600), sig. A2r, 59, 182–83, 211, 522–23, etc.).

[89] As Celeste Chamberland argues, the "relationship between rules, decorum, and the transgression thereof became the primary matrix through which London's largest body of licensed practitioners [barber-surgeons] fashioned a corporate social status that demonstrated their compliance to larger conventions of honor and reputation while highlighting the fusion of learned traditions and artisanal skill unique to their occupation" ("Honor, Brotherhood, and the Corporate Ethos of London's Barber-Surgeons' Company, 1570–1640," *Journal of the History of Medicine and Allied Sciences,* 64.3 [2009]: 300–332; 332). Chamberland builds on Cook, *The Decline of the Old Medical Regime.* For the question of surgery and terminology, see Marie-Christine Pouchelle, *The Body and Surgery in the Middle Ages,* trans. Rosemary Morris (New Brunswick: Rutgers University Pres, 1990).

[90] Important recent work includes Kathryn Hunter, *Doctors' Stories: The Narrative Structure of Medical Knowledge* (Princeton: Princeton University Press, 1991), Julia Epstein, *Altered Conditions: Disease, Medicine, and Storytelling* (New York: Routledge, 1995), A.G. Gross and W.M. Keith, *Rhetorical Hermeneutics: Invention and Interpretation*

One significant example is the advertisement hydrotherapy and balneology in the sixteenth and seventeenth centuries. The trend began in the mid-1500s with the publication of *De balneis omnia quae extant* (1553) and Andrea Bacci's *De Thermis* (1571).[91] Although recourse to baths and mineral waters was an ancient, pan-European practice, the early modern English case is instructive, as Jean Dietz Moss argues, for it points up the relationships between civic and national pride, medical advertisement and tourism, as well as questions of professional authority. As one writer suggests in 1572, "before ye seeke the ayde, fo the Bathes," a patient was to "co[n]sult, with your Physicions thereof." Although drinking and bathing in spa waters were widely recommended, physicians urged caution: determining the "virtues and uses of our Baths," Edward Jorden writes, belongs "properly to the Physician, and cannot well be intimated to the patient without dangerous mistaking."[92] As practitioners jockeyed for authority in determining the employment of waters, questions about their benefit divided physicians from empirics. Indeed, the scarcity of physicians at Bath, John Jones reports, left patients prey to apothecaries, charlatans, and ignorant purveyors of cures, including wise-women. To protect and widen their purview, to increase the revenues of the baths, and to draw patients from competing spas, physicians retailed the benefits of the waters as well as precise instructions for proper bathing and drinking. Moss' analysis of William Turner, Jones, Tobias Venner, Edward Jorden, Thomas Guidott, and Robert Pierce demonstrates that, in advising and advertising the waters at Bath, "rhetoric and science became inextricably intertwined." We might take the recent proliferation of scholarship on early modern anatomy as another exemplary case in the which the claims of 'science' were tested and contested rhetorically.

---

*in the Age of Science* (New York: SUNY Press, 1997), Jeanne Fahnestock, *Rhetorical Figures in Science* (New York: Oxford University Press, 1999), Anne Hawkins, *Reconstructing Illness: Studies in Pathography*, second edition (West Lafayette, Indiana: Purdue University Press, 1999), Alan Gross, James Harmon and Michael Reidy, "Argument and 17th Century Science: A Rhetorical Analysis with Sociological Implications," *Social Studies of Science* 30.3 (2000): 371–96, Kathryn Hunter, *How Doctors Think: Clinical Judgment and the Practice of Medicine* (Oxford: Oxford University Press, 2005), Robert Veatch, *Disrupted Dialogue: Medical Ethics and the Collapse of Physician-Humanist Communication 1770–1980* (New York: Oxford University Press, 2005), Rita Charon, *Narrative Medicine: Honoring the Stories of Illness* (New York: Oxford, 2006), and Alan Gross, *Starring the Text: Tthe Place of Rhetoric in Science Studies* (Carbondale: Southern Illinois University Press, 2006).

[91] Richard Palmer, "'In This Our Lightye and Learned Tyme': Italian Baths in the Era of the Renaissance," in *The Medical History of Waters and Spas*, ed. Roy Porter, *Medical History*, Supplement No. 10 (London: Wellcome Institute, 1990), 14–22.

[92] John Jones, *The Bathes of Bathes Ayde* (London, 1572), ff. 6v-7r and Edward Jorden, *A Discourse of Natural Bathes and Mineral Waters*, third edition (London, 1669 [1631]), 163, 166, both quoted in David Harley, "A Sword in a Madman's Hand: Professional Opposition to Popular Consumption in the Waters Literature of Southern England and the Midlands, 1570–1870," in *The Medical History of Waters and Spas*, 48–55; 48, 49–50.

The majority of early modern physicians and surgeons celebrated the benefits of both anatomy and post-mortem dissection.[93] Yet, as Thomas Sydenham and John Locke argue in their *Anatomie* (1668), anatomy reveals only "more superficies … to stare at,' adding little or nothing to the preservation of health or to therapeutics. It is unlikely to "assist a man in the findeing out and establishing a true method."[94] Although another contemporary insists that physicians must learn anatomy, "*Anatomy* is of the greatest fame and repute, tho not of much real use to the curing [of] Mankind."[95] Crucial to this debate is an early modern intellectual and publishing sensation—Vesalius' *Fabrica*, which Andrea Carlino re-situates in humanist circles of the 1530s and 1540s. One curious effect of this new attention to anatomy is the recognition, in recent inquiry, that medical images and metaphors, particularly those connected with dissection, were exceptionally well-travelled, popular, and precise. In this collection, Richard Sugg casts his net widely in order to capture the richness of early modern anatomical rhetoric. His exploration of titles and phrases, "sections" and "openings" demonstrates the rising popularity of dissective and anatomical terms and concepts in the work of divines, controversialists, playwrights, and poets from 1560 to 1640.

Complementing his work on the 'anatomical season' in *Murder After Death*, Sugg suggestively proposes that the increase in terms associated with public dissection in the period results from the ways in which both public and post-mortem anatomy impinge on the English imagination. Wisely leaving the question open, Sugg notes that either textual precedent or increased anatomical activity spurred writers as diverse as Castiglione and Lyly, Thomas Nashe and Robert Burton, to employ anatomical terms and metaphors. As Sugg argues, "writers seem to covertly transpose the limits of real bodies onto the potentially unlimited subject matter they address," and in the process claim to have probed "all the recesses, joints, and cavities of that particular topic." The body provided, in Barbara Stafford's formulation, "the ultimate visual compendium, the comprehensive method of methods, the organizing structure of structures."[96] Indeed, more and more authors in the late sixteenth and early seventeenth centuries turned to the "non-lying book of the body," to use Vesalius' phrase, as a way of organizing and presenting knowledge and engaging in polemic. The relationship between anatomy, dissection and discourse, between cutting into the human body and

[93] On post-mortem dissection and its differences from theatrical anatomical demonstration, see David Harley, "Political Post-Mortems and Morbid Anatomy in Seventeenth-Century England," *Social History of Medicine* 7 (1994): 1–28.

[94] Thomas Sydenham and John Locke, *Anatomie* (1668), PRO 30/24/47/2, ff. 60–67, printed in Kenneth Dewhurst, *Dr. Thomas Sydenham (1624–1689): His Life and Original Writings* (London: Wellcome Historical Medical Library, 1966), 87–8, 91, 79.

[95] Christopher Merrett, *The Character of a Compleat Physician, or Naturalist* (1680), 1.

[96] B.M. Stafford, *Body Criticism: Imagining the Unseen in Enlightenment Art and Medicine* (Cambridge, MA. and London: MIT Press, 1993), 12. See also David George Hale, *The Body Politic: A Political Metaphor in Renaissance English Literature* (The Hague: Mouton, 1971).

applying "a rude hand" to "launce" and "cut through skin" in satire, for example, was commonplace.[97] Early anatomists, too, were keenly aware that their incisions had philosophical, discursive analogues.[98] Dissection, Matthias Curtius writes in 1540, may be performed "in one way really or actually, in another way through description, e.g. in writing or lecturing." Anatomy "embraces the art of dissection, both performed actually and by description." In Galen's works, Curtius continues, dissection means "description by lecturing, not dissection actually performed."[99] According to Harvey, anatomy is "philosophical, medical, mechanical," revealing bodies real or intellectual.[100]

In 1613, the English physician and controversialist Helkiah Crooke insisted that anatomy had at least a "double acceptation": either "it signifieth the action which is done with the hande; or the habite of the minde, that is, the most perfect action of the intellect. The first is called practicall Anatomy, the latter Theoretical or contemplative."[101] The first is historical, and depends on "Section and Inspection"; the second, more "profitable" scientific anatomy, scrutinizes causes and parts, their structures and uses. The first or the "way of Historie" is more certain, the second less so but carries "more grace" since it concerns intellection. Opening the flesh affords access to the "motions of the hidden and secret parts"; those parts and functions not "subjected to sense," "must be sought out by dissection."[102] By 1640, Francis Glisson could define anatomy as "an artificiall dissection of [a certayne] objecte in such maner as may most conduce to the perfect knowledg

---

97 The phrases are Robert Burton's, "Democritus Junior to the Reader," *Anatomy of Melancholy* (1621), ed. Thomas C. Faulkner, Nicolas K. Kiessling and Rhonda L. Blair, 3 vols. (Oxford: Clarendon Press, 1989), 1.113.

98 See Thomas Willard, "Donne's Anatomy Lesson," *John Donne Journal* 3 (1984): 43.

99 Baldasar Heseler, *Andreas Vesalius' First Public Anatomy at Bologna, 1540, an Eyewitness Report*, ed. and trans. Ruben Eriksson (Uppsala and Stockholm: Almquist and Wiksells, 1959), 47.

100 Medical anatomy had five aspects: narrative description of the body and its parts, the actions, uses and ends of the part, the observation of pathological conditions of the organs, the resolution "of the problems of authors" (an assessment of medical and anatomical authorities) and the "skill or dexterity in dissection and the condition of the prepared cadaver" (Harvey, *Lectures on the Whole of Anatomy*, 22–3, 27).

101 Helkiah Crooke, *Microcosmographia: A Description of the Body of Man, Together with Controversies Thereto Belonging* (London, 1615), 26. On Crooke's life and career, see C.D. O'Malley, "Helkiah Crooke, M.D., F.R.C.P., 1576–1648," *Bulletin of the History of Medicine* 42 (1976): 1–18. Of late, Crooke has received keen attention in literary historical scholarship on the early modern body. See, for example, Gail Kern Paster, *The Body Embarrassed: Drama and the Disciplines of Shame in Early Modern England* (Ithaca: Cornell University Press, 1993), and *idem.*, "Nervous Tension: Networks of Blood and Spirit in the Early Modern Body," in *The Body in Parts*, 107–125 and several of the essays in *Sensible Flesh: On Touch in Early Modern Culture* ed. Elizabeth D. Harvey (Philadelphia: University of Pennsylvania Press, 2003).

102 *Microcosmographia,* 17–18.

of the same and all its parts." This "artificiall dissection implyes not the manuall dissection only but in especiall maner the mentall … which maynely denominats the artiste an anatomist, and hath use in livinge as well as dead bodys."[103] As John Hall writes in 1649, lamenting that England had fallen behind the continent in anatomical investigation, things unfolded are best understood; the anatomical exploration of the body epitomized reason itself—"if the veynes of things were rightly and naturally cut up."[104] These figurations were part of an overall shift to material explanations for various phenomena. During the seventeenth century "the reduction of psychic phenomena to somatic states … became increasingly explicit in medical writings and was taken up by speculative writers with various reformist religious intentions."[105] Sir Kenelm Digby calls metaphysicians "spiritual Anatomistes" and Bacon "opened … those peccant humours" that impeded the advancement of learning.[106] As Sugg deftly argues, by the early seventeenth century, the conception of anatomy and dissection as manual, discursive, and analogical activities was popular, indeed: both in discourse and in the flesh, anatomy addressed the relationship between parts and wholes, cause and effect, matter and spirit. But it may be that anatomy was first and foremost a rhetorical exercise, a "'science' that knows its own dependence on rhetoric."[107]

A monument both in the history of print and in the history of anatomy, Andreas Veslius' *De humani corporis fabrica* (1543) is a product of the ferment of humanist textual and cultural activity in Italy in the early to mid-sixteenth century. But it is also, of course, a product of discourse. Andrea Carlino restores Vesalius to his humanist context: as a member of various groups of virtuosi concerned with developing and refining classical scholarship, many of whom were devoted to resurrecting the ancient relationship between discursive and medical intervention, to exploring the construction—the fabrication —of bodies and texts, and to illuminating the broad affinities between medical theory and practice and the arts of discourse, especially logic and rhetoric. As Carlino argues, medical humanism is defined, in part, by the essential, and frequently neglected, relationship between

---

103 *Anatomia Hepatis* (1654), in BL Sloane MS 3315, ff165–69.

104 John Hall, *The Advancement of Learning*, ed. A.K. Croston (Liverpool: Liverpool University Press, 1953), 38, quoted in Sawday, *Body Emblazoned*, 231. Barbara Lewalski suggests that Donne in the *Anniversaries* is "an anatomist first of all in the general rhetorical sense of the term—one who undertakes to analyze a subject methodically, rigorously, point by point" (*Donne's* Anniversaries *and the Poetry of Praise* [Princeton: Princeton University Press, 1973], 226).

105 John Henry, "The Matter of Souls: Medical Theory and Theology in Seventeenth-Century England," in *The Medical Revolution of the Seventeenth Century*, ed. Roger French and Andrew Wear (Cambridge: Cambridge University Press, 1989), 90. See also Katherine Park, "The Organic Soul," in *The Cambridge History of Renaissance Philosophy*, ed. Charles B. Schmitt et al (Cambridge: Cambridge University Press, 1988), 464–84.

106 Digby, *Two Treatises* (London, 1644), 143; Bacon, *Works*, 3.295.

107 Devon Hodges, *Renaissance Fictions of Anatomy* (Amherst: University of Massachusetts Press, 1985), 17–18.

medicine and speech. Vesalius' various senses of the term for the structure of the human body, *fabrica*, are drawn from Cicero, for example, and were developed in the human circles in which he travelled. The affinities between Vesalius' thinking about structures and bodies and those of his contemporaries, particularly Serlio and Camillo, Varchi and the members of the *Accademia degli Infiammati*, suggest that the broadly transdisciplinary investigations of the humanists present a tradition alternative to what scholars have seen as the defining characteristic of demonstrative science: the separation of *res* and *verba*. Instead, the *fabrica* of the body and the *fabrica* of discourse point to the intimacy of words and things in early modern thought: bodies were flesh and blood, but flesh and blood mediated by, and materialized in, textual and interpretive communities.

## Pathology and Vulnerability

The reconfiguration of anatomy as a master discourse of inquiry is parallelled by a new 'anthropology,' a rethinking of the human and of the human sciences. According to Michel Foucault, medicine has a privileged status in the history and "architecture" of the human sciences. At the end of the eighteenth century, and throughout the nineteenth, "medical thought is fully engaged in the philosophical status of man," for it is central to the structures and processes that sustain disciplines dedicated to probing and charting, illuminating and envisioning 'the human.'[108] Via somatic mapping, the clinical practice and pathological anatomy of Bichat and Pinel, Corvisart and Tissot offered sick bodies, their signs and symptoms, even the etiologies of disease, to a new, piercing medical gaze. At the same time, according to Foucault, clinical description triumphs over the stilted *historiae* of a former age, and "clinical experience," made possible by the spatialization of disease,[109] trumps ancient prohibitions about a science of the particular—in this

[108] Michel Foucault, *The Birth of the Clinic: an Archaeology of Medical Perception*, trans. Am. M. Sheridan Smith (New York: Vintage, 1975 [1963]), 197–98. Further references included in the text. See the special issue of *The Journal of Medicine and Philosophy* 34.4 (2009) for a reevaluation of Foucault's work and its influence in contemporary medical thought.

[109] See Barbara Maria Stafford, "Voyeur or Observer? Enlightenment Thoughts on the Dilemmas of Display," *Configurations* 1 (1992): 95–128 and *idem*, *Body Criticism*, 12, 104. Several scholars have noted the particular affinity of logic and anatomy, and of the relationship between the representation of dissected bodies and epistemological shifts; see, for example, Walter Ong, who suggests that medicine contributed to a spatial model of knowledge with its presentation of "bodies" of learning. This tendency, in turn, led to the "related fad" of performing intellectual anatomies (*Ramus, Method, and the Decay of Dialogue* [Cambridge: Harvard University Press, 1958], 314–18). On the relationship between logic and anatomy, see John H. Randall, *The School of Padua and the Emergence of Modern Science* (Padua: Antenore, 1961), 35ff. and Thomas Joseph Arthur, "Anatomies and the Anatomy Metaphor in Renaissance England" (Ph.D. Dissertation, University of Wisconsin-Madison, 1978), chapter one. In *The Body Emblazoned*, Jonathan Sawday makes much of this point (135–37) as does Piero Camporesi, *The Anatomy of the Senses:*

case, febrile, consumptive, or distempered bodies (xiv). Idiosyncratic periodization aside, *The Birth of the Clinic* proposes a particular relationship between seeing and saying in the history of medicine, one in which the clinic operates as a proxy for the state. By the early nineteenth century, Foucault argues, bedside encounters between physicians and patients were little concerned with lengthy narratives of symptoms, which included the passions, habits, and fantasies of the sufferer; they were exercises in redescription, founded, in part, on the tact of the practitioner, that dissolved the particular in the general, in the medicine of "organs, sites, causes," and in "a clinic wholly ordered in accordance with pathological anatomy" (107–123; 122).

Daniel Gross questions this narrative, as he does Foucault's history of the human sciences in *The Order of Things*. The first human sciences—law and pedagogy, psychology and political science, theology, philosophy, rhetoric, and medicine—offer 'the human' as both the process and the result of self-transformation. Gross argues that the German humanist and reformer Philip Melanchthon reformulated the human sciences, grounding them in the "classical homology between rhetoric and medicine." The human sciences were at once exploratory and remedial: humans are active, engaged beings but ones that need therapy in the face of their own, potential depravity. Thus the intrication of scripture and natural philosophy, areas of doctrine and inquiry that describe, precisely, humankind, speaks to a kind of "curative medicine for the soul." These insights allow the emergence of "protreptic arts" devoted to both individual remediation and civic, corporate rectitude, both dependent on managing the passions. Rhetoric and medicine ballast particular interventions with the contours of time and place. We train up children in eloquence, but a training in eloquence would be incomplete without alerting our pupils to its communal valences and, indeed, its dangers.

Gross' investigation of the "early modern physics of persuasion" suggests the interrelationship between individual, passionate subjectivity and the life of the polis. After Francis Bacon, Keckermann, and Vossius loosened the relationship between rhetoric and occasion, insisting instead on mooring rhetoric to affect and the will, more and more thinkers examined the 'pathology' of rhetoric.[110] Indeed, analyses of the self in early modernity must necessarily explore "how souls are changed by institutions of state," and Gross offers Hermann Conring's "social technology" as a condign instance that posits rhetoric's role in managing the passions and occasioning civic prudence. To Conring, medicine is central to the "mutating body politic," relevant to sciences both moral and political; early modern 'political pathology,' as Gross calls it, combines the resources of physicians and

*Natural Symbols in Medieval and Early Modern Italy*, trans. Allan Cameron (Cambridge: Polity, 1994), 99. As Nancy S. Struever has argued, every change "in the notion of what is worthwhile to investigate is at the same time a change in the notion of worthwhile presentation, of discursive practice" (*Theory as Practice*, 199).

110 For early examples, see Johannes Dannhauer, *Pathologia rhetorica sive disputatio de affectibus* (Strasbourg, 1632) and Valentin Thilo, *Pathologia oratoria* (Königsberg, 1647).

moral philosophers, rhetoricians and political theorists (frequently in the same person) in order to prepare both individual and corporate bodies for intervention. Wielded by doctors of the body and of the soul, in the service of describing the (e)motions that pulse through moral and civil life, rhetoric serves, and surely embodies, political purpose: its pragmatics celebrated, its interventions calqued, its ambivalence muted. Describing and controlling the flows of individual and corporate bodies was all the more urgent in the light of individual vulnerability.

Amy Schmitter's chapter on Descartes and Baruch Spinoza offers a new and engaging reading of individual somatic fragility, finitude, and vulnerability. Her exploration of connections between vulnerability and finitude, somatic and psychic disruption, argues that rhetoric is prominent in the therapies both Descartes and Spinoza envision: their responses have "rhetorical interest," they urge various forms of intervention, and they embrace the "special province of rhetoric," the passions. In part, both thinkers acknowledge passivity as an essential human condition; we find ourselves in the midst of things and other beings, "in nature," and these act on, overwhelm, perhaps destroy us. What should condition our response? The 'medical engineering' advocated by Descartes, predicated on our 'interior,' individual vulnerability, epitomized by illness or vehement passion, or the political amelioration Spinoza both urged and embraced, founded as it was on the always contested relationship between singular things and their corporate nexes? In either case, we are never immune to breakdown, for our singular modes of finite being are part of, and dependent on, unending and conditioning causes, a continuum which includes the infinite. As part of this larger whole, singular things like human beings are identified by their *conatus*, by their striving toward self-preservation, by an increase in the radius of their volition, their "power of action." Spinoza imagines political solutions—including redescribing passive responses as active—as remedies against external causes of disruption or disintegration, while Descartes grapples with vulnerability from the inside: the finest ballast, for Descartes, is the quasi-Stoic, felt autonomy habitualized as generosity—what might be called autonomy watching, and taking pleasure in, itself. As Schmitter argues, this autonomy is dependent imaginative practices that habituate the mind to sovereign, rationally endorsed responses, responses not determined by the roiling spirits or the unpredictable alterations of our bodies. While both Descartes and Spinoza share concern with vulnerability, for Spinoza, the dynamic demarcation of individual identity is the issue, since we are forced, quite literally, to accommodate other bodies, other identities, other things; autonomy is the goal. For Descartes, autonomy suggests a problem of management rather than essence: 'medical engineering' and rhetorical therapy restore and sustain our identities over and above our basic vulnerability.

## Physician Rhetoricians

In a world beset with vulnerability and violence, deception and greed, rhetoric is a social prophylactic, protecting one's self and one's reputation, yet self-delusion and political disorder accompany the "canny and unscrupulous use of words." Guido Giglioni explores the physician Girolamo Cardano's ambivalent attitudes toward rhetoric: both rhetoric and medicine share "a fundamental critical attitude" that enables, on the one hand, somatic and psychological cure and, on the other, forms of social inquiry, the exploration and evaluation of sometimes distrait, always passionate human beings. Like medicine, rhetoric demystifies; it functions as armature or ornament, a means through which the self is preserved, even in its misrepresentation. For, as Cardano avers, it is generally more advantageous to appear happy, even if most consider themselves "less happy than they are." Civil interaction depends on one's circumstances and aims, so moderate dissimulation is occasionally enabling; but, because of "the discrepancy between thoughts, words, and deeds," one should exercise care and discretion, and conform to "mutually stipulated rules of practical wisdom" in all activities, including conversation, comportment, even walking. This version of the self both urges and excoriates hypocrisy.

Cardano's *Antigorgias* impugns Socrates' arrogance on these and other grounds. For Cardano, the philosopher is covetous of fame, arrogant and elitist, prone to fatuous wrangling, while Gorgias, demonstrating his facility with dialectic, defends wisdom, proper conduct, and "a favourable disposition towards mankind." As Giglioni argues, one of the central concerns of the dialogue is virtue, which is measured by both the actuality of individual appetite and the "social implications of public good." Cardano's Socrates focuses on abstract notions, and hollow moral generalisations, while Gorgias accounts for concrete situations, circumstances, and the consequences of particular ways of acting, with *aestimatio* in mind—here understood as "delicate balance" of self-judgement and the evaluation of appearances. Thus Cardano reinvigorates Gorgias' position by applying sophist techniques to Socrates' inflexible moralising. Yet his Socrates recognises the necessity not only of virtue and honour, but of "subtle cavils" in order that those in charge of "dispensing the *pharmakon* of truth . convince their audiences to buy their goods." Thus the diffuse therapeutic powers of rhetoric interest Cardano: *inventio*, for example, subvents healing via what Giglioni calls "controlled alienation," or distancing ourselves from ourselves by occupying the mind with light-hearted concerns, another's counsel, or creative activity. Rhetoric is "medicine" for the affects, and philosophers, treating both the active ingredients of truth and the 'excipients' of social, subjective values, are what Giglioni calls "apothecaries of the will."

The rise of voluntarism is central to the reevaluation of the passions in the sixteenth and seventeenth centuries. Recent work on the passions has emphasised the ways in which the humours impinge on, even dominate early modern conceptions of what I have called elsewhere "moral nosology."[111] In her chapter

[111] See Stephen Pender, "Subventing Disease: Anger, Passions, and the Non-Naturals," in *Rhetorics of Bodily Disease and Health in Medieval and Early Modern England*, ed. Jennifer Vaught (Aldershot: Ashgate, forthcoming 2010).

on the passions, Julie Robin Solomon adjusts this view. Indebted as we are to scholars who have explored the spirits, passions, and humours in the period, we must nevertheless resist the temptation to fully materialize the soul in the fluids and flows of the body. Contemporary scholarship's reliance on Galenic hygienic regimes distorts our sense of the political and rhetorical constituents of early modern embodiment. If we explore the passions and their ability to "respond to sensation, will, imagination, and reason," Solomon argues, if we follow sixteenth and seventeenth century theorists and locate the passions in the sensitive soul—responsible for perception and response, susceptible to reason and suasion—then we cannot simply resolve the soul into matter, whether humours or the attenuated spirits. The rich, robust accounts of psyche and soma that Solomon investigates focus our attention on reason and rhetoric instead: from Aristotle through Aquinas to Melanchthon and Vives, the history of the sensitive soul is in one sense the history of persuasion. Confecting Galen's and Aristotle's views offers early moderns both hylomorphism and various accounts of the influence of temperaments, spirits, and humours. The latter impinge on cognition and will, especially during sickness or emotional paroxysm, in which they produce 'seeming' or 'pseudo-passions,' but passions arise first in the soul, and are moored to questions of opinion, conviction, and belief. The body and its humours and spirits are mustered in response to the passions of the soul: that is, matter is activated in response to forms, to representations, or the ways in which passions 're-frame' information gleaned from the senses. These representations are us: our perspective on the world, conditioned by states of being, temperaments, habits of thought and action; they are perspectival, rhetorical, and thus subject to alteration, distortion, and error. Yet the rational soul was thought capable of "seizing the reigns, rectifying the passions, and re-establishing representational hegemony." Despite the fact that occasionally we mis-represent either the world or ourselves to ourselves, reason and prudence rectify; they can cure the passions via a delicate but firm grasp of the economy of volition and representation in the sensitive and rational souls. The cures are multiple: self-control, counsel, diversion, oratory. Solomon ends her paper with a Shakespearean excursion: *Macbeth*, she argues, proposes theatre as the "most potent instrument for rectifying these troubling forces of the sensitive soul." Plays "titillate" the soul, Descartes wrote, and when we "read of unusual adventures in a book or see them represented on stage," we take pleasure in having our passions excited, since there is little prospect of immediate harm.[112]

Both Gross and Solomon focus attention on the passions as media for medical and rhetorical investigation and cure, and they build on a growing body of scholarship initiated by Anthony Levi in the mid-1960s.[113] As both scholars confirm, rhetoric is perhaps the most important part of therapeutics: moving and managing spirits, souls, and wills trumps the care of the body, notably in extreme

[112] *Passions of the Soul*, arts. 94, 147, 187.

[113] Levi's ground-breaking *French Moralists: The Theory of the Passions 1585 to 1649* (Oxford: Clarendon Press, 1964) did much to open up new areas of inquiry.

states, like frenzy or melancholy, and especially in light of the increasingly voluntarist conceptions of psychology detailed by J.B. Schneewind.[114] But was rhetorical therapy effective? Certainly, sufferers resisted such consolation, as did Kenhelm Digby.[115] Perhaps we find exceptions to the efficacy of the 'therapeutic word.'

In his chapter on Robert Burton's *Anatomy of Melancholy*, Grant Williams notes the rich "ordering potential" of Galenic disease categories, but argues that, for melancholy and for Burton, this structuring miscarries: melancholy's symptoms are infinite, analogous to the "confusion of tongues" yielded by the tower of Babel. The body is a semiotic machine, akin to the discursive variety and infinitude of language itself, a common analogy in medical and intellectual history, as Williams suggests. Indeed, 'endless semiosis' defines both the distemper and the text: the "common Renaissance challenge of submitting nosology to a methodological order" is impugned by what Williams calls the "Babel event," which typifies not only a sufferer's experience of melancholy but the exfoliating text itself. Burton's treatise "tenaciously accumulates its encyclopedic girth as though melancholy were the core of nosology, the genus of all diseases, the only real medical problem." Yet, for all this effort, we are still lost in melancholy's "symptomological maze." Burton fails at accommodation, perhaps one of the central tasks of hermeneutics: the 'home' he has built in the *Anatomy* is unwelcoming, alien, foundationless, a spiralling out of signification, not the incisive dissection for which he had hoped. The book, like the distemper, is a "tireless" production of symptoms and signs. In some sense, then, he refuses to occupy the role of a physician. There is no *crisis*, no moment in the disease susceptible to application, to remedy. Surveying the state of learning and the hypertrophic growth in publishing, Burton loosely embraces a mild, "reluctant" scepticism, a scepticism about absolutes, in the face of a "labyrinth of intricable questions, unprofitable contentions," not least about melancholy itself and its roiling, irreconcilable explanatory voices. Thus the wrangling about symptoms, the consternation with semiosis, Williams argues, is reflected in the writing itself: inconsistency, piling phrases on phrases, periphrasis, etc., mark —some might suggest mar—Burton's prose. He identifies himself with a "failed anatomist," Democritus, who could not, as it were, make the cut. This is

---

[114] *The Invention of Autonomy: A History of Modern Moral Philosophy* (Cambridge: Cambridge University Press, 1998) and see also Arthur P. Monahan, *From Personal Duties Towards Personal Rights: Late Medieval and Early Modern Political Thought, 1300–1600* (Montreal and Kingston: McGill-Queen's University Press, 1994).

[115] Faced with the untimely death of his wife, Venetia, Sir Kenhelm Digby refuses the "helpe of other pleasing thoughts to drive" him from his grief (Lawrence Babb, *The Elizabethan Malady: A Study of Melancholia in English Literature 1580 to 1642* [East Lansing: Michigan State College Press, 1951], 39). Digby's and many others' poetic and visual responses to Venetia's death are well-documented (*Death, Passion, and Politics: Van Dyck's Portraits of Venetia Stanley and George Digby*, ed. Ann Sumner [London: Dulwich Picture Gallery, 1995]).

parallelled by Burton's "tropes of linguistic disorientation," which spell out "the breakdown of efficacious, healthy communication" in the public sphere.

Medicine in the public sphere, the "politics of cure," is the focus of Nancy Struever's contribution, one that centres on the "essentially contested" concepts that spur the intractable debate about the dualities governing theory and practice, physicians' reputations, and the status of medicine as a discipline. The tendency to 'bad theory' in medicine is funded by continual, amorphic changes in practice: as Anton Francesco Bertini recognizes, medicine transpires in the domain of the probable, so theory and practice are always, sometimes beneficially, at odds. This conflict is inflected with concerns shared by both physicians and rhetors: when Bertini describes the "particular, lived experience of cure," he focuses on an "observed manifold of affects, attitudes, beliefs, desires, temperaments," which define "the rhetorical domain of argument." Experience both underwrites and undermines medical authority, and its alignment with practice means that defending medicine may be only a "prolonged exercise in the description of obduracy." Yet this uncertainty courts ambivalence: on the one hand, it allows detractors to impugn medical theory and practice; on the other, it spurs self-consciousness about modes, methods, and authority. The "future epistemological essence of the humane sciences was already being formulated in these discussions on the 'uncertainty' of medicine."[116]

## Medicine and Experience

Ancient medical thought has an unexpected and under-explored legacy, one that speaks to the historical intimacy of medicine and rhetoric: hermeneutics and literary criticism. As Wesley Trimpi and Douglas Lane Patey have argued, thinking about signs and symptoms, effects and causes in medicine produced the kinds of sensibility, tact, and sagacity essential to other disciplines, including textual interpretation.[117] In fact, like all human sciences, literary inquiry and medicine share a method, an "evidential paradigm," defined by sign-inference and practical judgement.[118] Central to the epistemology and 'architecture' of the human sciences, medicine offers potent ways of thinking about aesthetics and ethics, cause and effect, particulars, universals, and experience—the latter a

[116] Carlo Ginzburg, "Clues: Roots of an Evidential Paradigm," in his *Myths, Emblems, Clues*, trans. John and Anne C. Tedeschi (London: Hutchinson Radius, 1990), 144. The entire essay is germane.

[117] Wesley Trimpi, "The Ancient Hypothesis of Fiction: an Essay on the Origins of Literary Theory," *Traditio* 27 (1971): 1–78 and "The Quality of Fiction: the Rhetorical Transmission of Literary Theory," *Traditio* 30 (1974): 1–118; Douglas Lane Patey, *Probability and Literary Form: Philosophic Theory and Literary Practice in the Augustan Age* (Cambridge: Cambridge University Press, 1984).

[118] See Ginzburg, "Clues," and Gadamer, *Truth and Method*, second edition, trans. Joel Weinsheimer and Donald G. Marshall (New York: Crossroad, 1989), 3–42.

contested concept thoroughly explored in early modernity.[119] While 'experience' in the later seventeenth century was transformed into experiment— events accompanied, determined by their explanations[120]—earlier explorations of experience suggest an attention to embodiment, and thus to both medicine and rhetoric.[121] This is clear in Montaigne. Investigating experience through the lens of medicine, Montaigne's conclusion to the *Essais* uses the non-naturals as a way of probing the self. He moves freely between the general, theoretical aspects of medicine he excoriates and particularity, impugning universalizing medical theory with the tractable experience of his own embodiment. As one scholar suggests, his "congenital antipathy toward medicine's proscriptive practices" obscures his "very real affinity with its descriptive function."[122] In effect, in "Of Experience," Montaigne uses the non-naturals—air, food and drink, evacuation and repletion, exercise and rest, sleep and waking, the passions of the soul—as templates for self-knowledge, for redirecting resources, and for rubbishing physicians. He composes his own *historia*, arguing that participatory, useful, and therapeutic knowledge of the self issues from the body: "it is necessary that our body, aided by our judgement, become itself the *subject* of its own knowledge."[123] To adjust Dilthey's famous formulation, there is real blood flowing in the veins of the vulnerable self fabricated by Montaigne—and by the physicians and philosophers examined in this volume.[124]

Knowledge of the embodied self is found at the intersection of medicine, philosophy, and rhetoric: the patient-physician encounter—the moment that focuses Elder's attention—thus stands in for a constellation of sometimes effective, sometimes rebarbative interaction between sufferers and healers, physicians and critics, centred on the sick, living body, on therapies and remedies, on text and tissue. Time, place, "the strength of the Patient, and other Circumstances" determine the encounter, but so does "a certain practical judgement, which is not got in the Universities."[125] This 'practical judgement,' a sensibility about the

---

[119] Martin Jay, *Songs of Experience: Modern American and European Variations on a Universal Theme* (Berkeley: University of California Press, 2005).

[120] Peter Dear, *Discipline and Experience: the Mathematical Way in the Scientific Revolution* (Chicago: University of Chicago Press, 1995).

[121] For embodiment as an ongoing concern of early modern science, see *Science Incarnate: Historical Embodiments of Natural Knowledge*, ed. Christopher Lawrence and Steven Shapin (Chicago: University of Chicago Press, 1998).

[122] George Hoffmann, "The Investigation of Nature," in *The Cambridge Companion to Montaigne*, ed. Ullrich Langer (Cambridge: Cambridge University Press, 2005), 169.

[123] As Jean Starobinski has shown, the non-naturals organise Montaigne's exploration of self in "Of Experience"; see "The Body's Moment," *Yale French Studies* 63 (1983): 273–305; quotation from 276.

[124] Wilhelm Dilthey, *Introduction to the Human Sciences: An Attempt to Lay a Foundation for the Study of Society and History*, trans. Ramon J. Betanzos (Detroit: Wayne State University Press, 1988), 73.

[125] Abercromby, *Discourse of Wit*, 224.

right moment and correct manner of intervention, is developed in the study and practice of rhetoric, nuanced by a course of licit reading and, of course, refined by interaction with suffering bodies. In these shared habits of thought, emotion is privileged: at the bedside, remedying 'hurtful conceits,' urging a 'merry heart' as tonic, recognizes discourse as essential to cure. As several contributors argue below, managing suffering is, in part, controlling 'what flows,' the passions and the spirits that may either mollify or exacerbate individual or civic distemper. Both medicine and rhetoric are forms of rheology, occasioning or assuaging, exciting or calming the spirits and the passions: both manage 'what flows' using the methods and means to hand. They are disciplines and practices dedicated to intervention, its exigencies and its urgency, as Aristotle recognised. With respect to "rhetoric and medicine and faculties of that kind," he insists, practitioners—puzzling over a discipline and its constituents, its principles and practices—must embrace all of the "available means," and must inquire "on both sides of a subject," in order to adequately grasp a 'science' (101b5–101b10, 101a35). So should we.

# Chapter 1
# Between Medicine and Rhetoric

Stephen Pender

To physician, *idéologue*, and reformer Pierre-Jean-Georges Cabanis, writing in 1788, medicine was the "basis of the only good rational philosophy."[1] Medicine, Cabanis argues, comprehends the "organic states" (*états organiques*) and "physical sensibilities" (*sensibilités physiques*) essential to intellection and emotion, action and reaction. That the intellect and the passions hold sway over the body is "an incontestable general fact" (*un fait général incontestable*); so too do physical processes condition moral operations.[2] Cabanis' "physiological monism," his assertion that "the moral is only the physical considered under certain more particular points of view," is central to his and others' efforts to establish a secure, material foundation for moral philosophy in the late eighteenth and early nineteenth centuries.[3] To Cabanis, moral philosophy cannot rest solely or comfortably on its theological substrata; instead, it should be investigated under the lissom rubric 'physiology,' envisioned as a "science of man" encompassing ethics, politics, and healing. Thus armed, physicians might form a 'new priesthood,' its liturgy medical, moral, and social reform.[4]

---

1 "The Author's Preface," *An Essay on the Certainty of Medicine*, trans. R. La Roche (Philadelphia, 1823), 25 (emphasis in La Roche's translation of Cabanis' third edition, 1819); *Du degré de certitude de la médicine* (written in the late 1780s, published 1798) in *Oeuvres Philosophiques de Cabanis*, ed. Claude Lehec and Jean Cazeneuve, 2 vols. (Paris, 1956), 1:36; see also 2:94–7.

2 Rapports du physique et du moral de l'homme (1802), in Oeuvres Philosophiques, 1:105–631, 604.

3 See *An Essay*, 84; *Oeuvres Philosophiques*, 1:78 (this notion is pursued at length in *Rapports*). In his introduction to *Oeuvres Philosophiques*, Cazeneuve claims that Cabanis thought "la matière ....est pénétrée d'énergie vitale; le corps est animé; le monde est habité par une volunté intelligente et providentielle," that Cabanis' world, "comme celui de Spinoza, est 'plein de Dieu'" (1:XXXVIII). Cabanis' views were adopted by "the majority of medical men" in France by about 1830, according to L.S. Jacyna, "Medical Science and Moral Science: The Cultural Relations of Physiology in Restoration France," *History of Science* 25 (1987), 111–146, esp. 113–14, 118.

4 Jacyna, "Medical Science and Moral Science," 116, 127, drawing on Cabanis, Gall, and Saint-Simon; Ludmilla Jordanova, "Reflections on Medical Reform: Cabanis' *Coup d'Œuil*," in *Medicine in the Enlightenment*, ed. Roy Porter (Amsterdam, 1995), 166; Martin S. Staum, *Cabanis: Enlightenment and Medical Philosophy in the French Revolution* (Princeton, 1980), *passim*; Dorinda Outram, *The Body and the French Revolution: Sex,*

If medicine was to be the "basis" of a new, rational philosophy, its theory and practice required substantial renovation. In *Du degré de certitude de la médicine* (1798), Cabanis moors this reformation to the recovery of Hellenistic medical thought. Consonant with late eighteenth-century neoclassicism, Cabanis insists that medicine's ancient legacy offered its inheritors a substantial repertoire of theories and practices as well as "all the means necessary to lead to their attainment." Attempting to rescue medicine from "an uncharted sea" (*une mer inconnue*) of uncertainty, combing ancient texts for resources that might assist his project, Cabanis proposes precise, detailed clinical observation as the engine of reform in contemporary nosology, medical epistemology, and therapeutics.[5] "The true knowledge of our art," Cabanis argues in *Du degré*, "is constituted of a more or less *correct assemblage* of sensations derived from clinical observations."[6] 'Sensations' are the physician's perceived or recalled impressions, "traces dans les organes de la pensée," raw material assembled for judgement.[7] For Cabanis, the solution to medical uncertainty hinges on the putative relationship between careful clinical observation, its extension by analogy (what ancient physicians called "transition to the similar"), and induction.[8] Cabanis sifts these sensations with tools drawn from the history of rhetoric:

> Noting with care all the circumstances capable of seducing, agitating, or convincing in discourse, in images, or in the form of reasoning, the ancient rhetors [*les anciens rhéteurs*] were soon convinced that these beauties, or rather

*Class, and Political Culture* (New Haven, 1989), 106–123; and see also A. Levin, "Venel, Fourcroy, Cabanis, and the Idea of Scientific Revolution: The French Political Context and the General Patterns of Conceptualisation of Scientific Change," *History of Science* 22 (1984), 303–320. Cabanis echoes Descartes who, in his *Treatise of Man*, wrote that "the mind is so dependent on temperament, and on the dispositions of the organs of the body, that if it is possible to find some way to make men wiser and more clever than they have been thus far, I think it must be sought in medicine" (trans. Thomas Steele Hall [Cambridge, MA, 1972], 86, n113); see also Henk Ten Have, "Medicine and Cartesianism," *Theoretical Medicine* 8 (1987), 235–46 and Stephen Gaukroger, *Descartes' System of Natural Philosophy* (Cambridge, 2002), esp. 215ff.

5 *An Essay*, 74; *Oeuvres Philosophiques*, 1:71. Cabanis was a "neo-Hippocratic" who attempted to "establish medicine as an observational science" (Staum, *Cabanis*, 102–103). He was an admirer of "le sage et bon" Sydenham, to whom Cabanis attributed "une véritable révolution dans la médicine" (*Oeuvres Philosophiques*, 1:102, 2:137–38). He has been called a "theoretician of a barely reformed classical medicine" (Georges Canguilhem, "Cabanis, Pierre-Jean-Georges," *Dictionary of Scientific Biography*, ed. Charles C. Gillispie et al., 16 vols. [New York, 1970–1980], 3:2).

6 *An Essay*, 111n (my emphasis).

7 *Oeuvres Philosophiques*, 1:537, 2:272.

8 For "transition to the similar" (reasoning from one case to a more or less similar case, from observable to observable) and related issues, see Mohan Matten, "Empiricism and Ontology in Ancient Medicine," in *Method, Medicine, and Metaphysics*, ed. R. J. Hankinson, *Apeiron* 21 (1988), 99–121, esp. 110–113.

> the means by which they are produced, are far from being as numerous as at first sight they would seem to be; and that by uniting under the same title all those that resemble each other, they are all reducible to a very limited number of heads, or of common results.... The preceding remarks are equally applicable to those objects which the study of diseases presents to our minds. Each new case is at first believed to present new facts – but these, however, are only new combinations or shades of the same circumstances.

While physicians must continue to pursue the particular "spirit" [*génie*] of an illness and inquire into the effects of specific remedies, by focussing on "common results" and by drawing on the methods of ancient rhetors, this "méthode symptomatique" simplifies the observation, history, and treatment of disease.[9] Cabanis' enthusiasm for this symptomatic method is tempered by his recognition that diseases "are various, and susceptible of infinite complication," that medical semiotics "or the art of recognising different states of the animal economy, by their characteristic signs, is without doubt the most difficult, as well as the most important branch of medicine." Faced with misprision, in practice physicians must content themselves with "certitudes practiques," practical certainties, which are nevertheless sufficient to ensure "conservation et ... bien-être."[10]

Nor does Cabanis' engagement with its history exhaust his attention to rhetoric; elsewhere, investigating the relationships between medicine, "belles-lettres et arts," he concluded that "the cultivation of letters and of fine arts can be moored to the more severe work of the art of healing." As Ludmilla Jordanova observes in relation to Cabanis' *Coup d'œuil sur les révolutions et la réforme de la médicine* (1804), it "should not be thought that literature and art were peripheral to medicine – quite the contrary, they constituted its very core, provided its languages, and were its basic tools of thought." While Cabanis nowhere suggests that physicians declaim in grand style, even his attentiveness to Hippocrates was in part stylistic.[11] Cabanis' recourse to *les anciens rhéteurs* also sharpens the focus on individual skill; he urges discretion and sagacity, recommending the study of art for refining the physician's tact.[12] As we shall see, these strictures draw on residual notions of what might be called 'medical prudence.'

Cabanis' turn to rhetoric as a model for thinking through contingency and probability in medical experience exemplifies the form of loose, eclectic reasoning

---

[9] An *Essay*, 75–6; *Oeuvres Philosophiques*, 1:72–3. In *The Birth of the Clinic: An Archaeology of Medical Perception*, trans. A.M. Sheridan Smith (New York, 1975 [1963]), Michel Foucault argues that Cabanis' "medicine of symptoms," which was "essentially expressive" and in which "experience was rightfully science," was soon eclipsed by a medicine concerned with "organs, sites, causes ... [and] pathological anatomy" (117, 122).

[10] *An Essay*, 66, 100–101; *Oeuvres Philosophiques*, 1:65, 91 (my translation).

[11] Jordanova, "Reflections," 171. *Oeuvres Philosophiques*, 2:250; Staum, *Cabanis*, 51. Diderot celebrates Hippocrates as the "father of semiology" (Ian Maclean, *Logic, Signs and Nature in the Renaissance: The Case of Learned Medicine* [Cambridge, 2002], 277).

[12] Physicians must develop and combine "beaucoup de sagacité, beaucoup de discrétion et de tact" (*Oeuvres Philosophiques*, 1:100n; cf. 1:225–6, where tact is explained with examples from Renaissance art).

– seeking out common forms from variable, particular data; reasoning about causes from the probable evidence of effects; and turning to the trivium for assistance in doing so – that has characterised medical thought since early modernity.[13] Gravely susceptible to error, medical reasoning relies on signs and examples, both gleaned from experience and both the subject of rhetorical inquiry; like rhetoric, medicine reaches plausible conclusions from probable premises.[14] As Nancy Struever has argued, from the fourteenth century, particularly in the work of Pietro d'Abano, rhetorical figures were used to explain medical theory, and both rhetoric and medicine are pragmatic and interventionist: one devoted to the body, the other to the body politic. Struever has investigated this "rhetorical-medical mind set," the intrication of therapy and cure, in d'Abano, Petrarch, Descartes, and others; and she has proposed a dual history of rhetoric and medicine in order to account for these habits of thought.[15] Indeed, rhetoric is a "method for dealing with … domain[s] apparently beyond method" – ethics, politics, and medicine.[16] In order to find viable means for inflecting normative medical theory with particulars and experience, ancient and early modern physicians settled on rhetorical and ethical tools – analogy, exemplarity, prudence. They enlisted a "rhetorised logic," or that aspect of rhetoric in the Aristotelian tradition that involved interpreting signs, essaying probability, and establishing proofs;[17] in Francis Bacon's resonant phrase, the subject of rhetoric is "Imaginative or Insinuative Reason."[18] And since both rhetors and physicians must intervene, they must embrace *certitudes practiques*.

An examination of the antecedents of Cabanis' 'symptomatic' method emphasises, if it does not solve, one of the central problems for the human sciences: how might general rules (about judgement, practice, intervention) be formed from the knowledge of particular cases? How might we attain 'practical certainty' in any inquiry devoted to the thinking, feeling human subject? How might a habit of thought, immured in one discipline, dwell productively in another? Early modern medicine is a fecund testing-ground for this inquiry; as Carlo Ginzburg notes in what is now a famous essay, the "future epistemological

13 Maclean, *Logic, Signs and Nature*, 136–45, 340, *passim*.

14 *Oeuvres Philosophiques*, 1:617; 3:384, perhaps with Plato's *Philebus*, 18b–d, 62a–b in mind.

15 Nancy S. Struever, "Petrarch's *Invective contra medicum*: An Early Confrontation of Rhetoric and Medicine," *Modern Language Notes* 108 (1999), 659–79 and *idem*, "Rhetoric and Medicine in Descartes' *Passions de l'Āme*: The Issue of Intervention," in *Renaissance-Rhetorik / Renaissance Rhetoric,* ed. Heinrich F. Plett (Berlin, 1993), 196–212.

16 Eugene Garver, *Aristotle's Rhetoric: An Art of Character* (Chicago, 1994), 41.

17 Nancy Struever, "Vico, Valla, and the Logic of Humanist Inquiry," in *Giambattista Vico's Science of Humanity*, ed. Giorgio Tagliacozzo and Donald P. Verene (Baltimore, 1976), 174. As Maclean suggests, in medical semiology there is a "smudging of the line between fact and non-discursive interpretation, and a penetration of hermeneutics into logical analysis" (*Logic, Signs and Nature*, 312).

18 *The Works of Francis Bacon*, ed. James Spedding et al., 14 vols. (London, 1857–74), 3:383.

essence of the humane sciences was already being formulated in … discussions on the 'uncertainty' of medicine."[19]

I focus on this moment in a very complex work – part of Cabanis' broad and controversial programme of medical reformation based on "speculative physiology"[20] – in order to isolate a constellation of ideas that has ancient roots and early modern branches, perhaps even contemporary foliation. In *Du degré*, Cabanis conjures the history of rhetoric as an entrepôt from which physicians might draw methods and models for reasoning about symptoms, for negotiating the relationship between the general (conceptions of illness) and the particular (individual cases). For physicians struggling with the variable, conflicting medical theories and a frangible, uncertain practice, rhetoric offers methods for reducing phenomena to their common forms, for placing these forms within emergent systems, and for practical intervention devoted to agitation, comfort, or cure.

Here, I explore some of the less obvious affinities between rhetoric and medicine – not solely to better understand Cabanis' ruminations, but to suggest that rhetoric is a significant, and sorely neglected, aspect of medical thought from antiquity through to the early modern period. Both rhetoric and medicine are concerned with embodiment and with the passions, of course; since all accounts of perception and emotion must be 'enmattered,' as Aristotle insists, rarely was either treated in isolation from medical thought. This association between medicine and rhetoric is quite clear in both Cicero and Quintilian, for example, who enlist medicine in their inquiries into the passions.[21] However, my purpose here is to suggest that rhetoric and medicine share forms of inference and reasoning as well as areas of inquiry and, in passing, to argue that these intersections should have more purchase in intellectual history.[22] While early modern physicians for the most part reject persuasion, the affinities between medical thought and 'rhetoricised logic' are clear; sound conjecture was acceptable, while arguing both sides of a particular

19 "Clues: Roots of an Evidential Paradigm," in his *Myths, Emblems, Clues*, trans. John and Anne C. Tedeschi (London, 1990), 114. In *The Birth of the Clinic*, Foucault argues for the "fundamental place of medicine in the over-all architecture of the human sciences" because "it is closer than any of them to the anthropological structure that sustains them all" (197–8).

20 Jean Starobinski, *Action and Reaction: The Life and Adventures of a Couple*, trans. Sophie Hawkes (New York, 2003), 157.

21 See Quentin Skinner, *Reason and Rhetoric in the Philosophy of Hobbes* (Cambridge, 1996), 126. The *locus classicus* is Quintilian, *Institutio oratoria*, trans. H.E. Butler, 4 vols. (Cambridge, MA., 1996), books 6 and 11.

22 I depart slightly from Ian Maclean's magisterial *Logic, Signs and Nature* in order to focus on the ways in which physicians borrow from rhetoric rather than logic; rhetoric, as Aristotle reminds us, is about proof. Maclean mentions that reasoning in Renaissance medicine belongs as much to language theory and to rhetoric as it does to logic, but he does not explore either of the former at length (149, 328, 340). There is very little work on the contribution of medicine to intellectual history; the latest and most comprehensive treatment of intellectual history, Donald Kelley's *The Descent of Ideas: The History of Intellectual History* (Aldershot, 2002), scarcely mentions medicine.

case was consistently vilified.[23] If, as Ian Maclean has amply demonstrated, logic was central to medical thought, what, then, about rhetoric, which in early modern medical discourse, and in contemporary historiography, often appears as a questionable spirit, urging misprision, folly, the fustian? In pursuing these questions, I range from Cabanis to Plato and Aristotle and alight on a resonant early modern example, the English physician John Cotta.

## Distinguishing Marks: Rhetoric and Medicine in Plato

While ancient Greek philosophy is not "unthinkable" without medicine, as Werner Jaeger claims, the 'cure of the soul' depends in part on terms and concepts developed and refined in medical thought.[24] Philosophy and medicine have a long history of mutual influence; not only do they traffic with one another in metaphor, some of the first 'scientific' treatments of epistemology, ontology, causality, and the philosophy of language were medical, and semiotics, of course, was developed and refined in classical thought.[25] Ancient medicine is a repository of metaphors and methods applicable to history and political theory, literary criticism and ethics.[26] In Plato, a healthy body is the primary analogue for both the 'good' human being and ideal justice; the skilled doctor is a model for the virtuous man; and the 'upright' soul clings to knowledge as "a sick man does to a doctor."[27] Like

---

23 Maclean, *Logic, Signs and Nature*, *passim*, esp. 96–7, 104ff.

24 Werner Jaeger, *Paideia*, trans. Gilbert Highet, 3 vols. (New York, 1939–44), 3:3.

25 Jacques Jouanna, "The Birth of Western Medical Art," in *Western Medical Though from Antiquity to the Middle Ages*, ed. Mirko D. Grmek (Cambridge, Mass., 1998), 47, 50ff. As G. E. R. Lloyd argues, the "undertaking and recording of careful observations in the context of clinical medicine provide our best early examples of sustained observation and research" ("Observation and Research," in *Greek Thought: A Guide to Classical Knowledge*, ed. Jacques Brunschwig et al., trans. Catherine Porter et al. [Cambridge, MA., 2000], 226).

26 On the ancient associations of history, rhetoric, and medicine, see Arnaldo Momigliano, "La Storia tra Medicina e Retorica," *Tra storia e storicismo* (Pisa, 1985), 1–24.

27 *Alcibiades*, 146e, quoted in Joel Warren Lidz, "Medicine as Metaphor," *Journal of Medicine and Philosophy* 20 (1995), 529. Plato frequently compares the virtues of the soul (wisdom, courage, justice, temperance) with the virtues of the body (health, strength, beauty) (*Republic* 591b1–7, *Laws* 631c1–d1, *Philebus* 26b5–7). D.S. Hutchinson argues that Plato is profoundly concerned with medicine ("Doctrines of the Mean and the Debate Concerning Skills in Fourth-Century Medicine, Rhetoric and Ethics," in *Method, Medicine and Metaphysics*, ed. R. J. Hankinson, *Apeiron* 21 (1988): 17–52), and Jouanna notes that "Among the arts (*technai*) that served as models for the thought of Socrates and Plato, medicine occupied a considerable position" ("The Birth of Western Medical Art," 68). For an early modern example, see *John Rainolds's Lectures on Aristotle's Rhetoric* [c.1570s], ed. and trans. Lawrence D. Green (Newark, 1986), 107: "Plato [says] that justice is the 'analogue' of medicine." Analogies between physicians, lawyers, and orators pervade ancient Greek philosophical and medical writing; see G.E.R. Lloyd, *Polarity and Analogy: Two Types of Argumentation in Early Greek Thought* (Cambridge, 1971).

medicine, jurisprudence is an uncertain art. In the *Republic*, Plato draws an explicit analogy between a judge and a physician, both of whom, in order to practice well, must cultivate long experience, and hence the most prudent judgement, of their respective subjects. Like the judge, the physician cures in part with his soul and thus requires a command of rhetoric (in order to convey prognoses to the friends and family of the sufferer, at least). For Plato, a physician treats patients by "going into things thoroughly from the beginning in a scientific way, and takes the patient and his family into his confidence."[28] The best physician is "in contact with the greatest number of sick bodies," has experienced every illness and, surprisingly, is "not very healthy by nature."[29] The health of the body, the soul, and the polity are inextricably linked; one of their ligatures is the "therapeutic word."[30]

The *locus classicus* for the relationship between medicine and rhetoric in Plato is the *Phaedrus*. "The method of the science of medicine," Plato writes, "is, I suppose, the same as that of the science of rhetoric."[31] The rhetor and the physician share a single method, its success determined by the aptitude with which

---

28 *Laws* 720c–e, 857d1–4. On medicine in Plato, see William Osler, *Physic and Physicians in Plato* (Boston, 1893). Lidz, "Medicine as Metaphor," identifies four ways in which Plato employed medical metaphors, terms, and models (529–30).

29 *Republic*, 408d–e. Here, Plato seems to deepen the analogy between the physician's body and the body of his patient. This analogy is rehearsed by Montaigne in the *Essays* (trans. Donald M. Frame [Stanford, 1958], 3.13; 827) and George Herbert in *The Country Parson*: "And it fares in [preaching] as it doth in Physick: He that hath been sick of a Consumption, and knows what recovered him, is a Physitian so far as he meetes with the same disease, and temper; and can much better, and particularly do it, then he that is generally learned, and was never sick. And if the same person had been sick of all diseases, and were recovered of all by things that he knew; there were no such Physitian as he, both for skill and tendernesse" (*The Works of George Herbert*, ed. F. N. Hutchinson [Oxford, 1941], 278–9).

30 "Whenever our body is unduly loosened or overstrained by diseases or other mishaps, it is a necessary result that the soul be at once destroyed" (*Phaedo*, 86c). Compare Aristotle's assertion that "all the affections of the soul involve a body – passion, gentleness, fear, pity, courage, joy, loving, and hating; in all these there is a concurrent affection of the body" (*De anima*, 403a16–18; cf. *Physiognomics* 805a1–18, 808b11 15). On this connection in antiquity and the seventeenth century, see Pedro Lain Entralgo, *The Therapy of the Word in Classical Antiquity*, trans. L.J. Rather and John M. Sharp (New Haven, 1970) and Susan James, *Passion and Action: The Emotions in Seventeenth-Century Philosophy* (Oxford, 1997).

31 *Phaedrus*, 270b1–9. There is "a close parallel between medicine and rhetoric" in the *Phaedrus* (Entralgo, *Therapy of the Word*, 123). As Galen comments, "Plato thinks it proper to use in the investigation of the soul the same method as employed by Hippocrates in the case of the body" (*On the Therapeutic Method, Books I and II*, trans. R.J. Hankinson [Oxford, 1991), 1.2.8; p. 9). The passage from the *Phaedrus* is treated at the beginning of Neil W. Gilbert's *Renaissance Concepts of Method* (New York, 1963). Gilbert discusses Galen's readjustment of both Plato and Aristotle (16ff.) and the afterlife of his division of inquiry into analysis and synthesis in the Renaissance (80). See also David A. White, *Rhetoric and Reality in Plato's* Phaedrus (Albany, 1993), Chapter 8, esp. 238–240.

effects (passions aroused in oratory or symptoms of illness) are sutured to causes (the nature of an auditor's soul or the character of illness). Plato's model for a competent rhetor is an Hippocratic physician. In order for a rhetor to understand the soul as a physician comprehends the body, the soul must be "taken as a whole" (270c1–10); that is, a rhetor must inquire into the soul's composition, the nature and means of its actions and reactions, and its "natural capacity" (270d1–10).[32] Arguing against 'hacks' and 'empirics' (268a-269c), Socrates insists that a rhetor must shun mere "empirical routine" and, like a physician, cultivate natural talent (*physis*), knowledge (*epistēmē*), and practice (*meletē*).[33] Hack rhetoricians, who merely assume talent and the ability to practice and focus on the rudiments of rhetorical knowledge (tropes, figures, schemes, etc.), are deficient; to Socrates, a rhetor must have knowledge of the workings of the soul, since it is obvious that the art of rhetoric 'influences' souls through language (261a7–8). Indeed, in the *Gorgias*, medicine is set apart from the impoverished oratory of Plato's contemporaries, particularly the sophists, because it "has investigated the nature of the subject it treats and the cause of its actions and can give a rationale [*logos*] of each" (501a1–3). To follow the model of the learned physician, then, the rhetor must "classify the types of discourse and types of soul, and the various ways in which souls are affected, explaining the reasons in each case, suggesting the type of speech appropriate to each type of soul, and showing what kind of speech can be relied on to create belief in one soul and disbelief in another, and why" (*Phaedrus*, 271a5–b9). Since the "function of oratory is in fact to influence men's souls," Socrates continues, "the intending orator must know what types of souls there are" (271c10–d2). These are "of a determinate number," which in turn correspond to a "determinate number of types of discourse" (271d3–6). Like discourse, souls appear to have "distinguishing marks" (263b8).

Unlike talent, knowledge, and practice – reading the 'distinguishing marks' of souls or discourse – depend on learning, experience, and inference. Not only do common rhetoricians lack the knowledge that affords discrimination between souls, they lack the learning and experience that join theory with practice. They cannot determine the proper *application* even of their limited knowledge and are thus ignorant of "the right occasions for speaking and for keeping quiet" (271d7–272b5). For a physician, proper application is crucial: since each individual possesses a particular nature, diagnosis, prognosis, remedies, and the "therapeutic word" must be accommodated and attuned to the character of a patient.[34] Thus

32 See *Charmides*, 156b–157c for comments on treating 'the whole.' Plato seems to be drawing on the Hippocratic *Regimen*, 1.2; see Hutchinson, "Doctrines of the Mean," 23.

33 G.R.F. Ferrari, *Listening to the Cicadas: A Study of Plato's* Phaedrus (Cambridge, 1987), 74.

34 Lidz, "Medicine as Metaphor," 537 and Entralgo, *Therapy of the Word*, Chapter 3, esp. 124ff. As Plato writes in the *Statesman*, "The differences of human personality, the variety of men's activities, and the inevitable unsettlement attending all human experience make it impossible for any art whatsoever to issue unqualified rules holding good on all questions at all times" (294b). Plato distinguishes between the more and less exact arts (*Philebus*, 56bff.).

Socrates proposes the distinction between the quack and the Hippocratic physician – the quack knows only symptoms and the effects of certain remedies, while the physician inquires into the causes of illness (268a–c, 270b–d) – as an analogue of the disparity between dilettante and reformed rhetors: the former are merely aware of the effects of a limited constellation of rhetorical techniques (267c7ff.), while the latter understand the psychological bases of fear, hope, anger, pity, and approval; the former are indiscriminate in their application of these techniques, while the latter – who possess a knowledge of their subject, the soul – adjust their practice to particular contexts, audiences, and inquiries. Behind this distinction is Socrates' insistence that dialectics should be the foundation of a reformed oratory.[35]

Although physicians appear frequently in the Platonic corpus,[36] in the *Phaedrus* and the *Gorgias*, the relationship between rhetoric and medicine forms the basis of Plato's evaluation of oratory in general: the ideal rhetor is a skilled, 'rational' physician of words.[37] In the *Phaedrus*, as we have seen, Socrates argues for an intimate kinship between theory and practice, knowledge and occasion (*kairos*), employing the Hippocratic physician as a model for his ideal rhetor. The Hippocratic physician, who represents a potent admixture of knowledge, acumen, and experience, is, like a knowledgeable rhetor, distinguished by his understanding of causes, his diligent attention to occasion, and his facility with symptoms and signs.[38] Both are required to know the whole in order to know the part, both require long experience and familiarity with myriad examples, and both trade in effects.

For example, in *The Science of Medicine* Hippocrates insists that what "escapes our vision we must grasp by mental sight, and the physician, being unable to see the nature of the disease nor to be told of it, must have recourse to reasoning from the symptoms with which he is presented." Through 'mental sight' the absent is made present, the invisible disease made visible. Physicians 'weigh' the "the significance of various signs" and thus "deduce" the type of illness, its history,

---

35 See Ferrari, *Listening to the Cicadas*, 77–8. The allusion to the Hippocratic physician is controversial; see Jouanna, "The Birth of the Western Medical Art," 69, n. 194.

36 Of course Plato's attitudes toward medicine vary; as Hutchinson argues, "Plato's views seem to have changed from an earlier phase, in which medicine is an exemplary skill, suitable for emulation by the highest ideals of virtue (as in the *Gorgias*, *Phaedrus*, and *Charmides*) to a later phase, in which he is more interested in what is precisely true and free of the fluctuations found in experience, with reference to which medicine is defective" ("Doctrines of the Mean," 47); see also Jouanna, "The Birth of the Western Medical Art," 68–71.

37 See Entralgo, *Therapy of the Word*, 93. The "close structural and genetic connection" between medicine and rhetoric, Entralgo notes, is explained with clarity by Plato at *Gorgias*, 464b, 465a, 501a and *Phaedrus*, 270a–d (164).

38 Although Celsus argues that Hippocrates, "notable both for professional skill and for eloquence," is the rightful founder of medicine, since he separated medicine from philosophy (*De medicina*, trans. W.G. Spencer, 3 vols. [Cambridge, 1940], 1.proemium.8), Galen regarded Hippocrates as the ideal philosopher-physician (Jouanna, "The Birth of the Western Medical Art," 71).

and its prognosis.[39] Raw (subjective) symptoms are translated into meaningful (objective) signs; probable sign inference becomes the main constituent of diagnosis, prognosis, and retrospection. Like Cabanis' symptomatic method, Hippocratic case-taking involves the scrutiny of concordances and discordances of signs until "a single concordance is derived from the discordances," until an array of signs points to a syndrome.[40] Hippocrates calls this process 'deduction.' Yet Hippocratic practice, including the *historia*, also employs 'rhetoricised logic' and, in particular, relies on exemplarity and analogy, 'transitions to the similar.' Training 'mental sight' on an individual case necessitates drawing analogies between sufferers if a physician is to build on practice and experience, as we shall see; in turn, this process relies on semiotics.

Thus for Plato the Hippocratic ideal establishes rational knowledge and understanding, over and against mere experience, as the distinctive characteristics of a skilled physician; one must "know the whole in order to know the part."[41] While Hippocrates epitomises a learned physician who inquires after causes and who has a sure command of medical theory, there are still problems with practice, with application and intervention, all of which are necessarily conjectural. Now, perhaps, we might begin to understand Cabanis' turn to the history of rhetoric for prophylaxis against medical imprecision: just as the reformed rhetor is able to reduce the teeming diversity of souls and discourses to a 'determinate number' by means of 'distinguishing marks' or signs, so too the physician should be able to reduce myriad symptoms of disease to "combinations or shades of the same circumstances." Both should know the whole in order to know the part.

## Boundless Guesswork: Rhetoric and Medicine in Aristotle

Aristotle discerns similar parallels between rhetoric, ethics, and medicine.[42] Where Plato argues that the philosophical and 'scientific' knowledge epitomised

---

39 *The Science of Medicine*, in *Medical Works*, trans. John C. Chadwick and W.N. Mann (Oxford, 1950), 87–9; compare, for example, the *Prognosticon*, 15, 25. Entralgo, *Therapy of the Word*, claims that one of the innovations offered by Hippocratic medicine was the "formation of a *logos iatrikos* or 'medical reason'" (148). See also Louis Bourgey, *Observation et expérience chez les médicins de la collection Hippocratique* (Paris, 1953), esp. 109–188 and Bernard Vitrac, *Médicine et philosophie au temps d'Hippocrate* (Saint-Denis, 1989). Owsei Temkin puts the issue at stake here precisely: "The speculative element cannot be eliminated from medicine. It is both possible and necessary to penetrate beyond the visible, because what is visible does not account for the elements of which things are composed" (*Galenism: Rise and Decline of a Medical Philosophy* [Ithaca, 1973], 16).

40 See Entralgo, *Therapy of the Word*, 148–155; quotation from Hippocratic texts at 150.

41 Hutchinson, "Doctrines of the Mean," 42.

42 Rainolds, *Lectures*, recognizes the relationship between the *Phaedrus* and Aristotle's writings on rhetoric in the 1570s: "[In c. 1469, Johannes] Bessarion ... shows that Aristotle's *Rhetoric* is patterned after the rhetorical precepts which were sketched in Plato's *Phaedrus*.

by the Hippocratic physician is essential for medical practice, and that it parallels the knowledge required by a skilled rhetor, Aristotle endorses experience as the principal ground for medical theory and medical practice. We aim to *be* healthy, Aristotle writes, not to know what *health* is.[43] Arguing for a profound renovation of Platonic medical thought, Aristotle subverts the Hippocratic ideal: while Plato insists on a 'knowledge of the whole' in order to cure a part, Aristotle assumes that there can be no precise ('scientific') knowledge of the variable, suffering human subject. Mathematics and demonstrative, 'hard' sciences are certain; they have internal ends (knowledge and understanding). In contrast, medicine has an external aim, healing a sick body, and thus its effectiveness is determined by an individual physician's experience, skill, and sagacity, not his knowledge of physics.[44] But in medicine ends and means do not always agree: physicians frequently misunderstand the specific nature of illness and their curative means may be ineffective, even harmful. Medicine is "boundless guesswork."[45]

As a confected ensemble of theories and practices devoted to pragmatic intervention in human affairs, medicine exemplifies the necessity of probable reasoning and practical wisdom (here its affinities reside with rhetoric and ethics), the complexities of signification and interpretation (in relation to hermeneutics), and the relative uncertainty of disciplines concerned with human experience.[46] In the

---

This is evident in the work itself" (97). Hutchinson argues that both Plato and Aristotle "compared ethics with medicine" ("Doctrines of the Mean," 17, *passim*). The hierarchy of disciplines is set out at *Nicomachean Ethics*, 1094b12–27; see Maclean, *Logic, Signs and Nature*, 115. See also Janet M. Atwill, *Rhetoric Reclaimed: Aristotle and the Liberal Arts Tradition* (Ithaca, 1998), esp. 70–82 and Werner Jaeger, "Aristotle's Use of Medicine as a Model of Method in His Ethics," *The Journal of Hellenic Studies* 77 (1957): 54–61.

43 *Eudemian Ethics*, 1216b22–25.

44 Although those who study health and disease 'philosophically' begin with "a consideration of nature" (*De sensu et sensato*, 436a17–21), "it is for the doctor to know the fact that circular wounds heal more slowly, and for the geometer to know the reason why" (*Posterior Analytics* 79a1.15, 129).

45 *Politics* 1331b34–35; Hutchinson, "Doctrines of the Mean," 42–3.

46 Book 6 of the *Nicomachean Ethics* deals largely with the questions of art, knowledge, practical wisdom, judgement, and understanding (1138b18ff.). Practical wisdom (*phronesis*) consists of deliberation about 'things which might be otherwise,' the contingent and mutable. Also called temperance (1140b11) or prudence (*Rhetoric*, 1366b20–23), practical wisdom is confined to "things human," to particulars, and to opinion. Its constituents are experience, foresight and, in relation to jurisprudence, "the right discrimination of the equitable" (1140b20–1143a25). The literature on practical wisdom is large; for my purposes, the most useful treatments are Eugene Garver, *Machiavelli and the History of Prudence* (Madison, 1987), Victoria Kahn, *Rhetoric, Prudence and Skepticism in the Renaissance* (Ithaca, 1985), and Kathy Eden, *Poetic and Legal Fiction in the Aristotelian Tradition* (Princeton, 1986). Eden writes: "Aristotelian probability is empirical rather than mathematical, qualitative rather than quantitative, relying less on calculation and more on experience" (70). The best contemporary treatment of *phronesis* and the *phronimos* (the prudent deliberator) is C.D.C. Reeve, *Practices of Reason: Aristotle's Nichomachean Ethics*

*Ethics*, for example, medicine underwrites Aristotle's claim that moral philosophy is inexact and contextual: "matters concerned with conduct and questions of what is good for us have no fixity, any more than matters of health." Moral deliberation does not fall within "any art or set of precepts, but the agents themselves must in each case consider what is appropriate to the occasion, as happens also in the art of medicine or of navigation."[47] As he writes in the *Rhetoric*, most "things about which we make decisions, and into which we inquire present us with alternative possibilities."[48] All such inquiry requires equitable, 'Lesbian' rules.[49] Medicine is Aristotle's "perennial" example of probable reasoning; his "primary analogon to rhetoric is not virtue but medicine."[50]

Although he denigrates the use of persuasion by physicians (a "physician is not expected to persuade or coerce his patients"), Aristotle recognises that physicians share with orators forms of inference and reasoning common to practical, probable deliberation.[51] As one early modern commentary on the *Rhetoric* suggests, a rhetor "does not create probabilities, but instead perceives them;" so too "a doctor does not create healthful things, but instead perceives them."[52] The perception of probabilities and of 'healthful things' occurs in the interstices, as it were, between variable, individual cases and broad conceptions of disease. In both disciplines, general knowledge is forged from particular cases. Rhetoric's potency resides in its flexibility; it is "the power of observing the means of persuasion on almost any subject presented to us." Like the rhetor, who must "discover the persuasive facts in each case," the physician must assemble and apply the appropriate heuristics in

(Oxford, 1995), 67–98. On equity in Aristotle, see N. Sherman, *The Fabric of Character* (Oxford, 1989), 13–28, and on Aristotelian hermeneutics, see Hans-Georg Gadamer, *Truth and Method*, trans. Joel Weinsheimer and Donald G. Marshall (New York, 1997), esp. 19–21 and 383–491.

47 *Ethics*, 1104a3–5, 14–19. As Aristotle writes later in the *Ethics*, "individual education has an advantage over education in common, as individual medical treatment has" (1180b7–8; cf. 1104a11–b3, 1106a26–b7). "For to get anyone whatever – anyone who is put before us – into the right condition," he continues, "is not for the first chance comer; if anyone can do it, it is the man who knows, just as in medicine and all other matters which give scope for care and practical wisdom" (1180b26–29). On the importance of *phronesis* to medicine, see Eugenie Gatens-Robinson, "Clinical Judgement and the Rationality of the Human Sciences," *Journal of Medicine and Philosophy* 11 (1986), 167–178 and Kathryn Montgomery Hunter, "Narrative, Literature and the Exercise of Practical Reason," *Journal of Medicine and Philosophy* 21 (1996), 303–320. The *phronimos* and the ideal rhetor have much in common; see Reeve, *Practices of Reason* 29, 67–98 and Lois S. Self, "Rhetoric and *Phronesis*: the Aristotelian Ideal," *Philosophy and Rhetoric* 12 (1979), 130–145.

48 *Rhetoric*, 1357b124–25.

49 Aristotle, *Ethics*, 1137b26–32.

50 Pierre Pellegrin, "Medicine," in *Greek Thought: a Guide to Classical Knowledge*, 414–32; Eugene Garver, *Aristotle's Rhetoric: An Art of Character* (Chicago, 1994), 41; compare Entralgo, *Therapy of the Word*, 171, 176.

51 *Politics*, 1324b30.

52 John Rainolds's *Oxford Lectures on Aristotle's Rhetoric*, 161.

order to heal.[53] Yet both rhetors and physicians must address a "class" of people. Although rhetoric, as Aristotle confirms, "is not concerned with any special or definite class of subjects," it is also not concerned with "what seems reputable to a given individual … but what seems so to men of a given type." So medicine "does not theorize about what will help to cure Socrates or Callias, but only about what will help to cure any or all of a given class of patients: this alone is subject to technique – individual cases are so infinitely various that no knowledge of them is possible."[54] In other words, while both medicine and rhetoric are devoted to 'discovering' the appropriate means of treating, discursively or remedially, the individual human subject, both aspire to traffic in classes, inferring from individual cases probable rules for a class (the feverish, the rash). As Owsei Temkin has pointed out, medicine suffers from a fundamental contradiction: its practice treats individuals while its theory can only grasp universals.[55] Both rhetoric and medicine propose experience as the ground of probation, but if there can be no demonstrable science of things 'enmattered,' and if inference from experience is the main constituent of medical thought, how does one reason from heterogeneity of particulars to universals? How are particular experiences compared with one another? How does practice relate to theory? In both rhetoric and medicine, these questions are answered using examples and enthymemes (arguments based on probable grounds), rhetorical techniques for treating "what is for the most part capable of being otherwise," or things uncertain, like health.[56] Again, in both rhetoric and medicine, 'discovery' (of the means of persuasion or of healing) is dependent in part on the tracking and deciphering of signs: the rhetor and the physician sift experience, hierarchise effects and 'accidents,' read symptoms and signs, and discriminate between apparent and real causes. The problem of course is that semiotics is complex, freighted with uncertainty, and more than occasionally vexing.

To detractors and supporters alike, medicine is an uncertain art founded on reason, experience, and examples.[57] As a weaker form of persuasion, examples are employed only when enthymemes are unsuited to an argument or audience. Examples are "supplementary evidence."[58] Furthermore, exemplarity seems not to allow for the construction of universal principles from particular cases; instead, examples treat the relationship between parts and parts, not parts and wholes. As Aristotle writes, an example relates "part to part, when both are subordinate to

---

53 *Rhetoric*, 1357b32–33, 1355b110–35.

54 *Ibid.*, 1356b30–33.

55 "The Scientific Approach to Disease: Specific Entity and Individual Sickness," in his *The Double Face of Janus and other Essays in the History of Medicine* (Baltimore, 1977), 446.

56 *Rhetoric*, 1357a14–15.

57 The most concise formulation is Montaigne's: "Medicine is based on examples and experience; so is my opinion" (*Essays*, 2.37; 579; cf 3.13; 819). See my "Examples and Experience: On the Uncertainty of Medicine," forthcoming.

58 *Rhetoric*, 1394a10ff.

the same term, and one of them is familiar."[59] Yet examples have their place in reasoning; they are "a variety of induction which brings out the meaning of a thing by comparing it with one or more other things which are like it *but clearer or better known*."[60] Thus in practice, they *function* similarly to enthymemes.[61] Indeed, examples are artificial or technical proofs, equivalent to induction in dialectic: they have the "nature of induction, which is the foundation of reasoning." When "we base a proof on a number of similar cases, this is induction in dialectic, example in rhetoric."[62] The key term here is 'similar,' for examples serve to draw out, as Aristotle explains, similarities between variegated particulars, to sort out their relevance to a general principle or concept, without involving the middle term of a proposition.[63] Examples are effective means of persuasion, Aristotle implies, because they evacuate middle terms; they are links between concepts and particular experiences that might be subsumed under that concept.[64] This 'part-to-part' inference is natural, intuitive, and leads to *archai*; since "the method by which even sense-perception implants the universal is inductive," universals are grasped – because they are always already present – in particular cases.[65] As Gerard Hauser suggests, this process describes, precisely, the dynamics of argument, particularly epideictic argument. [66]

Where the use of an example entails inducing the common characteristics of a person or thing based "on a number of similar cases," an enthymeme involves deduction from commonly held, culturally-accepted opinion.[67] Equivalent to the *syllogismos* in dialectic, an enthymeme is a deductive, rhetorical argument from a

59 *Prior Analytics*, 69a14–16; cf. *Rhetoric*, 1357a27–30.

60 Gerald F. Else, *Aristotle's Poetics: The Argument* (Cambridge, MA., 1957), 19.

61 "Where we are unable to argue by enthymeme, we must try to demonstrate by this method of example, and to convince our hearers thereby" (*Rhetoric*, 1394a10–11); see also Aristotle, *Problems* 916b25–34. As Aristotle makes very clear, narrative, analogy, inartificial proofs, and similitudes are essential to learning. On inartificial proofs, which are deduced from outside the oratory, see *Rhetoric*, 1355b36–1356a1 and Quintilian, *Institutio oratoria*, 5.1.1–3.

62 *Rhetoric*, 1393a26; 1355b35–40, 1356b14–18.

63 *Prior Analytics*, 69a16–19.

64 See John D. Lyons, "Circe's Drink and Sorbonnic Wine: Montaigne's Paradox of Experience," in *Unruly Example: On the Rhetoric of Exemplarity*, ed. Alexander Gelley (Stanford, 1995), 87.

65 Gerard A. Hauser, "Aristotle's Example Revisited," *Philosophy and Rhetoric* 18.3 (1985), 171–81; the quotation is *Posterior Analytics*, 100b5.

66 *Rhetoric to Alexander*, 1429a22–28; *Rhetoric*, 1368a30–32.

67 *Rhetoric*, 1356b1–1357a7. On the enthymeme and example, see Garver, *Aristotle's Rhetoric*, 162–71, 232–48. The enthymeme has recently received close scrutiny in two articles by Myles F. Burnyeat, "Enthymeme: the Logic of Persuasion," in *Aristotle's* Rhetoric, ed. D.J. Furley and A. Nehemas (Princeton: Princeton University Press, 1994), 3–55 and "Enthymeme: Aristotle on the Rationality of Rhetoric," in *Essays on Aristotle's* Rhetoric, ed. A.O. Rorty (Berkeley: University of California Press, 1996), 88–115.

likelihood (*eikos*), an example, evidence (a necessary sign or *tekmērion*), or a sign (*sēmion*). As Aristotle explains, enthymemes based on probabilities or likelihoods "argue from what is, or is supposed to be, usually true"; those based on examples "proceed from one or more similar cases, arrive at a general proposition, and then argue deductively to a particular inference"; those based on signs are rather more complex.[68]

A "sign is meant to be a demonstrative proposition either necessary or reputable; for anything such that when it is another thing is, or when it has come into being the other has come into being before or after, is a sign of the other's being or having come into being."[69] In contrast to probabilities or likelihoods (*eikota*), which derive from experience and are related only in general ways to the instances they condition, signs are either necessary or non-necessary, convertible or non-convertible.[70] Although there was some blurring between *tekmērion* and *sēmion* in his period, Aristotle distinguishes signs which might form the middle term of a demonstration (necessary signs), and from which a class of objects might be inferred, from those related to the 'enumerative' induction which characterises exemplarity.[71] Although Aristotle's definition of enthymemes is supple enough to include inference from effect to cause using both *tekmērion* and *sēmion*, signs technically "yield no deduction" and are treated with circumspection along with

---

68 *Rhetoric*, 1402b13–21. Wesley Trimpi succinctly defines the enthymeme: "The enthymeme, the orator's 'demonstration' of what he wishes to persuade his listeners, reaches a probable conclusion from probable premises with the same logic as the syllogism reaches a certain conclusion from certain premises" ("The Ancient Hypothesis of Fiction: An Essay on the Origins of Literary Theory," *Traditio* 27 [1971], 1–78, 17). The most perspicacious writing on the enthymeme is by M.F. Burnyeat, "Enthymeme: Aristotle on the Logic of Persuasion," in *Aristotle's Rhetoric: Philosophical Essays*, ed. David J. Furley and Alexander Nehamas (Princeton, 1994), 3–55, citing Renaissance examples at 50–51. See also the collection, *Essays on Aristotle's Rhetoric*, ed. Amélie Oksenberg Rorty (Berkeley, 1996). Thomas Hobbes discusses the relationship between enthymemes and probabilities, and proposes a distinction between fallible and infallible signs; see *A Briefe of the Art of Rhetorique*, in *The Rhetorics of Thomas Hobbes and Bernard Lamy*, ed. John T. Harwood (Carbondale, 1986), 103–104.

69 *Prior Analytics*, 70b3ff. Compare the *Rhetoric to Alexander*: "One thing is a sign of another thing, but one thing taken at random is not a sign of something else taken at random, nor is everything a sign of everything else; but the sign of a thing is that which usually occurs before, or simultaneously with, or after it. That which has happened is a sign not only of what has happened but of what has not happened; and similarly what has not happened is a sign not only of what does not exist but also of what does exist" (1430b30–36). This formulation is remarkably similar to sixteenth- and seventeenth-century definitions of a symptom.

70 W.M.A. Grimaldi, "*Semeion, Tekmerion, Eikos* in Aristotle's *Rhetoric*," *American Journal of Philology* 101 (1980), 383–98.

71 On the blurring of signs, see Carlo Ginzburg, "Aristotle and History, Once More," in his *History, Rhetoric, and Proof* (Hanover, 1999), 38–53; on the demonstrative sign, see Maclean, *Logic, Signs and Nature*, 126ff.; and on the enumerative, see *Rhetoric*, 1393a22ff.

pseudo-deductive arguments from accident, consequence, or synecdoche.[72] Yet signs might allow a 'practically certain' knowledge of things, Aristotle claims, because it is easy to obtain an "abundance" of signs from any one body.[73] As they accumulate, signs become indicative. The pseudo-Aristotelian *Physiognomics*, for example, proposes that inferences from "several signs" allow for confidence in concluding aspects of character from parts of the body, especially the face. But we should recall that reasoning from signs, as the *Physiognomics* makes clear, requires "expert understanding" and sagacity.[74] But as the number of signs increases, so too do the complexity and the plausibility of interpretation.

Sick bodies people Aristotle's treatment of signs; illness serves as a central illustration of sign-inference. Differentiating between necessary and non-necessary signs, Aristotle offers the following examples: suppose, he writes, one were to say that "[t]he fact that Socrates was wise and just is a sign that the wise are just." Even though this proposition is true, the argument is refutable (in other words, there are those who might be wise and unjust), since one cannot reason from particulars to necessities. Against such a non-necessary sign, Aristotle offers arguments that employ a "deductive" or necessary sign, one of which is "The fact that he has a fever is a sign that he is ill." In this statement, if the premise is true, the conclusion is irrefutable. Although other somatic – in this case pathological – signs might speak to the relationship between the universal and the particular, they are refutable:

> The other kind of sign, that which bears the relation of the universal to the particular, might be illustrated by saying, 'The fact that he breathes fast is a sign that he has a fever.' This argument also is refutable, even if true, since a man may breathe hard without having a fever.[75]

The signs of fever cannot function as evidences (irrefutable, necessary signs that reveal an invariable condition or quality) since they merely point up but do not demonstrate "the relation of universal to particular." That Aristotle's example of probable reasoning is drawn from medicine is not surprising, as we have seen; and as Douglas Lane Patey has argued, in the "schematizations" of inference from effects to causes, ancient and early modern rhetors and logicians frequently borrowed from medicine, especially Galen.[76] The language of sign-inference, and

---

[72] *Rhetoric*, 1401a1-b27; see also see *Prior Analytics*, 70a3–70b38.

[73] *Rhetoric*, 1430b37, 1430b39–1431a4.

[74] *Physiognomics*, 806b33–807a2, 809a2–6. On the importance of this text to early modernity, see Maclean, *Logic, Signs, and Nature*, *passim*, esp. 315–319.

[75] *Rhetoric*, 1357b2–21.

[76] Indeed, as recent scholarship has shown, Galen was acutely attentive to rhetoric in his public demonstrations and his autobiographical writings. See Heinrich Von Staden, "Anatomy as Rhetoric: Galen on Dissection and Persuasion," *Journal of the History of Medicine and Allied Sciences* 50 (1995), 47–66; *idem*, "Science as Text, Science as History: Galen on Metaphor," in *Ancient Medicine in its Socio-Cultural Context*, 2 vols. (Amsterdam

thus the ensemble of terms on which probable reasoning rested, was drawn from ancient medicine and, by the time of Quintilian, wholly absorbed into rhetoric; this sharing of methods, monikers, and metaphors is reciprocal.[77] Cabanis' suggestion that *les anciens rheteurs* are fecund resources for medical reasoning draws, in fact, on the insights of rhetoricians themselves. Perhaps Cabanis had Cicero, or Quintilian, in mind. To the latter:

> Just as men discovered the art of medicine by observing that some things were healthy and some the reverse, so they observed that some things were useful and some useless in speaking, and noted them for imitation or avoidance, while they added certain other precepts according as their nature suggested. These observations were confirmed by experience and each man proceeded to teach what he knew.[78]

*Observatio* is the origin of oratory, just as observation and experience are central to medicine. Like rhetoric, the art of medicine developed, and was refined, according to the principles of its own reasoning: observation, analogy, exemplarity, and induction.

According to Plato and Aristotle, then, medicine utilises enthymemic reasoning and exemplarity, which are both forms of probable inference. The former relies on a *consensus gentium*, while the latter, crucial to medical thought, involves intuitive, inductive, part-to-part thinking which compares similars and dissimilars. While both are conjectural (and interventionist, for as Aristotle insists we aim to *be* healthy, not to know what *health* is; like rhetoric, medicine means very little unmoored to practice, which is perforce about particulars), we should recall that the true and the approximately true, the demonstrable and the probable, are apprehended by the same faculty.[79]

## Artificiall Conjecture: Rhetoric and Medicine in Early Modern England

This attention to probable reasoning and sound conjecture is revivified in the early modern period, an aspect, it seems, of a renewed concern for particulars,

---

and Atlanta: Rodopi, 1995), 2:499–518; and *idem*, "Galen and the 'Second Sophistic,'" in *Aristotle and After: Bulletin of the Institute of Classical Studies*, Supplement 68, ed. Richard Sorabji (1997), 33–54. I thank Nancy Siraisi for suggesting this material.

[77] *Probability and Literary Form: Philosophic Theory and Literary Practice in the Augustan Age* (Cambridge, 1984), *passim*, esp. 35–74; see Quintilian, *Institutio oratoria*, 5.9.8–10.

[78] *Institutio oratoria*, 3.2.3.383. All arts that depend on "conjectura" and *opinabilia*, Cicero argues, and are beset by problems of prediction; medicine is no different, then, than rhetoric, since all 'divination' depends on the observation of signs (*De divinatione*, in *De senectute, De amicitia, De divinatione*, trans. W.A. Falconer [Cambridge, MA., 1923], 1.14.24).

[79] *Rhetoric*, 1355a14–15. On practice and particulars, see *Ethics* 1141b14–16.

for history, and for *symptomata*. In fact, there was a "general conviction" in the period that "the human mind can safely reason from effects or *symptomata* to their hidden causes." This conviction developed in part due to humanist critiques of natural history, revisions to Hippocrates' and Galen's teachings, and a renewed emphasis on the empiricism of Aristotelian thinking.[80] And as Nancy Siraisi has demonstrated, physicians were thoroughly attentive to history in general and to the history of medicine in particular; it would be mistaken, she argues, to imagine physicians divorced from any sphere of intellectual life in the Renaissance.[81] Early modern English medicine reflects this diversity of interests; in addition to those now well-known in contemporary scholarship, like John Caius, one might educe numerous early modern English examples of medical eclecticism. Thomas Cogan, for instance, published not only one of the most popular health manuals in early modern England, he also edited an epitome of Cicero's familiar letters and selected orations and compiled a book of "sayinges" from the Old Testament.[82] Although it seems that among physicians the term *grammaticus* was an insult,[83] surely the concerns of the trivium are not far from figures, like Cogan, who were writing and editing both medical and non-medical texts.

Although Charles Schmitt claims that sixteenth-century physicians agreed that rhetoric was insignificant to medical practice, this intimate association of medicine and rhetoric persists in early modern European thought.[84] Rhetoric's role in propagandising medicine and medical discoveries was clear: changes in theory and practice (as well as professional authority) were secured rhetorically and, then as now, rhetoric was an essential component to shifts in styles of investigation and scenes of inquiry. Against Robert Burton's insistence that Galen held that many "have been cured by good counsel and persuasion alone,"[85] and following Celsus (although Schmitt does not point to this borrowing), early modern physicians

---

[80] William A. Wallace, "Traditional Natural Philosophy," in *The Cambridge History of Renaissance Philosophy*, ed. Charles B. Schmitt and Quentin Skinner (Cambridge, 1988), 201–235; 207.

[81] Nancy Siraisi, "Anatomising the Past: Physicians and History in Renaissance Culture," *Renaissance Quarterly* 53 (2000), 1–30; *idem*, "Medicine and the Renaissance World of Learning," *Bulletin of the History of Medicine* 78 (2004), 1–36. See also Brian Nance, *Turquet de Mayerne as Baroque Physician: the Art of Medical Portraiture* (Amsterdam, 2001).

[82] Thomas Coghan, *The Haven of Health* (1584, 1588, 1589, 1596, 1605, 1612, 1636); *Epistolarum familiarium M. T. Ciceronis epitome secundum tria genera ...* (Cambridge, 1602); *The Well of Wisdome, Conteining Sayinges Gathered out of the Olde Testament* (London, 1577).

[83] Maclean, *Logic, Signs, and Nature,* 104.

[84] "Aristotle among the Physicians," in *The Medical Renaissance of the Sixteenth Century*, ed. A. Wear, R.K. French, and I.M. Lonie (Cambridge, 1985), 1–15, esp. 14.

[85] *The Anatomy of Melancholy,* ed. Floyd Dell and Paul Jordan Smith (New York, 1927), 475; 2.2.6.2.

generally attest that remedies, not eloquence, cure.[86] Medicine, they claim, is founded on reason, experience, and practice, not disputation. Perhaps this attitude is best summarised by Petrarch who, writing in 1352 to Pope Clement VI, claims that "while their patients are dying, [physicians] knit the Hippocratic knots with the Ciceronian warp," indulging in "the empty elegance of words."[87]

In both ancient and modern commentary, this turn from rhetoric obscures its central, structuring role in medical thought and medical practice. The notion that rhetoric, in Schmitt's opinion, "could claim little direct relevance for medicine" depends in part on a very narrow conception of rhetoric as trope and ornament. In contrast, past practitioners recognised rhetoric as a form of inquiry, as a flexible method for reasoning about signs and symptoms in the suffering body, and as a discourse of *kairos* and *krisis* with close parallels to medical thought. Several early modern physicians recognised the importance of rhetoric as a repository of techniques for reasoning about illness; here, I focus on John Cotta (c.1570 to 1650).

Although Cotta is well-known for his works on witchcraft,[88] there are few details available about his life.[89] A Puritan physician who practised in Northampton, by 1612 he reports that he was "above 40. years" of age and had been, for twenty years, an "observer and partaker of divers and different medicinall practise."[90] In *A Short Discoverie of the Unobserved Dangers of Severall Sorts of Ignorant and Unconsiderate Practisers of Physicke in England* (1612), which Burton seems to

---

86 "[I]t is not ... by eloquence but by remedies that diseases are treated" (Celsus, *De medicina,* prooemium 39). For early modern examples, see Maclean, *Logic, Signs, and Nature,* 104, though he also does not mention Celsus in this context.

87 Petrarch, *Rerum Familiarum* Libri I-VIII, trans. A. Bernardo (Albany, 1975), 279. On Petrarch and medical eloquence, see George W. McClure, *Sorrow and Consolation in Italian Humanism* (Princeton, 1991), esp. 49–54 and Struever, "Petrarch's Invective contra medicum."

88 "What seems to have preoccupied seventeenth-century English medical writers like John Cotta and William Drage was not witchcraft belief but witchcraft *knowledge*; Cotta's *The Triall of Witch-Craft*, in particular, is a sustained analysis of what it meant to know ('discover') witches in terms of a traditional epistemology of sense experience, reasoning, and conjecture" (Stuart Clark, *Thinking with Demons: the Idea of Witchcraft in Early Modern Europe* [Oxford, 1997], 155).

89 In Adam Winthrop's (1548–1623) annotated copy of *The Triall of Witch-Craft* (1616), he has written, after Cotta's printed name at the end of the dedicatory epistle, "the sonne of Peter Cotta an Italian." I thank Francis Bremer for sending along copies of Winthrop's thorough annotations of Cotta's text.

90 *A Short Discoverie of the Unobserved Dangers of Severall Sorts of Ignorant and Unconsiderate Practisers of Physicke in England* (London, 1612), 84. Further references are included in parenthesis. Cotta is clearly learned and contemporary; aside from the canonical ancient Latin and Greek sources, he refers to Jean Fernel, Jacques Houllier, and Jean Riolan, Senior and Junior.

have read with care,[91] Cotta devotes most of his energy, and his vitriol, to empirics, apothecaries, wise-women, astrologers, "conjectors by urine," and the like. I am less interested in his suggestions about the proper selection of a physician (e.g., 28), his warnings against unlettered surgeons (36), or his excoriation of those who merely mouth "aphorisms, maxims, and rules of ancient truth" (78) than in his careful efforts, both in *A Short Discoverie* and in *The Triall of Witch-Craft, Shewing the True and Right Methode of the Discovery* (1616), to enlist rhetoric, ethics, and logic in his description of the "true Artist" of medicine.[92]

Cotta begins both works by establishing the intricacy and difficulty of the art of medicine.[93] The uncertainty of medicine is symptomatic of "this life of mortalitie," in which "much more is that which is unknowne, then that which is knowne and revealed unto us." There is much that is obscure: "*Hoc tantum scio, quod nihil scio*, that is, so few are those things, which are demonstratively, truely, and certainely knowne" that they pale in comparison with those "onely probabble, or obscure or inscrutable."[94] Even what seems certain in medicine is, "by continuall accesse of different accidents and circumstances, ... begotten [with] uncertainties." Physicians have recourse to "reasonable likelihood," conjecture, and opinion, but not to certainty.[95] As in law, physicians can only know "by likely and artificiall conjecture."[96] Reacting to the popular notion that medicine is bad philosophy, worse practice, even the lowest of professions,[97] Cotta offers theoretical and methodological eclecticism, refined 'medical prudence,' and individual learning and sagacity as prophylaxes.

Facing diagnostic and prognostic uncertainty, physicians must multiply their means of inquiry; the true physician is eclectic, who "with impartiall and ingenuous desire free from sectarie affectation, doth from both [Galenic and chemical systems] draw whatsoever may in either seeme good or profitable unto health or physicke use." He disdains to follow in "strict & superstitious imitation" common

---

91 *The Anatomy of Melancholy*, 222; 1.2.3.2.

92 For a later, similar though less learned treatment of the same issues, see *The Character of a Compleat Physician* (London, 1680), which makes similar claims for medical prudence.

93 For example, he that "considereth the multitude of causes of in diseases, their infinite kindes, manners, and natures, the varietie of accidents, their sodaine and variable mutations, the soone lost occasions, and hardly gained opportunities, the wisedome which circumstances require, the care and vigilance which the subject exacteth, the doubts which repugnances bring, the resolutions which necessities urge; shall find the most exquisite powers of understanding, judgement, wit, discretion, and learning herein exactly sifted" (*A Short Discoverie*, 2).

94 *The Triall of Witch-Craft*, 101–102.

95 *A Short Discoverie*, 115, 29, 49.

96 *The Triall of Witch-Craft*, 17.

97 The story is, by now, familiar; as Montaigne avers, "the very promises of medicine are incredible" (*Essays*, 2.37; 587). See my "Examples and Experience: On the Uncertainty of Medicine," forthcoming.

rules and received customs (83–5). Instead, the true practitioner epitomises "the summe of art and prudence" (116) and combines his 'local' awareness of particular cases (*historia*) with a 'global' understanding of "essentiall propertie[s] ... belonging unto the generall" conception of health (117–118). Since God has mixed human knowledge with "much intricate difficultie and ambiguitie," Cotta urges theoretical and methodological diversity.[98]

Drawing out parallels between the good physician, the capable rhetor, and the *phronimos*, Cotta inflects his call for diversity with a paean to *prudentia* and discretion or decorum, both watchwords in *A Short Discoverie* and *The Triall of Witch-Craft*. For Cotta, prudence is the ability to reason with and act on probabilities; it is concerned with particulars, as Aristotle insists.[99] Cotta argues that prudence must guide physicians' actions "unto the schoole of contemplation of the world, and of the general revolution of all things therein." Learning and prudence allow a physician to "know and distinguish what is in nature, and the ordinary vicissitude of things, according to several seasons, circumstances and subjects, meanes, measures, and manners variously, now true, now false; now necessarie, then casuall ...". The ability to "forecast and husband occasion and opportunitie, that ill haps harme not, vaine hope deceive not, time beguile not, advantage escape not, uncertaintie prejudice not" is the "summe of art and prudence" (115–116). Cotta proposes prudence as a master skill, the property of the sagacious in various pursuits, from pedagogy to medicine to natural philosophy. For Cotta, all natural occurrences are perceived in one of three ways, either as certain and demonstrable, as probable, or as "contingence and good hap." With the first, the learned and the prudent cannot be deceived; with the second, they rarely err; and with the third, they "may be deceived, but not so readily as the unlearned." In all situations, the learned have either knowledge or "right probability and artificiall conjecture" as guides and thus are "seldome found erring" (41–2). The learned and the prudent share tact and sagacity, notably with respect to particulars. As Cotta writes, echoing Aristotle and citing Galen, "that which is probable cometh neare unto truth, and he that industriously exerciseth himselfe in discerning rightly true probabilitie, shall alway more wisely walke, and most seldome erre or be deceived." Those who are prudent, who read widely, "are generall readers or scholars" have "somewhat more advantaged conjecture" (130). Physicians who lack prudence and discretion have brought the profession itself into disrepute, "casting the excellent facultie .... almost behind the most inferiour science" (123)

The "true Artist" is prudent then. In the light of medical uncertainty, "there remaineth no other refuge, but prudent and artificiall conjecture, narrowly looking and searching thorow probabilities, unto the neerest possibilitie of truth and certainty" (4). Probabilities here are mute symptoms, "likely markes" (8); artificial conjecture is probable sign-inference, which cuts through "clouds

98 *The Triall of Witch-Craft,* 101–102.

99 *Nicomachean Ethics,* 1141b14–16; see also 1143a28–35 and my "'The Open Use of Living': Prudence, Decorum, and the 'Square Man,'" forthcoming.

and mists of ambiguities."[100] With recourse to "true trials and just estimates," physicians adhered to the "idea of prudent deliberation" in order to "judge rightly of the causes and differences of … diseases."[101] To "distinguish and discerne the validitie,…difference, and right use of probabilities," Cotta, among others, recommends that physicians draw on the opinionative arts and the trivium. As one of Cotta's contemporaries, Eleazar Duncon, insists, empirics are to be condemned for their lack of training in letters.[102]

In doubtful or uncertain cases, Cotta writes in *The Triall of Witch-Craft*, the man with "Sagacitie, exquisitnes of judgement, Prudence, Art" prevails and is able to "perswade and settle discreete resolution and disposition in all affaires." Persuasion, it seems, is key. In *The Triall*, two figures epitomise the skills of conjecture exhibited by the true artist: the logician, who produces precepts consonant with truth; and the orator, who, fitted with "his conjecturall state [*status*] or questions," and working through "mature, acute, and seasonable pressing, and urging," discovers what is "most equall, upright, and worthy to be credited, respected" in uncertain circumstances. While the logician uses "mature disquisition, and ratiocination," the orator urges "that which is most like[ly], most reasonable, and constant with right, with law and equitie." "What evictions of truth and right," Cotta concludes, "what convictions of guilt and errour doe dayly issue from hence, common experience doth prove and demonstrate."[103] 'Evictions' in this case means probation, or trial by argument. Cotta engages rhetoric in an attempt to assert the authority of the physician based on his negotiation of the perilous straits of conjecture. That authority is based on Cotta's efforts to link probable inference with ethical probity, rectified reason, and informed practice; it is founded, in part, on the notions of *vis aestimativa* and *ingenium*, to which Cotta refers several times in both books.[104]

To Cotta, the logician, the orator, and the true physician are defined by "the power and skill of right and true conjecture." In diseases not readily evident to the senses or reason, the true artist, with "prudent, artificiall, and exquisite perpension,"

---

[100] *The Triall of Witch-Craft,* 13.

[101] Cotta, *A Short Discoverie,* 2–3, 17, 118, 121–2; *The Copy of a Letter written by E. D. Doctour of Physicke to a Gentleman, by Whom it was Published* (London, 1606), 22–5, 33. The necessity that a physician developed a "setled perfection and generall idea of prudent deliberation" was clear; early logical and rhetorical texts often contained references to and examples of medical cases, medical problems, and semiotics.

[102] *The Copy of a Letter,* 24–5.

[103] *The Triall of Witch-Craft,* 4–5, 86–7.

[104] On the importance of ingenium to the history of rhetoric, see Ernesto Grassi, *Rhetoric as Philosophy: The Humanist Tradition* (University Park, 1980). "'Aestimatio' was the apprehension of the inwardness of a thing together with its external appearance." It might be defined, writes David Summers, "as the activity of the first faculty by means of which the spiritual or inward could be intuited in particular things" (David Summers, *The Judgment of Sense: Renaissance Naturalism and the Rise of Aesthetics* [Cambridge, 1987], 206–210, quotation at 208; see also his chapter on prudence).

> doth exactly valew and esteeme all the different manners, quantities, qualities, positions, and situations of pains; likewise accidents, motions, times, manners of motion, caracters, orders, and all other both substantiall and circumstantiall considerations.[105]

All three must enlist prudence, which is, as one contemporary put it, "the Arte of our life, as Physicke [is] the arte of our health."[106]

For early modern English physicians, it is not only reputation, character, and status that rhetoric helps to secure; if I might generalise from Cotta's example, rhetoric – as a practical, prudential interpretation of probable signs directed toward intervention in a given situation – is at the heart of medical practice. Sign-inference, exemplarity, and analogy – and the shared attention to the probable, to 'what might be otherwise,' that lies at the heart of rhetoric – enable the physician to conjure, to grasp through 'mental sight,' the absent presence of disease. In fact, rhetoric makes the absent present. To Thomas Wilson, who echoes Quintilian in the most popular book of rhetoric in England in the sixteenth and early seventeenth centuries, "Rhetorique at large paints wel the cause" which logic speaks in "but a worde."[107] Physicians do not only employ 'rhetoric' in "discipline formation, in distinguishing science from society, or in medical encounters with the sick"; rhetoric does not only structure the experience of sickness and healing.[108] Through probable sign-inference and analogy, through 'prudent perpension' and exemplarity, rhetoric enables early modern physicians to heal.

If one accepts that the human sciences can rarely offer an assured, normative portrait of humankind, rhetoric is indispensable to the interpretation of experience.[109] As Cicero makes clear, in situations where certainty is unavailable, the "need for eloquence becomes paramount."[110] Rhetoric is a logic of discovery, a practical philosophy related to topical reasoning, and a theory of probability, not simply a judicious disposition of words; it is more "a philosophy of human life

---

105 *The Triall of Witch-Craft,* 11.

106 Pierre Charron, *Of Wisdome,* trans. Samson Lennard (London, n.d. [1607]), 350. For another meditation on prudence and discretion, see Joseph Hall, *Salomons Divine Arts, of 1. Ethics, 2. Politickes, 3. Oeconomicks* (London, 1609), 21ff..

107 Quoted in W. S. Howell, *Logic and Rhetoric in England, 1500–1700* (New York, 1961), 14. This is a common conception of rhetoric in seventeenth-century philosophy. See James, *Passion and Action,* 218–19, who cites Bacon, Donne, Walter Charleton, Descartes, and Hobbes.

108 Ivan Dalley Crozier, "Social Construction in a Cold Climate: A Response to David Harley, 'Rhetoric and the Social Construction of Sickness and Healing' and to Paolo Palladino's Comment on Harley," *Social History of Medicine* 13 (2000), 535–46; 540.

109 Timothy Reiss, *Knowledge, Discovery and Imagination in Early Modern Europe: The Rise of Aesthetic Rationalism* (Cambridge, 1997), 87.

110 Skinner, *Reason and Rhetoric in the Philosophy of Hobbes,* 99.

as determined by speech than a technical doctrine about the art of speaking."[111] When rhetoric was exhausted by taxonomies of tropes and figures, it ceased to live "under the watchful eye of philosophy."[112] The merit of ancient rhetoric, as Cabanis realised, was its attention to the links between reasoning, persuasion, and probability; and the ancient cross-pollination of rhetoric, hermeneutics, and philosophy, the result of which was the "philosophical justification of probability," owes much to medical thought. [113] As I have argued for the intersection of medicine and rhetoric, it should be clear that I propose more continuity than change in medical thought. From Hippocrates on , reasoning about the living, suffering body depends upon analogy, exemplarity, and probable sign-inference, all of which find their home in the history of rhetoric. Then, as now, medicine cannot be immured from the pressures and pulsions of rhetorical inquiry.[114]

[111] Hans-Georg Gadamer, "Hermeneutics as a Theoretical and Practical Task," in his *Reason in the Age of Science*, trans. Frederick G. Lawrence (Cambridge, Mass., 1981), 113–38; 119. For a contemporary account of these issues, see Thomas M. Conley, *Rhetoric in the European Tradition* (Chicago, 1994).

[112] For the notion that rhetoric is wan when it is artificially separated from philosophy, see Paul Ricoeur, *The Rule of Metaphor: Multi-Disciplinary Studies of the Creation of Meaning in Language*, trans. Robert Czerny (Toronto, 1977), 9–64.

[113] Wesley Trimpi writes: "The adoption of terms from medicine, politics, ethics, dialectic, and rhetoric by those who first discussed the purposes and deficiencies of literature suggests how a theory of literature may have been forming in its borrowed vocabulary prior to the recorded documents as well as the ways in which later theorists would perceive, define, and defend their critical principles" ("Ancient Hypotheses of Fiction," 3). Aristotle, in particular, defending the mimetic arts against Plato, established a philosophical justification of probability (11, 16).

[114] I thank Christoph Lüthy, Suzanne Matheson, Stéphanie Nadeau, Nancy Siraisi, and an anonymous reviewer for *Early Science and Medicine* for their patient reading of an early draft of this essay. Research for this paper was supported by a Standard Research Grant from the Social Sciences and Research Council of Canada. This paper is slightly revised from its first publication.

# Chapter 2
# The Promotion of Bath Waters by Physicians in the Renaissance

Jean Dietz Moss

Bath's fame in the eighteenth and nineteenth centuries as a premier social resort owed a considerable debt to the promotion of its medical benefits by physicians of the previous two centuries. These physicians were encouraged to publish accounts extolling the spa's healing power by Bath's city fathers, who sought to increase revenue, and also by peers and prelates whose seats were nearby. At that time, the city could not boast the elegant accommodations or the opulent entertainments offered at the peak of its fame. In fact, Bath was a rather dreary place. Its lodgings were few and unprepossessing. The baths themselves were dilapidated, frequented by the very poor, lepers, and tennis players who merely sought a dip after exercise. And the roads leading to the city, three days journey from London, offered slow, muddy progress. The legends of healing springs at Bath would not have been enough to draw visitors. Only after renovations were underway and the campaign to draw visitors had begun would men of quality and "honest women" seek to journey there. They did so in increasing numbers, with only a slight decline in the mid-seventeenth century, until enthusiasm resumed when the purveyors of health united with the leisure industry to create the Bath spa of the Georgian era.

The waning of the cloth trade and the dissolution of the Benedictine monastery that stood in the centre of the city spurred the city council to turn to the most obvious means of increasing trade—the hot springs that the Romans had once developed. The effort was also supported by the Crown, which hoped to persuade citizens to repair to English spas and avoid the Catholic influences that might be encountered abroad. This sentiment was shared by the Bishop of Bath and Wells, Gilbert Berkeley, and the Dean of Wells, William Turner, both of whom wished to forestall any resurgence of Catholicism.[1]

[1] The Bishop persuaded Robert Lesse to write a promotional piece extolling the virtues of the baths some twenty years after Turner's account. A copy of the little manuscript, *A brief view of all baths*, is in the Folger Shakespeare Library's rare book collection. (Indeed, most of the rare books referenced herein are housed in the Folger. I am grateful for the gracious assistance of its librarians.) Primarily, the manuscript is an English translation of Gabriel Fallopius's advice on using the waters, *De medicatis acquis*. It does not seem to have been published. Phyllis Hembry mentions Berkeley's efforts to publicize the spa, *The English Spa 1560–1815: A Social History* (London: Athlone Press, 1990), 28. Her extensive study describes the variety of forces at work behind the scenes in this period, especially in Chapters 1–2.

The print publicity for Bath was spearheaded by resident physicians who hoped to draw more patients to the baths, particularly people of means who could reward them appropriately. After all, cities and resorts were for physicians the best sites for making a good living.[2] A recent study by Katherine Park shows that English physicians were not unusual in this kind of publicity campaign, for Italian physicians excelled as promoters of spas during the early modern period.[3] That is not to say that some physicians were not believers in Bath's waters as the most salutary aid for sufferers who had exhausted all other medical efforts.

A growing national pride in the country's natural endowments lent itself to this economic and political agenda. "The baths of Bath," one eloquent physician exclaimed in a hyperbolic metaphor, were "the principall jewels" of the country, and so obviated the need for more expensive travel to continental spas.[4] The physicians in this campaign, however, were always intent upon undergirding such obvious rhetorical appeals with the philosophical medicine that characterized the science of the day. The relationship of rhetoric and science revealed in these texts furnishes further evidence of the larger transformations taking place in both of these disciplines during the period.

The most popular foreign spa was Spa, whose name became synonymous with healing baths. Its location in the Low Countries near Liège made it accessible, but that destination became impolitic after 1567 when the Duke of Alba arrived in Brussels with a large Spanish army. In 1571, fearing English Catholics' collusion with this powerful adversary, Privy Council moved to control travel, requiring passports for those seeking to embark for such visits abroad.[5]

Bath also had some competition in England. It was not the only site of hot springs, although it could boast the hottest water. Early on, Buxton became Bath's principal rival. But, at 159 miles northwest of London, it required longer travel for those living in south and central England. Furthermore, its popularity had suffered somewhat because of its association with Catholic causes in Queen Elizabeth's reign. Mary Queen of Scots visited it nine times and, not surprisingly, rumors arose of plots being hatched there against Queen Elizabeth. Fifty miles closer to London, Bath had been more successful in sloughing off its Catholic associations.[6]

---

[2] Anne Digby notes that, next to hospital towns and London, spas offered the most lucrative livings, *Making a Medical Living: Doctors and Patients in the English Market for Medicine 1720–1911* (Cambridge: Cambridge University Press, 1994), 187.

[3] Katherine Park, "Natural Particulars: Medical Epistemology, Practice and the Literature of Healing Springs," in *Natural Particulars: Nature and the Disciplines in Renaissance Europe*, Anthony Grafton and Nancy Siraisi, eds. (Cambridge: MIT Press, 1999; 347–67. See also Roy Porter, *Disease, Medicine and Society in England: 1550–1860* (London: Macmillan Press, 1987), Chapter 2.

[4] Edward Jorden, *A Discourse of Naturall Bathes, and Mineral Waters* (1631), preface.

[5] Hembry makes this point (9–10). But she also notes that the Elizabethan government was not entirely successful in stemming the tide of visitors to Spa (302).

[6] Hembry, 27.

(Phyllis Hembry lists 60 spas as having been developed by 1699 as the spa fad grew.[7]) After the Restoration, Tunbridge Wells in the southeast, much closer to London than Bath, became the most popular drinking spa for royal visitors. The chalybeate waters, considered a healthful tonic, were imbibed by the hale and the ailing. However, Bath soon regained its popularity with royalty, partly through the efforts of its publicists, and partly through the city's improvements in sanitation and living accommodations. Political strife also accounted for some shifts of clientele, but these changing sentiments are too complicated and varied in effect to describe here.

## The Baths and Their Physician Propagandists

The ailing who journeyed to Bath found the baths' structures open to the air, limiting their use to temperate weather. Five separate baths were developed during the Elizabethan era. Two stood in the centre of the town, adjacent to the old Abbey Church—the King's Bath, which had been the prime site of the Roman spa, and beside it, the New Bath. The latter drew its water from the spring feeding the King's Bath. Built primarily for women, the New Bath boasted an enclosed changing room that protected users from the eyes of curious bystanders. The name morphed into the "Queen's Bath" when Queen, Anne of Denmark, used it in hope of curing dropsy in 1613 and again in 1615.[8] Today, the Queen's Bath has disappeared, but the King's remains, viewable from the windows of the elegant Pump Room, constructed in the early eighteenth century. About one city block away, the Cross Bath (named for the cross erected in its centre) still stands on its own corner site. Across from it once stood the Hot Bath whose water reached 120° FWater from it fed a smaller bath, the Leper's Bath, long since demolished. The Hot Bath has today been replaced by the thoroughly modern Thermae Bath Spa.

Five eminent physicians, and one of mixed reputation, who practiced at Bath from the mid-sixteenth through the seventeenth century published a variety of persuasive descriptions of the efficacy of drinking the water and bathing in Bath's hot springs.[9] Each was a graduate physician: William Turner (1503?-1568) took his doctoral degree from Ferrara; John Jones (fl. 1562–79), probably from Cambridge; Tobias Venner (1577–1660), Oxford; Edward Jorden (†1632), Padua. Thomas Guidott (1638–1706) received his MB from Oxford but never completed his MD. The last contributor described here, Robert Peirce (1622–1710), graduated with an MD from Oxford.

7 Hembry, 356. The sites are noted on maps on the inside covers of her book.

8 Percival Rowland James, *The Baths of Bath in the Sixteenth and Early Seventeenth Centuries* (Bristol, England: Arrowsmith, 1938), 55–7; Hembry also describes the visits (39–40).

9 James turns to the works of the physicians treated herein for much of the information he includes about the use of the baths in the period.

All of these physicians demonstrate a considerable knowledge of the art of rhetoric, imparted, no doubt, from grammar school through university. They used it as educated people of the early modern period did, not with studied application, but in customary manner, having been constantly exposed to its power in speech and writing. Moreover, rhetoric came (and still comes) naturally to physicians who must constantly deal with uncertainty in treating illnesses and yet want to persuade patients to follow the course of treatment they recommend. In this way, rhetoric and science became inextricably intertwined in their writing as in their practice.

Beneath rhetoric's concern with style, figures of speech, schemes and tropes, is its basic terrain—opinion. Students in early modernity learned to canvas the most probable answers to questions through the topics (*topoi*), a method shared by dialectic and rhetoric.[10] Rhetoric, unlike dialectic (the logical method of exploration and proof of the sciences), demanded attention not only to the problem but to the audience. Besides the logic of their arguments, authors, such as our physicians, relied on professional ethos and pathos to inspire belief. We can see traces of all of these tactics in the writings of physicians as they recommended Bath's waters for the suffering.

In their advertisements for the spa, the authors prominently displayed their learning, seeking to instill confidence and, at the same time, to educate their readers—potential patients—by providing a kind of primer in the theory and practice of spa medicine. In general, the physicians still adhered to the rubrics of presentation in natural philosophy derived from Aristotle. Dialectical arguments ideally led to "demonstrations" of the true cause or causes of the effects perceived. The physicians did not need to disclose these in full syllogistic style, simply a nod to a demonstration's existence was sufficient for their purposes.

For readers of the twenty-first century, the writings offer rare glimpses of the patients who placed their hopes in the water cures. The discussions of specific illnesses and treatments, however, rarely attend to gender-related problems, except in the case of Peirce's book in which women's ailments merit a separate chapter. He includes also a chapter on children's maladies, broadening his book's appeal.

The physicians transparently wooed patients of quality and wealth through their dedications to influential patrons and through the accounts of cures enjoyed by notable patients. They claimed to be the best purveyors of treatment and advertised the kind of attention referring physicians could expect for their patients.

[10] The topics most frequently used by physicians described here are definition (genus and species), difference, property, accident, relationship, cause, effect, testimony of authorities, more or less, possible or impossible, past fact or future fact. The first four of these are the predicables of dialectical logic; the next three permutations of the Aristotelian predicables used both in rhetoric and dialectic; the remainder are the "common" topics of rhetoric. For a detailed explanation of terms and logical theory see my *Novelties in the Heavens: Rhetoric and Science in the Copernican Controversy* (Chicago: Chicago University Press, 1993), Chapter 1; and for tutelage in the period see Jean Dietz Moss and William A. Wallace *Rhetoric and Dialectic in the Time of Galileo* (Washington, D.C.: The Catholic University of America, 2003), 12–21.

In addition, they saw themselves as aiding in the instruction of physicians less knowledgeable about the effects of the waters. The part each physician played in the campaign is addressed chronologically herein, to place it within the context of the spa's development.

## Beginning of the Print Campaign

By the mid sixteenth century, miraculous cures claimed for "holy" springs and wells were disparaged as superstitious. Instead, the physician publicists of Bath based their claims for the waters on the curative powers attributed to the particulars of the mineral content of the waters. Demonstrating their mastery of the scientific method of the day, they mounted dialectical arguments, citing numerous authorities whose definitions and distinctions were buttressed by their own observations. These arguments might be expected to resonate well with their peers. In the next century, as classical theories of medicine began to dissolve, the scholastic style also gradually disappeared, replaced by case histories and accounts of experiments. The classical art of rhetoric lost some of its luster as well. The attitudes expressed by Francis Bacon in the early seventeenth century and Thomas Sprat some sixty years later regarding rhetoric and science were to influence medical writing as well.[11] The cumulative effects are most marked in Peirce's work.

Despite their citations of authorities and evidence, all of the authors firmly declared that the waters were divinely bestowed. But they believed that God expected man to find the best way of putting these terrestrial gifts to use. The most trustworthy knowledge of the spa's benefits, they declared again and again, would be found in the medical expertise dispensed by resident graduate physicians and ordered to each patient's needs.

The first publicist of Bath's benefits was William Turner, physician, naturalist, Anglican priest, and Dean of Wells.[12] Although he did not live in Bath, his residence at nearby Wells and his on-site descriptions, class him with our Bath physicians. Turner was also an irrepressible Protestant reformer, who fled to the continent during the reign of Henry VIII, having been too zealous in his preaching. There he pursued his naturalist studies, wrote polemics against English Catholic prelates, and acquired a doctoral degree in medicine, probably from the University of Ferrara. In the second and third editions of his *Herball* (1562, 1568), he included a little book on baths, an appendix of seventeen folio sized pages that he first penned

[11] Francis Bacon had begun the reform of rhetoric in his *Advancement of Learning*, 1605, ed. Brian Vickers (Oxford: Oxford University Press, 1996 ), 2.215–44; but Thomas Sprat declared rhetoric off limits for scientists in his *History of the Royal Society*, 1667, eds. Jackson I. Cope and Harold W. Jones (St. Louis: Washington University Press 1958), 111–113.

[12] For a biography of Turner, see Whitney R.D. Jones, *William Turner, Tudor Naturalist, Physician and Divine* (London: Routledge, 1988).

in 1557. Turner's observations led him to term the chief ingredient of Bath's springs brimstone (sulfur). He is scrupulous in naming the authorities whom he follows.[13] The waters are useful "to heat and drye the cold and moyst joyntes and to scoure them from fleme." They are also "good for the palsey for the colick for the flixe [flux] and for the stone in the kidnees". They "warme a womannis mother [womb], wherefore they will make woemaen fruytfull, if the[y] be let blood in the mother veyn before, and be wel purged of suche humores as are the hinderance of conception" (sig. B3r).

Dismayed by the condition of the baths, he pleads for their renovation. He calls particularly for separate facilities for women, deploring the "bestly filthiness" of permitting male and female to bathe "together like unreasonable beastes to the destruction of both body and soul of very manye" (sig. B2r). The simile drives home the enormity of the bathers' sins. To remedy that situation, he suggests that lofts could be built over the principal bath. That would permit buckets of fresh water to be conveyed up to "honest Weomen" who otherwise would not come to the baths (sig. B2).

Employing the topical argument of the more and the less to acid effect, Turner excoriates the wealthy who spend money liberally "upon cockfightinges, tenesplayes, parkes, bankettinges, pageantes and playes," that bring brief pleasure to only a few. They spend not "one grote in twinty yeres.[for] these noble bathes beyinge so profitable fore the hole comon welth of Englande" (sig. B4). Turner's pleas for funding were obviously prompted by altruism rather than mendacity, for as Dean of Wells he would not be situated so as to profit by practice at Bath.

Unlike later physicians in this series, Turner criticizes more than he praises, but his claims for the potential cures offered by the waters may have sparked a rebuilding project. Not long after his death in 1568, the bath for women was constructed.

Dr. John Jones, who flourished ten years later, carried on Turner's effort. The long title of his book declares his medical expertise and his philosophical method: *The Bathes of Bathes Ayde: Wonderful and most excellent agaynst very many Sicknesses, approued by authoritie, confirmed by reason and dayly tryed by experience: with the antiquitie, commoditie, propertie, knowledge, use, aphorismes, diet, medicine, and other thinges thereto be considered and obserued* (1572). After such a title, employing *incrementum* and *articulus* exhaustively, one might expect more than 34 quarto sized folios.[14] But the book was only the fourth

[13] Turner's treatment of foreign baths in this appendix are derived from various sources. Some of the spas he visited himself, but he credits many authorities for the descriptions of their powers, among them, he names Conrad Gesner, Michael Savanarola, Anthonius, Fumanellis, Bolderius, Aleardus, and Agricola.

[14] Jeanne Fahnestock describes the ubiquity of these figures in science, *articulus* being "a simple listing of words or short phrases in tandem syntactically" and *incrementum*, also a list but one that builds from the least to the most important; see her *Rhetorical Figures in Science* (Oxford: Oxford University Press, 1999), 91.

part of a volume that included a philosophical treatise on nature, his translation of Galen's *Elements*, and a book on the baths of Buxton.

Jones had been recruited by two nobles, the Earl of Shrewsbury, who asked him to write a book praising the baths of Buxton, a part of his estate, and the Earl of Pembroke, lord lieutenant for Somerset (the county in which Bath lies) and Wilton, who suggested that he similarly address the wonders of Bath.[15] Should the reader not be impressed by the title page, Jones's treatment of Bath contains remarkable framing. It boasts a dedication to the Earl of Pembroke and laudatory poems—two in Latin and two in English.[16] The flyleaf's list of classical and contemporary authorities from Aristotle to Melanchthon further underwrite his erudition.

The work is divided into four books; the first deals with the ancient origin of England and the baths, noting the opinions of authorities regarding the efficacy of taking the waters and refuting those who had spoken against drinking them. The second and longest reviews diverse opinions concerning the causes of the waters' heat and its properties. The length of these two books—more than half the whole—seem strangely out of proportion to the purpose announced in the title, but Jones probably thought that such an examination of history and philosophy revealed the providential source of Bath's origin and buttressed his medical claims. The history of Bath and its legendary founder was to occupy several of the physician-authors. The inclusion of historical narrative in medical discourse had become a common feature of physicians' writings during the Renaissance, as Nancy Siraisi has shown.[17] The narratives also attest to the authors' acquaintance with the special *topoi* of epideictic rhetoric (the rhetoric of praise and blame). Adapted from persons to things, it might include positive or negative accounts of origins, circumstances of nature, description, comparison, development of natural assets. In the case of Bath, authors of its publicity meant to inspire audiences by reminding them of their shared heritage of values.

The third part of Jones's book describes the beneficial effects of the waters, and the last offers aphorisms for the proper preparation and use of the baths, prescriptions for clisters (enemas), distillations, and other medicaments. He states that this material is intended for physicians, surgeons, students of medicine, and others who would like to be better informed about the efficacy of the waters. But, obviously, he hoped that readers who were moved by his words to come to Bath would not fail to consult the author himself.

In the introduction to his treatise, Jones crisply describes his method as dialectical, using the topics of definition and distinction. To which he adds a promise to pay no mind to Momus and omit all "the colours of Rhetorique to avoid

---

15 Hembry, 10–13.

16 The authors of the Latin poems are Christopher Carlyle and John Ludus (Archdeacon of Nottingham); the English verse is by Thomas Churchyarde and Thomas Lupton.

17 "Anatomizing the Past: Physicians and History in Renaissance Culture," *Renaissance Quarterly* 53.1 (Spring 2000): 1–30.

prolixity," since "*Veritatis oratio simplex*" (aiiv). Forgetting his promise almost immediately, he proclaims the fame of Bath, as attested to by "the authoritie of the most sage Philosophers, most renowned Physicyons, and most auncient Historiographers, as by reason it selfe, aproued by arte, confirmed by vse, and dayly tried there by practise for these 2460 yeares, or thereabout" (aiiv–aiiir).

Jones' history of the city of Bath describes first the contribution of its legendary founder King Bladud from whom Bath's name was derived. The king discovered the value of Bath's waters when his leprosy was cured after he fell into one of the springs. Bladud, he explains, was the ninth king of Britain and a philosopher who studied in Athens. Jones traces his lineage back to Israel, and beyond that to Adam and Eve. The historical account, Jones notes, is meant to demonstrate the nobility and antiquity of Britons as well as the baths. Here, again he forgets his anti-rhetorical stance as he makes explicit his use of epideictic *topoi.*

After his historical summary, he employs dialectical topics, debating the causes of the waters' heat and its properties, airing the opinions of authorities. Shifting from the dialectical mode, he turns to the particulars of Bath's waters, which he bases, not on written authorities, but on his own observations and on consultations with chemists and finers in London and elsewhere. In agreement with Turner, he concludes that the main element is brimstone, but finds traces of copper, iron, and marquisite also.[18] Today, chemists describe Bath's spa waters as 65 per cent calcium and sulphate, by weight, sodium and chloride next, iron, and other trace elements.[19]

Jones goes far beyond Turner, however, in what follows—his description of accidents and ailments that could be aided by the baths. His recital of 51 maladies would surely attract interest, for the list includes many of the most common and vexing: scales, scabs, scurvy, ulcers, ringworm, leprosy, pocks, gout, palsy, apoplexy, the falling sickness, cramps, coughs, ringing in the ears, diabetes, constipation, wasting of seed, sleeping sickness, swelling of the matrix (womb), and memory loss. Here, again, lists are used to magnify the marvelous power of the waters.

To further corroborate his professional expertise, Jones inserts elaborate tables of humoral medicine that other physicians might use in analyzing sickness and health.[20] He suggests that "a wise and learned patient" should apply to a physician

18 This preoccupation with the particular elements of the water and the causes of its heat were also concerns of continental physicians (Park 350–354).

19 W.M. Edmunds and D.L. Miles, "The Geochemistry of Bath's Thermal Waters," in G.A. Kellaway, ed., *Hot Springs of Bath* (Bath: Bath City Council, 1991) 143–56, analysis at 151.

20 A table of taste in Latin and English provides the definition, description, and object of the organ, as well as kinds of taste based on Galen and on Melanchthon's *De anima*, (18r–v). Another table treats the waters' heating, concocting, piercing, dissolving, attracting, cleansing, binding, drying, stopping and consolidating effects (21r). The text also includes a folded insert of humoral concepts: "A Table of the vii Naturals, out of the Which the Actions according to Nature doe spring." Its headings are defined along the left

so instructed, lest more, rather than less, suffering be the result. One reason for the pointed advice becomes apparent in the plea that follows for a benefice, stipend, or prebend to support a "graduate physician" (23r). The scarcity of physicians at Bath, Jones reports, has left patients prey to apothecaries, charlatans, and such ignorant purveyors of cures as "goodwyfe Marjerie, and dame Siblie" (33r). Even when physicians became more numerous, other physicians also voiced the fear that the sick might try to economize and yield to the appeals of quacks. Some of these, readers are told, are hired by the owners of rooming houses who seek clientele.

As do the rest of the physicians, Jones provides precise instructions for patients taking the waters. His description of the attentive and elaborate regimen must have been meant to inspire confidence in the programme. It also provides the modern reader with a general picture of patients' treatment. He advises visitors to come to the baths in the warm months, rest for a day after travel, be purged, and follow a light diet while there. On the day deemed right for entering the baths, patients should rise an hour after sunrise, drink the spa water, fast, take a gentle walk, empty the bowels, and void. Upon entering the water, they should seat themselves farthest from the spring, drawing nearer little by little. They should be careful to immerse the body with regard to where the problem lies—above or below the navel. They may be able to stay in the water as long as two hours in the morning, and an hour and a half in the evening. Upon leaving the water, patients should cover their bodies to avoid a chill, then walk, or be taken in sedan chairs, to their beds. There they should sweat for an hour. After drying off and donning warm clothing, they might walk in a protected place. The same regimen should be followed for the second immersion, four or five hours after dinner. Jones adds that however long one stays at the baths, one must avoid copulation (29v). Other physical activities are permitted—bowling, tennis, and dancing. Pregnant women should not use the baths. If not with child, they can take the waters, but should be aware that if their wombs swell or ache, become hot and then cold, these are dangerous signs (30v).

Accidents, Jones warns, can sometimes occur in the baths: fainting, sleepiness, thirst, headaches, heavy sweating, burning urine, loss of appetite, rheum, and fever. The treatment recommended for headaches, termed "bucketing," may have caused some of these accidents; it called for sturdy attendants to hoist full buckets of water to their shoulders and pour them repeatedly over the head of the sufferer or, in the case of some other localized pain, pour the water directly over that area. The treatment was superseded by "pumping," when pumps were introduced into the baths.

Some two years after the publication of Jones's book, Queen Elizabeth and the court visited Bath. From all accounts, however, she did not enter the water, being repelled by its heavy sulfurous smell. A later source of her displeasure was the

side and then subdivided with bracketed parts and explanations on the right. Jones notes that these enumerations are not as elaborate as usual, but enough so that an astute patient might consult about them with a physician.

reported bucketing of her cousin, George, Lord Hunsdon, in 1602. She wondered that he had not drowned from the continuous flow of water over his head.[21] The effect of the royal visit, however, was to increase the popularity of the spa, at least for a time.

## Renewed Persuasive Efforts

Fifty years after Queen Elizabeth's visit, the efficacy of spa treatment seems to have required additional validation, for two more physicians were prompted to add treatises to the publicity campaign. Their books disclose some further improvements in the baths but little change in medical philosophy or practices. The authors are, however, just as skillful in self-promotion. One of these physicians, Tobias Venner, gained considerable fame as a specialist in "balneology" through his book, *The baths of Bathe or a necessary compendiovs Treatise concerning the Nature, Vse, and Efficacie of those famous Hot Waters, with a Censure of the medicinable faculties of the water of* 'Saint Vincent's' *Rocks neere the City of Bristoll* (1620).[22] As a resident physician at Bath, Dr. Venner zealously denigrates the reputation of nearby Bristol, noting on the title page that his work is published for the patients that "yeerly for their health, resort to those Baths."

Like his predecessor Jones, Venner annexes his book on Bath to a longer work of philosophical medicine. Its title declares his competence as a Bath specialist: *Via Recta ad vitam longam, Or, A plain Philosophical Demonstration of the Nature, Faculties, and Effects of all such things as by way of nourishments make for the preservation of health.* His wide knowledge of spas and the curative effects of their waters allows him to claim the singularity of Bath. The facilities there are now "fairely built and fitted with such conveniencie for bathing, as the like. is not else-where to bee found." (311). Moreover, the waters of Bath cure illnesses that cannot be cured elsewhere (312). The presence and power of the minerals—sulfur with traces of niter and bitumen—can be judged by their effects: "they heat they dry, discusse, resolve, attract, mollifie, clense" (312).

The reasons behind this new burst in advertising are disclosed in remarks Venner makes concerning the reports of some of Bath's clientele. Although they have come in increased numbers to Bath in the spring and fall, some claim not to have received the benefits they expected, especially after great expenditures. Venner hopes to restore Bath's reputation by claiming a unique nature and efficacy of the waters. He does add a caveat, reminding his readers that "Sickness is a Symtome of Sinne," so patients should first make peace with their consciences before departing for the baths.[23] Although this reservation might seem to offer a

[21] Hembry 29.

[22] According to James, Venner's work was expanded in 1628 and merited three more editions (55–7).

[23] The belief is commonly expressed by most of the physicians in their works. Porter comments on the influence of Protestant theology in this regard (21).

convenient excuse for the failure of a physician's treatment, neither Venner nor any of the physicians described herein fall back upon that explanation.

Not surprisingly, Venner suggests that the cause of the decline in Bath's reputation may be attributed to the poor medical care given by inadequately trained physicians or to advice dispensed by non resident physicians or by charlatans. To counter the problem, he advises prospective patients to consult only graduate physicians resident at Bath. They alone have the requisite knowledge to provide *individual* prescriptions for patients' ailments. The classical appeal of *to prepon*, appropriateness or what is fitting, finds frequent purchase here. Even renowned physicians who live in London cannot prescribe effectively, for they do not have the daily contact necessary to observe and order the proper combination of bathing and drinking.

Another reason for the decline in Bath's patronage in the early seventeenth century may have been the popularity of the newly developed springs and spas closer to patients' homes that could offer more affordable relief, a problem alluded to in Venner's criticism of Bristol's claims. Seven additional spas were being frequented by the late sixteenth century.[24] Thus, if relief were not immediately forthcoming at Bath, some clients might have left in a huff, thinking that they could have saved considerable travel and expense by visiting a nearer spa. So it was imperative that publicists for Bath dwell on the particular and rare qualities of its waters. The rhetorical *topos* of the more and the less magnifies the importance of the right choice of site and practitioner.

Venner demonstrates his special knowledge of each of Bath's baths and his concern that individual patients receive careful attention. He stresses the need to choose the bath appropriate to a patient's malady, age, health, and strength. The King's bath is the hottest, he says, and the most effective for certain diseases: "a Kingly Bath indeed," best for "cold and moist bodies, and cold and moist diseases" (312). The Hot Bath he finds so similar that it can be used to treat the same sicknesses. The Queen's Bath, being separated by a partition, is less hot, making it attractive for those who are unable to stand the heat. And the Cross Bath, the mildest, is "a dainty Bath for young, weake and tender bodies." The temperate quality makes it best for "relaxing and mollifying … contractions of any member …[and for] obstructions of the brest, spleene, liver, and kidneys." (314). In fact, all of the baths prove quite effective for ailments of the head and sinews, which come from cold and moist causes, among these: "Rheumes, Palsies, Epilepsies,

24 Hembry lists these: besides Buxton in Derbyshire; there were St. Vincent's Well at Bristol; Horrogate, Yorkshire; Holy Well, Flintshire; King's Newnham, Warwickshire; St Neots, Huntingdonshire; Ratcliff in London; and Utkinton, Cheshire: schedule A, 355; see the discussion on 14–15, 18–19. She cites the work of William Harrison, *Description of England* (1577, 1587) for the use of these spas in the period, 18. The spas were located in places accessible to all inhabitants of the country, as if strategically sited. Hembry comments, "It seems that a traditional bath or well was allowed to flourish or a new one to develop in each region" (19).

Lethargies, Apoplexies, Cramps, Deafnesse, Forgetfulnesse, Trembling or weaknesse of any member, Aches and swellings of the joynts." (314).

Venner proceeds to reassure potential visitors that the baths can also help those who do not have a cold and moist constitution. Indeed "the plethoric or phlegmatick," suffering from swellings, pain, or numbness in the joints, or from liver and yellow jaundice, can expect relief. Even those who want to be slim and "fear obesitie" can benefit by attendance at the bath. Prescriptive bathing helps to "keep ther bodies from being unseemly corpulent" (314).

Women, Venner declares, can expect other benefits through bathing in the hot springs. Barrenness and ailments of the matrix can be cured. Skin problems, scabs, sores, and itches are greatly alleviated.

> All of which to be true, we daily find with admiration, to the exceeding great comfort of many, who with deplored diseases, and most miserable bodies resort to these Baths and are there, by the help of wholsome Physick, and vertue of the Baths, through the blessing of Almighty God recovered to their former health. (315)

Venner's impassioned claims regarding the effects of the waters on such a range of maladies surely heartened ailing readers, whether they understood the humoral basis for them or not. Venner continued to serve as a physician in Bath until his death in 1660.

## Broadening the Appeal

The medical expertise of Edward Jorden, the second physician who participated in this renewed campaign to attract more patients, seems to have been even more highly regarded; for, 37 years after his *A Discourse of Naturall Bathes and Minerall Waters* (1631) first appeared, Thomas Guidott published a third edition of the work and included a panegyrical biography of "the very learned and incomparable Doctor Jorden."[25] Guidott praises Jorden's accomplishments, which he declares stand in clear contrast to the "Empiricks, and juggling Medicasters" of the age who claim cures and offer medicaments for sale to support themselves. But a physician such as Jorden has studied not only "the praeliminary helps of the Tongues," but "Natural Philosophy, the structure and uses of the parts of the body; the virtues of Plants, the compositions of Medicines; the Nature, Causes, and Signs of Diseases." The biographer reports that Jorden was so respected by King James that he commended the Queen to his care on her visits to Bath. That such eminent practitioners reside at Bath would seem to argue implicitly for the superiority of its claims to offer the best in spa medical advice, but more on Guidott and his part in the publicity effort below.

[25] Guidott's biography, 54. The first edition of the work appeared in 1631.

An increased emphasis on erudition and application of theory noticeable in the writings of these Bath physicians in the mid- and late seventeenth century suggests that the authors may have believed that, in this way, physicians living outside Bath would be moved to refer their patients to them. The grounding in humoral theory shared by "graduate physicians" when coupled with the sharp localized observations of the authors would seem to recommend their care to practitioners weary of treating intractable cases. For most of these physicians, travel to Bath would be impractical and costly.

In the preface of his treatise, Jorden pleads with his dedicatee, Sir Francis Cottington, Chancellor of the Exchequer, to support improvements in the baths, which he says are "the principall jewels of your Country." He complains that they are now in a deplorable state, despite a petition sent by the City of Bath to King James, who died before it was acted upon. Jorden's admission that the baths have deteriorated is surprising, given the need to increase attendance and his later remarks. He may have decided that the potential of such a public appeal to Cottington outweighed its negative impression.

Reflecting his Paduan training, Jorden begins scholastically, defining a bath (a remedy applied to the body, consisting of liquids, solids, or vapor), and noting that he will treat only mineral waters used as a bath or a potion. He then regales readers with some entertaining history, declaring that the use of baths goes back to the ancients, particularly the Romans and the Turks. The Romans developed them because they went barelegged and the Turks because their clothes harbored lice (3). Since their diets consisted of many crudities—lettuce, asparagus, raw fruits—the Turks sought help in digesting them and, being forbidden wine, drank water. They bathed often, and their women, the most delicate creatures in the world, bathed twice a week. For them, baths were used "for pleasure and delicacy, and cleanlinesse" (3). Their baths generally were water baths, but mineral baths would have been far more efficacious because of their success in curing disease (4).

Jorden continues in this vein, offering other examples from authority, the ancients, sages, and scripture. He finds it strange that none of the Greeks wrote of the curative powers of drinking the waters, nor did they attend much to their mineral content. More importantly, recent authorities—Agricola, Fallopius, and others, who have added much to the knowledge of baths—have erred in their opinions regarding minerals. These errors he hopes to correct through his book. Indeed, Jorden reveals considerable knowledge and interest in the chemistry of the waters.

In summary, 15 of the 19 chapters of Jorden's book concern the content of mineral waters. These chapters seem designed both to instruct (or impress) inquiring minds and to inform his peers of his opinions in a curious mixture of scholastic and empirical study. Thus, he defines, distinguishes, and then provides explanations of the water's origins. Mineral waters "besides their own simple nature, have received and imbibed some other qualitie of substance from Subterranean Mynes" (8). He is careful to explain what he means by "simple" and "imbibed," distinguishing the latter from "confused" waters (11–13).

This discussion of simple waters has been introduced, Jorden explains, in order to judge mixed or "infected" waters. Having supplied the genus, he proceeds to provide the difference, not daring to use dichotomies, he adds, which neither Agricola nor Fallopius, nor others have done (26). (Guidott, however, is not to be so deterred. He offers a dichotomized table in a fold over leaf.)

The composition of the waters becomes an important topic in these works because Bath's claim of offering unique therapeutic benefits depends on the perception of the waters' actions on the body. Jorden argues from the effects of the waters on disease to conclude that these baths have bitumen in them. Here, he disagrees with Turner, who claimed that sulfur was the main mineral and copper next. Both assumptions are untrue, he claims. The heat of the water does not prove brimstone is there, nor does Turner's observation of marquisite (iron pyrite which may have a yellow tinge) in the hills mean that copper is present (43). He does admit that they do contain some nitre and sulfur.

Jorden deftly draws on his analyses of the nature of minerals to explain their use in Bath. Waters that contain niter, alum, virtriol, sulfur, bitumen, iron, and copper are good taken inwardly. But, since Bath's waters are not pure, he does not recommend drinking them "unreservedly" (150). The problem, he notes, is that the water for drinking is often derived from the baths rather than from a pump outside the baths (159). (Could this be intended as *litotes,* a deliberate understatement, here?) Jorden goes on to suggest that the drink be taken hot, since it penetrates more quickly and agreeably. Bath waters can be used to make broths, beer, and juleps. They can also be injected into the womb, urinary tract, and bowels (154).

Concerning external usage, Jorden suggests that both the water and the mud at the bottom of the baths can be used for body ailments such as palsies, contractions, rheums, cold tumors, aching, and skin problems. The baths heat is similar in all four baths, probably because they issue from the same "mine." Like Venner, he treats the effectiveness of each of the baths and their individual uses.

Announcing to his readers that the baths have the very latest equipment, he mentions that pumps in the King's and Queen's Baths permit more successful treatment, and that a "dry pump" installed above the Hot Bath enables patients to sit fully clothed while water is directed only to the affected part.

In his summary of the effects to be expected from the baths, Jorden finds bathing the most beneficial treatment. The baths

> warm the whole habit of the body, attenuate humors, open the pores procure sweat, move urine, cleanse the matrix, provoke womens evacuations, dry up unnatural humors, strengthen parts weakned, comfort the nerves, and all neutrous parts, cleanse the skin and suck out all salt humours from thence, open obstructions.ease pains of the joynts and nerves and muscles, mollifie and discuss hard tumors. (162)

Jorden then lists the many diseases, familiar to most of these accounts, which the baths can be expected to cure. He concludes with the most hyperbolic claim of all for Bath's hot waters:

> And whereas without the help of such Baths, these diseases could not be cured without tormenting the body, either by fire, or lancing, or casticks, or long dyets, or bitter and ungrateful medicines, &. In this course of bathing, all is pleasant and comfortable, and more effectual than the other courses, and therefore it is commonly the last refuge in these cases, when all other means fail (162).

He reminds readers that this information is intended for the prospective patient who will need a physician to carry out the best treatment.

This edition of Jorden's book provided the occasion for Guidott, who had come to practice medicine in Bath in 1667, to advertise his own competence as a physician, chemist, an antiquarian, and scholar, as well as to advance its announced purpose of praise for Bath and its hot springs. In addition to his biography of Jorden, which was inserted following the preface to the original work, Guidott inserts his *An Appendix concerning Bathe: Wherein the Antiquity Both of the Bathes & City I more fully discours'd; with a brief account of the Nature and Virtues of the HOT WATERS There.* In the first chapter, Guidott tediously rehearses Bath's history beginning with Bladud, whom he thinks was a contemporary of the prophet Elias. He includes a description of Bath by Alexander Necham [sic], "a Poet of our own, somewhat above 400 years ago," which he translates from the Latin into awkward English verse.

Guidott must have thought his additions to Jorden's text would supply further incentives to attract visitors: history, antiquities, and an appreciation of literature on the part of at least one of its doctors. Four chapters extol the history and antiquities of the city. The baths themselves receive three chapters, one devoted to the subject that had interested his admired predecessor, the mineral content of the water, which he holds to be chiefly bituminous, a point much criticized that he corrected in a later work. The effects of bitumen are similar to that of sulfur, he says, citing Turner and Venner to corroborate his views of its curative powers. But it is nitre that should receive much of the credit; it cools the baths from the effects of the sulfur and bitumen it possesses, quickly penetrating the body, entering into its passages and pores. Guidott ends the appendix, asking to be excused from providing further particulars "till a just amassment of Observations and Experiments and a rational deduction of Conclusions from them … shall either confirm me in the opinion I now have of the Nature and Vertues of the Baths of Bathe, or supply me with a better" (59–60). Guidott presents himself as a much more modern physician than Jorden, no longer content with theory, but rather placing his trust in empirical investigation.

Seven years later, Guidott honors his promise of recording further investigation by publishing a revision of the *Appendix*. In this much expanded and emended work, besides *A Discourse of Bathe and the Hot Waters There,* he included *Enquiries into the nature of the Water of St Vincent's Rock, near Bristol and that of Castle Cary; A Century of Observations, more fully declaring the Nature, Property, and Distinction of the Baths,* and *An Account of the Lives and Character of the Physicians of Bathe.* The book, more chauvinistic than any of the other physicians' writings, praised everything about Bath, from its buildings to its ancient artifacts, and extolled the talents of its physicians and the quality of its waters, while simultaneously describing the disadvantages of other spas.

Leaving no means of self-praise neglected, Guidott dedicates the book to Sir Edward Greaves, Baronet, and Fellow of the Royal College of Physicians, mentioning his post as Physician Ordinary to the king. He reminds Greaves of being an eyewitness to some of his experiments on the waters of Bath while Greaves himself was a physician there. What Greaves witnessed was the first discovery of many things unknown before, that the water has nitre in it, for example, and Guidott's advocacy of the "Rational use" of the water." No wonder Peirce remarks in his *Memoirs* that Guidott "arrogated to himself" all the credit for the therapeutic method of drinking the waters.

Guidott's revised *Discourse* seeks to correct an error for which he says he was roundly criticized–his conclusions that the waters contained bitumen and sulfur. On further experiment, he has found that there is sulfur, but not "proportionable in quantity to the Salts." Bitumen may also be there at times when it is forced upward in the summer and remains on the surface (10). He then devotes a chapter to a description with drawings of the salt crystals he has grown in experiments (22–5).

The history of the spa again occupies Guidott, but this time he leaves out Bladud, saying that new information has come to his attention. He notes ancient references to the spa but does not wish to attribute its founding to Julius Caesar, as some had done. Instead, he records ancient references to Bath's hot springs in Antoninus, who called them *Aquae Solis,* and in Ptolomy's *Thermae.*

By Chapter 12, his exposition finally turns to the baths themselves, detailing the measurements of each of the baths and computing the volume of water they hold. In the remaining two chapters, he takes up the advisability of drinking the waters. He approves that remedy, which Venner did not, declaring that Venner did not really understand its benefits. These Guidott describes, noting their effects on various parts of the body.

In his encomia of physicians' lives published with this revised work, Guidott extolls the deceased physicians of Bath who had brought such fame to the city, among these Dr. Jorden and Dr. Venner. When he describes the last of these medical benefactors, he chooses to do so in satiric verses. Guidott introduces his description of Mr. Somerschall, a chemist, with an aside, saying he composed it when he was in "a merry riming humour." There he mocks the pretensions of Somerschall whose search for the philosopher's stone exhausted his funds and his life's energy. This particular poetic effort brought Guidott such disfavour at Bath that he felt constrained to leave and set up practice in London. After a time, he returned to live part of each year in the city he had praised so highly, and to spend the rest in London.[26]

[26] In the entry for Thomas Guidott in the *Oxford Dictionary of National Biography* (2004), Mark S. R. Jenner notes that Thomas Hearne termed Guidott "'vain, conceited, whimsicall'"; and that Anthony à Wood in *Athenane Oxoniensis* 4.734, accused him of "'impudence, lampooning, and libelling.'".y

Nevertheless, Guidott continued to turn out publications promoting Bath. A volume that included several of his later works was published posthumously: *A Collection of treatises Relating to the City and Waters of Bath* (1724). It contains an encomium of Bath by Henry Chapman, mayor of the city, entitled *Thermae Redivivae or the City of Bath* (1673), dedicated to Charles II. The collection attests to the value accorded Guidott's contribution to Bath's publicity; it reprints Guidott's revised *A Discourse*, and his last work *An Apology for the Bath* (1705).

## Demonstrated Cures

Guidott's *The Register of Bath,* the last of the irrepressible physician's works described here, is puzzling. In it, he lists the names, ailments, treatments, and benefits for patients, most of whom he says were his own. But the publication date, 1694, mystifies because it conflicts with the account given by Peirce in his *Memoirs*, of 1697, described below. Peirce claims that he is the first to publish accounts of cures with all of the particulars, such as names and dates, even though for some time, people had suggested that the information be published yearly. Since Peirce's case book bears a date three years later than that of Guidott's *Register*, one might conjecture, based on contemporary assessments of Guidott's character, that he got wind of Peirce's projected work and tried to upstage him. The long title of Guidott's *Register,* which highlights the length of his observations, *XXVII Years last past,* increases the suspicion that he wished the work to be seen as comparable to Peirce's *three and forty years* of case notes. Moreover, Guidot may have hoped his readers would later bear in mind the differences between his and Peirce's work when, after mentioning that he hopes to publish a register each year, he adds:

> In the mean time, I hope, I have done enough to bespeak me a Friend, not so much to a private interest, as a publick Good; and having done mine Endeavour to use distributive Justice to all, and offend none, I may the better promise Freedom to myself from that Unhappiness of Censure, which some Writers of Cases have before incurred. Preface

Whatever the explanation may be for the discrepancy in claims of priority, Peirce's case histories provide far more information concerning patients, the circumstances, kinds of treatments, and effects than do Guidott's. Perhaps Peirce was, indeed, one of those criticized for his efforts, but he seems to have taken elaborate precautions.

The manner in which Peirce presents his observations underwrites his ethos as an expert medical practitioner and attests to a compassionate interest in his patients. Readers are apprized of his credentials by the long title of his book: *Bath Memoirs or Observations in Three and Forty Years Practice at the Bath, what Cures Have been There Wrought (both by Bathing and Drinking these Waters) by God's Blessing, on the Directions of Robert Peirce, Dr. In Physick and fellow of the College of Physicians in London, a constant In habitant in Bath from the year 1653 to the present Year 1697*. Further substantiation is provided in the text where mention is made of referrals from royal and other eminent physicians, consultations with other doctors, as well as the record of remarkable cures, detailed in the case notes.

Despite his credentials, Peirce, unlike his predecessors, claims neither great learning nor pretension to fame, saying that he aims simply to provide a manual of cures. He does note that previously patients had been reluctant to have their names published but that he was able to convince them that their case histories would provide credible evidence of the efficacy of Bath's waters for people with similar ailments. The boost that publication might give to the town's economy, and, not least, to physicians' incomes, he probably did not mention.

Peirce expects his readers to be aware of the new scientific age in which they are living. He makes clear his stand on theoretical medicine in the preface: "I shall only relate *Matter of Fact*, not medling much with *Theories*, or setting up new *Hypotheses*." Instead, he will apply the experience of successful practices to particular cases, not, he adds, in order to direct other physicians, nor to establish rules. He dismisses the need to offer an analysis of the waters, saying that "the useful knowledge of a Mineral water is sooner and better had a Posteriori, than a Priori, that Experience and long Observation, is the best and surest way of acquiring that knowledge"(C ir).[27] These remarks make clear that no demonstrations or dialectical arguments will be offered in his book. He relies instead on patients' narratives of their ailments, his examination, and close observation of effects.

Peirce's advocacy of the curative powers of the waters begins with his own case. He writes of the many debilitating illnesses that preyed upon him from childhood. Relief came only through visits to Bath, motivating him eventually to stay and develop his practice.

The *Memoirs* is divided into two books: "Of Bathing" and "Of Drinking". Each part contains chapters devoted to specific ailments, ranging from "Wandring Pains" to "Old Gonorrheas." He introduces each section with a general discussion of the disease or ailment, its frequency, and the kinds of treatment most often given. Then he begins to relate each case, including the following information: the patient's name, gender, social rank, occupation, place of residence, origin of the ailment or injury, previous treatment, date, circumstances of treatment, regimen prescribed, length of stay, and effects of treatment. Of the 197 patients whose

---

[27] In this opinion, Peirce, in part, echoes the view of Michaele Savonarola, stressed in Peirce's day, that in medical practice, observation precedes deduction. Ian Maclean places Savanarola's teachings in Renaissance medical education, *Logic, Signs and Nature in the Renaissance* (Cambridge: Cambridge University Press, 2002), 17, 56, 69. Katherine Park notes that Savanarola thought that the use of mineral baths is necessarily based on signs that are "not definitive or infallible," only probable. The physician must use his judgment on how to interpret these, "Natural Particulars" 360–61. Vivian Nutton finds that practice outweighed theory even in the views of prominent English physicians in the early Tudor period. And by 1580 the main focus of English medicine was on the practical not the theoretical–"medical rather than intellectual benefits" was the aim ("Introducing Renaissance Medicine to Tudor England," in *Natural Particulars*, 275–93, 287).

cases he describes, 91 of these were female and 106 male. Among them were farmers, butchers, tavern keepers, married and unmarried women, children, peers, a general, colonels, captains, and clergy. His descriptions of these cases are based solely on his own experience, although he occasionally consults other physicians.

Many of his patients are treated for scurvy, which often caused the wandering pains mentioned, and other more unpleasant symptoms—sore gums, loosened or lost teeth, swollen painful legs and feet. Other patients suffer from the "fixed" pains of sciatica and arthritis, and from gout, tumors and headaches.

Women's diseases are considered in two separate sections: virgins and married women. Children, too, merit special attention from Peirce. The illnesses he records range from lameness through crooked legs to rickets. All of these have found improvement from bathing in the mineral waters, and from medicaments prescribed, he reports. Drinking the waters is prescribed for patients with palsy, coughs, asthma, dropsy, palpitations, and diseases of the esophagus, stomach, spleen, pancreas, and urinary tract.

Pierce's book does for the last half of the seventeenth century what that of John Hall, Shakespeare's son-in-law, does for the early part, that of supplying detailed case notes.[28] Hall, however, does not treat spa medicine.

Peirce's fame as a practitioner brought him an illustrious patient, the third Duke of Hamilton, recommended, he relates, by Sir Alexander Fraizer, chief physician of King Charles II.[29] Peirce was delighted to treat this patient and expects his readers to be impressed. In the chapter on 'fixed" pains, he writes, "I shall begin with an eminent Personage, and a great Prince in his Country, Duke Hamilton" (19). His is the first person of "quality" named, of whom there were many to follow. The Duke, William Douglas (1634–94), came to see him in 1674, very ill and suffering from pains in the hip. After the usual preparation, Hamilton was given 200 strokes of the pump, rising by 100 to 1,000 strokes over the period of four to five weeks. He drank little water, except to quench his thirst. The treatment had a favorable outcome. The duke was able to walk without much favoring the bad leg. He came two more times over the year and was eventually pronounced "perfectly recovered" (20).

Another of such cases was that of Sir John Cloberly, described by Peirce as formerly a colonel in Scotland who served under General Monck and aided King Charles II in attaining the throne. He came in 1666 to Bath, suffering from sciatica, pains in the hip, and inability to stand erect. His illness derived from lying on

[28] Joan Lane introduces Hall's case notes in *John Hall and his Patients: The Medical Practice of Shakespeare's Son-in-Law*, Medical commentary by Melvin Earles (Stratford-upon-Avon: The Shakespeare Birthplace Trust, 1996). Lane claims that such case histories were quite rare in the early seventeenth century. After the Restoration more were published: those of Sir Theodore Mayerne, 23 volumes; and John Symcotts' notes (introduction, xiii).

[29] Elizabeth Lane Furdell's research confirms the importance of Fraizer in *The Royal Doctors 1485–1714. Medical Personnel at the Tudor and Stuart Courts* (Rochester, University of Rochester Press, 2001), 162.

snow covered ground in the Scottish campaign and from sleeping on a damp bed afterwards. He was bled and purged and underwent six to eight weeks of bathing and pumping. He left not completely cured, but after several months had passed, he reported that he was able to walk upright and was eased of his pain (21–3).

Peirce uses Cloberly's case to illustrate the need for the public to be better instructed concerning the delayed improvement that might follow treatment at the spa. His remarks address the declining reputation of Bath, noted above: "So true it is, that the benefits of the *Baths* appears not always presently, but some time after they have been used; and therefore needful it is to allow time for the Expectation of it, and not to be too hasty in the tryal of other means, but to give Nature leave to work after such an assistance. Had this Caution been well observ'd, the Bath had had more Reputation, and Patients had sav'd a great deal of Expence and Trouble" (23). Effects of treatment for Peirce require careful, prolonged study.

In the chapter devoted to women's diseases, Peirce records four cases under maladies of virgins and twenty under those of married women. Virgin's diseases are listed as anemia, hysteria, and cessation of menstruation; married women's as barrenness, miscarriages, spontaneous abortions, and uterine flows. Peirce gallantly states that in some cases he will omit names for "the Modesty of the Sex, and the Respect we owe them … And since God and Nature have given them the heavier end of the Staff, in bearing the Burthens of this Life" (187). The courteous attention and compassion he displays in passages such as these must have encouraged women to seek him out for treatment.

He argues in the introduction of the chapter that virgins were likely to suffer from "green sickness" or what was commonly called the "virgin's disease" (anemia). This illness causes them to be pale, often failing to menstruate, and exhibit hysteric passions or "fits of the Mother." For this he prescribes apperitive medicines, bathing and imbibing the waters.

In the mid-seventeenth century, many married women came to the baths to be cured of barrenness. The efficacy of the waters was so well regarded that it prompted the frequent comment, "she comes for the common Cause" (195). Even barrenness after miscarriages of previous full term pregnancies could also be treated by bathing in the waters. He cites the case of Mrs. Clement, who had not borne a child for nine years. After bathing for five weeks, she became pregnant and was able to give birth to twin boys.

Wives of kings also came for the cure, the most famous case being that of the wife of King James II, Mary of Modena, who gave birth nine months after her stay at Bath.[30]

In part two of the book, Peirce describes cases for which he has prescribed imbibing the waters, which, he says, has been less common than bathing, but is growing in popularity. He considers it very helpful for many diseases, devoting chapters to patients treated for many illnesses: palsy, palpitations, pectoral distempers, diseases of the lower body (particularly dropsy), diabetes, cachexies (obstructions of the spleen, liver, pancreas), diseases of the stomach, and difficulties

---

30 Croutier, 120.

of urination, rheumatism, and gout. "It corrects all saltiness, sharpness, sowerness of blood and Nervous Juices" (260–61). He cites other, more prominent, physicians who attest to its effectiveness, among them Sir Thomas Browne, who wrote to him commending a patient to his care in drinking the waters, and Sir Alexander Fraizer who, on Peirce's recommendation of the treatment, sent patients to him for the same purpose. On one of his visits to Bath, Fraizer suggested that a drinking pump be built in the middle of the King's Bath. It was erected as directed in 1674.[31]

Although other springs in England could offer healthful mineral waters for drinking, only Bath's physicians could coordinate that therapy with bathing and provide such informed and careful attention to individual patient's needs—that is the implication of Peirce's remarks. And a patient, under a physician's direction can continue to drink the waters and enjoy its "Balsamic Healing Virtue" any time of year (261).[32]

Most important for Bath's custom, and certainly not little for his own, Peirce describes a visit in 1663 of King Charles II and Queen Catherine, who actually stayed in his residence, Abbey House, adjacent to the Kings Bath. In fact, Sir Alexander Fraizer accompanied the royal couple. The Queen returned again in 1677 and 1686.[33]

The fact that Peirce writes so deferentially concerning the august people who come to him for care does not mean that he does not just as carefully examine and treat the farmers, servants, grocers, clerks, and their wives. They too merit detailed descriptions of their ailments and reports of their responses to treatment. By including them in his case histories, he could encourage similar patients with modest incomes to come to Bath.

Charity cases Peirce appeared to tend with less enthusiasm. He notes that after the death of Dr. Venner in 1660, he had the honor as well as the trouble to serve as "Physician to poor Strangers" for thirty years, an appointment made by the Council.

Cures predominate in Peirce's account; only occasionally does he note failure. Perhaps this may be partially explained by the practice of turning away patients deemed terminal. Peirce mentions a Mrs. Frisby sent to him by another physician, whom he persuaded to go home, "lest the great Bell should have rung out for her here: for then Enquiry would have been made whose patient she was: Not what Distemper she had Or whither a due Method had been used for her Recovery: But with the Vulgar (who measure all things by the Success) the Physitian that doth not Cure shall be sure to have the Reputation of Killing." (77).[34]

---

[31] Hembry, 88.

[32] Bottled water was available from Bath as well as seven other spas and wells; see Hembry 366 and Appendix D, which records the dates and sources.

[33] Peirce, 257. Hembry gives further particulars of the visits, 88.

[34] Andrew Wear mentions other reasons for physicians' reluctance to treat the dying. The prevalent view in the period was that such patients should be turned over to ministers and priests. They should have jurisdiction over those about to depart this world, when prayers and/or absolution might be needed. Moreover, Wear asserts, that physicians thought

How much patients in this period may actually have been aided by bathing in and drinking the waters of Bath, so highly touted by the resident physicians, is subject to debate today. Certainly, except for Peirce, the physicians discussed here did not voice doubts regarding the humoral theory passed on from the ancients, hallowed by Hippocrates and Galen. But they described no individual cases. Had they done so, they might readily have justified their curative claims by matching the particular complexion of the ailing patient to the humors, computed the efficacy of the water's mineral content, heat, and frequency of application. The other variables in spa treatment medicaments, period of stay, diet, and exercise, all could be used to explain the outcome. Peirce, for his part, narrates the particulars of the treatment applied and the success or failure as reported to him or as he perceived it. He fervently believed that the waters, if taken as he prescribed, were eminently curative. His own case supplied the evidence on which he built his practice.[35]

Whether cures were effected or not, the practice of visiting spas continued to grow in popularity. By the end of the seventeenth century, the social attraction of meeting the right people and the prospect of leisurely entertainments probably far outweighed any lingering misgivings concerning the health benefits of the visit.

---

it could harm their practice if they were to take money for incurable sicknesses, *Knowledge & Practice in English Medicine 1550–1680* (Cambridge: Cambridge University Press 2000), 34 and n. 67.

[35] See David Harley's persuasive essay on the rhetorical construction of cures, "Rhetoric and the Social Construction of Sickness and Healing" *The Society for the Social History of Medicine* 12.3 (1999): 407–435.

Chapter 3

# The Anatomical Web: Literary Dissection from Castiglione to Cromwell

Richard Sugg

In Baldasar Castiglione's *Book of the Courtier* the character 'Unico aretino' declares that, 'an ungrate woman', whose tongue 'never agreeth … with her minde … with a fained deceivable compassion, purposeth nothing els but to make anatomie of hearts'.[1] This brief statement shows that dissection was transferred into literary rhetoric some time before Andreas Vesalius published his monumental *De Fabrica Humani Corporis* in 1543. Castiglione's *Book of the Courtier* was published in 1528, and was probably in progress as early as 1513. Its author might have been influenced by the first recorded dissection of a human corpse, an event which took place in Rome on 22 March 1512 (with a second occurring on 14 February 1518).[2] He may also have known one of the earliest textbooks of this new anatomical culture, Alexander Benedetti's *Anatomice sive Historia Corporis Humani* (Paris, 1514).[3]

Castiglione's usage is sufficiently skilled to suggest that it was by no means the first literary exploitation of medical dissection. It employs metaphor, rather than simile. And it does so in order to imply that the metaphorical dissector is cold, calculating, and more or less inhumanly detached. Not only that, but she seems to

---

1 Baldassare Castiglione, *The Book of the Courtier*, trans. Sir Thomas Hoby (1561), ed. J.H. Whitfield (London: Dent, 1974), 25. Although *The Courtier* was published in 1528, it is supposed to have been written between 1513 and 1519 (Whitfield, vi; Julia Cartwright, *Baldassare Castiglione: The Perfect Courtier*, 2 vols (London: John Murray, 1908), 2:24–5). Hoby is here faithful to the original Italian: 'intende che a far anatomia de cori' (*Il Cortegiano*, ed. Vittorio Cian [Firenze: G.C. Sansoni, 1939], 30).

2 On the dissection, see Andrea Carlino, *Books of the Body: Anatomical Ritual and Renaissance Learning*, trans. John Tedeschi and Anne C. Tedeschi (Chicago: University of Chicago Press, 1999), 87. Castiglione seems to have been far from Rome on those dates in 1512, but he clearly had many Roman contacts by this time (see Cartwright, *Baldassare Castiglione*, 1:309–12, 2:24–8).

3 Other pre-Vesalian textbooks include Berengario da Carpi, *Commentaria* (Bologna, 1521); Joannes Dryander, *Anatomia Capitis Humani* (Marburg, 1536), *Anatomiae … corporis humani dissectionis* (Marburg, 1537). For more on da Carpi's work, see Roger French, 'Berengario da Carpi and the Use of Commentary in Anatomical Teaching' (1985), in *Ancients and Moderns in the Medical Sciences: From Hippocrates to Harvey* (Aldershot: Ashgate Variorum, 2000), 42–3).

use her minutely rigorous incisions not for any kind of 'public good', but purely for the sake of egotistical pleasure or conceited display.

What did it mean for non-medical writers to 'anatomise' their subjects during the early absorption of empirical dissection – a practice pioneered and promoted by men such as Berengario da Carpi, Andreas Vesalius, Helkiah Crooke, and William Harvey?[4] I will take a three-fold approach to this question. An opening section sets out the basic chronological frame of relevant events in medicine, along with statistics on the rise and growth of extra-literary anatomising. I will then argue, secondly, that the 'meaning' of any one act of literary anatomy is valuably illuminated if seen as potentially linked to all the anatomies preceding it, and to the associated range of terms which seems to have arisen (or significantly developed) around the same time. In doing so, I will show that a number of quite precise rhetorical habits co-existed alongside a considerable amount of loose imitation and broadly commercial opportunism. Finally, I will look in some detail at a familiar literary term in an unfamiliar way. In some of its early rhetorical uses, the once clearly dis-sective word 'section' seems to have been curiously poised between the abstract, formal qualities of dissection, and that edge of violence to which Castiglione has introduced us.

## The Pen and the Scalpel

It can be argued that anatomy was etched into the general consciousness most forcibly not by writers or dissectors, but by the painstaking labours of the wood-cutter's knife. Vesalius' *De Fabrica* boasted a quantity and quality of illustrations markedly surpassing any existing textbooks. Vesalius' rigorously conceived and executed presentations of the body, down through several layers of dissection, combine verisimilitude and vibrancy with an effect still breathtaking today. Perhaps the most convincing testimony to Vesalius' success in his own lifetime was the extensive plagiarism of these illustrations. Repeatedly borrowed, with varying degrees of accuracy or completeness, well into the seventeenth century, the Vesalian figures reached England as early as 1545, in Thomas Geminus' Latin epitome of *De Fabrica*, *Compendiosa Totius Anatomie Delineatio*, with English-language versions of this title appearing in 1553 and 1559.[5] A sense of that visual

4 For various reasons the distinction between medical 'professionals' and the 'non-medical' public was a much less definite one prior to the eighteenth century. I use the term here as a matter of convenience.

5 On the numerous thefts, see K.B. Roberts and J.D.W. Tomlinson, *The Fabric of the Body: European Traditions of Anatomical Illustration* (Oxford: Clarendon Press, 1992), 141. Crooke's *Microcosmographia* (1615) borrowed from Bauhin's *Theatrum Anatomicum* (Frankfurt, 1605), which had already produced hybrid, as well as exact, representations of Vesalius' original figures. The 1532 *De Indiciis et Praecognitionibus opus apprime utile medicis* of David Edguard is notable for its titular advertisement (*Eiusdem in anatomicen introductio luculenta et breuis*) but is also significantly un-illustrated.

power is conveyed by John Dee, at a time when figurative anatomy was itself still rare: 'To what artificer, is not picture, a great pleasure and commoditie …? … Our lively Herbals, our portraitures of birdes, beastes, and fishes: and our curious Anatomies, which way, are they most perfectly made, or with most pleasure, of us beholden? Is it not, by picture onely?'[6]

In the 1560s, notes in the Barber-Surgeons' Annals suggest an increasing emphasis on dissection, and this appears to grow in the following decade.[7] 1565 saw the appearance of *A Most Excellent and Learned Woorke of Chirurgerie*, an English version of Lanfranco of Milan's thirteenth-century surgical textbook, published by John Hall (1529–1568).[8] As Jonathan Sawday notes, it was in 1564/5 that the Royal College of Physicians was granted the right to dissect four bodies per year; and by this point Caius College was also receiving two bodies annually for anatomy.[9] In 1577 the surgeons of St. Bartholomew's hospital reissued the *Anatomie* of Thomas Vicary (d.1561), sometime surgeon to Henry VIII.[10] Though both Lanfranco's and Vicary's works were themselves unillustrated and outdated, the former contains important new additions by Hall, who was self-consciously presenting his work as superior to that of Vicary. Moreover, the respective efforts of Hall and the surgeons at re-publicising anatomy were compounded, in 1578, by John Banister's *The Historie of Man, sucked from the sappe of the most approved anathomistes, in this present age*. As Banister's title is at pains to stress, this substantial folio featured text from the contemporary Italian anatomist, Realdo Colombo, as well as four Vesalian illustrations. Significantly, Banister was not only surgeon to Elizabeth, but one of the first influential figures to strive for a closer union between empirical anatomy and the more purely conceptual medicine of the physicians.[11] This altered stance may itself have been partly responsible for

---

6 Preface to Euclid, *The Elements of Geometrie*, trans. H. Billingsley (1570), 23r.

7 See *The Annals of the Barber-Surgeons of London*, ed. Sidney Young, 2 vols (London: Blades, East and Blades, 1890), 1:315.

8 Rivkah Zim in the new *DNB* notes that Hall was commended by William Cunningham MD (reader in anatomy for 1563); but adds that, despite his strong interest in anatomy, there is no record of his admission to the Barber-Surgeons' company.

9 Jonathan Sawday, *The Body Emblazoned: Dissection and the Human Body in Renaissance Culture* (London: Routledge, 1995), 56. For evidence on the initially slow effect of the Lumleian lectures, see *Annals of the College of Physicians of London*, trans. J. Emberry, S. Heathcote, M. Hellings, 5 vols (London: Wellcome library, RCP), 2:26.

10 The 1548 edition of Vicary's book, the text used for the 1577 publication, is now lost.

11 D'Arcy Power, 'Notes on Early Portraits of John Banister, of William Harvey, and the Barber-Surgeons' Visceral Lecture in 1581', in *Proceedings of the Royal Society of Medicine*, 6 (1912), (repr. London: John Bale, Sons, and Danielsson, 1912), 6–7. For the College's evident resistance to Banister, see *Annals*, 2:49.

the physicians' new public anatomy lecture, the Lumleian, founded in 1582 and begun in 1584.[12]

Although I focus chiefly on events and publications in England, one continental publication deserves special mention here. Coeval with the first resurgence of anatomy in continental Europe, there arose a new printed form with a markedly popular appeal: the 'flap anatomy' or anatomical 'fugitive sheet'.[13] Male and female figures were 'dissected' on these images by means of paper flaps cut and pasted onto their bodies. While the relative cheapness of such productions meant that many examples were fairly crude, the extreme possibilities of the format are breathtakingly revealed in Johann Remmelin's *Catoptrum Microcosmicum*, unofficially published first in 1613, and again in 1619 and 1639.[14] The 1619 edition, a tall and broad folio, contains three plates, the first featuring a man and woman, and a central torso displaying the womb, and the latter two depicting male and female figures respectively. The anatomy itself is, allegedly, mediocre at best.[15] The plates nonetheless achieve an impression of depth and complexity arguably unrivalled by any other anatomy textbook of the period. The female figure, for example, has a total of sixteen different flaps (some of which are double-sided), and which can progress down into the body through as many as ten separate layers. Unfolding these with increasing wonder, the amateur anatomist is struck not only by the convincing mimesis of depth, but by the physical difficulty of replacing sometimes extremely minute paper flaps (the separate eye of plate 1, for example, has seven layers).[16] The sense of labyrinthine somatic immersion produced is in a way stronger than 'real' anatomy, owing to the artificially rapid speed at which so many stages of dissection are undergone.

Very shortly after Remmelin's book first appeared, two key events occurred in England. In 1615, William Harvey was appointed as lecturer for the Lumleian annual anatomies, and Helkiah Crooke published his anatomy textbook, *Microcosmographia*. While there is evidence to suggest that the Lumleian was poorly attended by physicians in its earliest years, it seems that from the time

---

12 It is not quite clear if the earliest lectures involved actual dissection or just oral delivery. For details, see Holinshed, *Chronicles* (1587), 2:1349; Gweneth Whitteridge, *William Harvey and the Circulation of the Blood* (London: Macdonald, 1971), 86; *Annals*, 2:24.

13 The most comprehensive overview of this format credits it with 'tremendous commercial success' (Andrea Carlino, *Paper Bodies: A Catalogue of Anatomical Fugitive Sheets 1538–1687*, trans. Noga Arikha, *Medical History* supplement No. 19 (London: Wellcome Institute, 1999) (3)). For early examples published in England, see *The Woman* (1540), *The Anathomy of the Inwarde Partes of Man* (1545), and *Interiorum Corporis Humani Partium* (1559).

14 Robert Burton, in his survey of prominent modern anatomists, includes 'Remelins' alongside the names of Vesalius and Fallopius *(Anatomy*, 1:140).

15 See Roberts and Tomlinson, *Fabric*, 64.

16 Although we cannot be sure just who these paper anatomists were, the initial piracy of Remmelin's book makes it clear that the work was thought to have a profitable market.

Harvey took up his post (carrying out his first dissection in 1616) its impact in medical circles and on the wider public was quite considerable. We now find that certain preachers appear to be responding to the broadly seasonal character of this event, which usually took place a few weeks before Easter, owing to its reliance on the Lenten assizes to supply criminal corpses as specimens. It is possible that in London a new 'dissecting season' came to overlay and partly merge with the existing penitential period of Lent.[17]

With hindsight it might seem whimsical to elevate the minor physician Helkiah Crooke alongside Harvey, who even at this stage was probably lecturing on his new theory of circulation, prior to the 1628 appearance of *De Motu Cordis*. But in terms of popularising anatomy, Crooke's influence may well have been much greater than that of Harvey. Although *Microcosmographia* was a thoroughly opportunistic work (borrowing not only Vesalian plates, but text from the French anatomists Caspar Bauhin and André du Laurens) it was arguably more imposing (at over a thousand folio pages) than Vesalius' original *Fabrica*. While this lavish format necessarily limited its market, the ever adaptable Crooke quickly had a much smaller and cheaper version issued the next year as *Somatographia Anthropine*. Here once again the visual power of anatomy loomed large. The new book was composed almost entirely of Vesalian plates and explanatory labels.

It seems probable that changing attitudes to anatomy spurred a rise in post-mortem autopsies – investigations which allowed physicians and surgeons further specimens and a potentially wider access to pathological conditions.[18] David Harley has argued that the post-mortem autopsy gained a new respectability after that which was performed on the assassinated French king, Henri IV, on 15 May 1610.[19] It may have been partly this royal precedent that prompted the autopsy made on the English Prince Henry in 1612, as well as the inspection of the body of his father, James I, in 1625.[20] Elsewhere we find John Donne referring to the 'opening' of 'one Swinburne, a clerk', who died very soon after a disastrous gambling bout. As far back as 1587 we hear of a horse being 'ripped' in order to discern the cause of its death.[21]

The very earliest Vesalian piracies did not seem to make much impact on the English literary imagination. Over on the continent we find the first known 'literary anatomy', Augustino Mainardo's *Annotomia della Messa*, published in

---

[17] For further details see Richard Sugg, *Murder after Death: Literature and Anatomy in Early Modern England* (Ithaca: Cornell University Press, 2007), 4, 217–18.

[18] In the late 1630s, the physician Edward May is still lamenting that it is chiefly the educated who permit such procedures (see *A Most Certaine and True Relation* (1639), 36.)

[19] 'Political Post-mortems and Morbid Anatomy in Seventeenth-century England', *Social History of Medicine* 7.1 (1994), 1–28, 6.

[20] In the first case, the sudden death of a young man was also an important factor; in the latter, the rumours of poisoning – aimed in particular at the Duke of Buckingham – must have been important.

[21] John Stowe, *The Annales of England* (1594), 719.

1553.[22] Tellingly, when translated into English in 1556 (by one Anthoni de Adamo) this required a cautiously explanatory title: *An Anatomi that is to say a parting in peeces of the masse* (Strasburg). Perhaps the first native English-language reference to anatomy by a non-medical writer comes, aptly enough, from William Baldwin's *Beware the Cat* – aptly, because this work has often been considered as marginal and *avant-garde* as early-modern anatomy itself.[23] Here the narrator tells of how he 'flaied my irchin [hedgehog] … wishing oft for … some expert phisition to mak the disseccion, for the better knowledge of the anatomy'.[24] In making this sideways, partly arbitrary reference, Baldwin demonstrates a tendency seen repeatedly in following decades: his reference to the 'expert phisition' sets the pattern for an intense, at times seemingly involuntary, fascination with anatomy, a practice soon to become a kind of imaginative centre of gravity for descriptions of corporeal invasiveness, surgical or otherwise. Baldwin seems to have composed his intriguing novelistic tale in 1553. It is therefore possible that he was influenced by the translation of Geminus' Vesalian piracy, published that same year.[25] A slightly stronger candidate for such influence would be the anonymous author of perhaps the earliest English literary dissection, 'An Anatomy of a Hand in the Manner of a Dial' – a piece evidently published within a larger book in 1554.[26]

But Geminus' publications clearly did little to promote anatomy as a rhetorical source in the following decade. Compared to the explosion of dissective inventions which would shortly burst from pens, pulpits and presses, the 1560s were all but pre-anatomical.[27] I have so far found no native English uses of the word in an

---

22 For a Catholic reference to this work, see Jean d'Albin de Valsergues, [*A Notable Discourse*] (1575), 22v.

23 On dating of this work, see *Beware the Cat: The First English Novel*, ed. William A. Ringler and Michael Flachmann (Huntingdon Library, 1988), xvi; 1, ll.6–9; John N. King argues convincingly that the work was complete by late 1552 (*DNB*). On the book's experimental nature and narrative complexity, see Edward T. Bonahue, Jr., '"I Know the Place and the Persons": The Play of Textual Frames in Baldwin's *Beware the Cat*', *Studies in Philology* (1994), 91:3, 283–300, 286.

24 [A Maruelous hystory intitulede, beware the cat] (1584), C5r.

25 Although the STC does not give an entry date for Geminus' 1553 translation, his preface is dated 9 July 1552.

26 See Devon L. Hodges, *Renaissance Fictions of Anatomy* (Amherst: University of Massachusetts Press, 1985), 127.

27 Even uses of 'anatomy' in its non-figurative sense are rarely made by English non-medical authors prior to the 1570s. Including 1570 itself the same search yields just six cases (Sir John Elyot, *Bibliotheca Eliotae Eliotis librarie* [1542], C6r; Thomas Lupset, *Tho. Lupsets Workes* [1546], Dd5v; John Stow, *A Summarie of Englyshe Chronicles* (1565), 242r; William Painter, *The Palace of Pleasure* (1566), 332v–333r; Robert Copland (fl. 1508–1547), *The Shepardes Kalender* (1570), H8r; John Dee, in Euclid, *Elements of Geometrie* (1570), 23r. Painter, who uses the word in something like the sense of a decaying corpse (or possibly 'skeleton') has newly introduced 'anatomy' to his translation of a continental tale (see Sugg, *Murder after Death*, 14–16).

extra-medical sense before 1563. As Sawday has pointed out, in that year John Foxe claimed to have 'anatomised' the Roman Catholic mass.[28] Two years later, the anatomically minded surgeon, John Hall, titled a poem in his *The Court of Vertu* 'The anotomy or particular description of a byrche broome or besome' (125r–v). Though similar to the English *Anatomy… of the Mass* in its careful qualification, this is nevertheless a thoroughly extra-medical usage – unlike that of Baldwin, which had not shifted far from the immediate operations performed on an animal body. At the same time, it is also notable that Hall is himself a surgeon, and thus has a very close professional association with dissection (almost certainly closer, at this stage, than that of the physicians).[29]

In 1572 the Bishop of Ross and Catholic conspirator, John Leslie, uses a marginal heading 'The true anatomie of the new religion' in a piece of anti-Protestant polemic.[30] The following year, the poet George Gascoigne, though using the word in a strikingly visceral context, seems also to register its more abstract sense. Describing the horrors of mutilated corpses which he personally witnessed after the Spanish sack of Antwerp in 1567, he notes how one 'might looke downe into the bulk and brest and there take an anatomy of the secrets of nature'.[31]

In 1576 the first two native literary anatomies appear in England: Thomas Rogers' *A Philosophicall Discourse, entituled, The Anatomie of the Minde,* and John Woolton's *A Newe Anatomie of Whole Man, as well of his body, as of his soule….* Both these works still show some degree of rhetorical hesitancy. Most obvious in the case of Rogers (who effectively introduces his modish new title as 'A Philosophicall Discourse') we find this also in Woolton, who – like Baldwin – clearly signals the corporeal basis of medical anatomy. For all that, it is still notable that these books (along with John Lyly's more enduring Euphues, the *Anatomie of Wit* [1578]) all appeared before the founding of the Lumleian anatomy lectures. What prompted them? It is possible that the increasing activity of the surgeons could have made itself felt in terms of dissections. But we must also consider an alternative possibility. The physicians were notoriously conservative, preferring established theories of medicine to the grubby empirical details of the body itself. In this sense, they may have responded to the textual dignity of Banister's 1578 textbook. Yet they may also have responded to the impression that anatomy had now been elevated to the level of metaphor. Did the growing prominence of literary dissection play some part in promoting empirical dissection, making

28 Sawday, *Body Emblazoned*, 2.

29 A 1565 use of 'anatomy' by the English Catholic exile John Rastell (*A Replie Against an Answer* [1565], 50v) may well reflect Rastell's continental residence (at Louvain) after fleeing Protestant England in 1560. (For this and other details, see Dennis Flynn in *DNB*.) For another early usage, see Andrew Kingsmill (d. 1569), *A Viewe of Mans Estate* (1580), J8v–K1r.

30 *A Treatise of Treasons against Q. Elizabeth* (1572), 141r.

31 *The Complete Works of George Gascoigne*, ed. J. W. Cunliffe, 2 vols (Cambridge: Cambridge English Classics, 1907–10), 2:596.

some physicians feel slightly embarrassed at finding their scalpels pre-empted by the pen?[32]

This early stage of what would become a thriving new genre in its own right suggests that issues of cause and effect must be treated with some caution. One instance of life affecting art, however, does seem quite clear-cut. Between 1576 and 1650 there appeared at least 120 English literary anatomies (including three instances preserved only in manuscript form). Before the 1640s, only nine of these titles involved verb forms ('anatomised', 'anatomising', 'dissected'). But as Britain spiralled ever deeper into the vortex of civil war, the statistics dramatically reversed. In the 1640s there are 33 verb form anatomies against 25 titles employing noun forms. In either case, the works are almost all political or highly polemical ones.[33] In general terms, it is unsurprising that a period of such extreme social chaos should have produced a fondness for a term promising a certain kind of abstract order. But the verb form anatomies in particular seem especially well-suited to that active polemical vigour of literature which is so often a substitute for real physical violence.

## The Anatomical Web

In his own *Anatomy of Criticism*, Northrop Frye states of Robert Burton's famous *Anatomy of Melancholy*: 'The word "anatomy" in Burton's title means a dissection or analysis, and expresses very accurately the intellectualised approach of his form'. Frye's definition is an extremely partial one. His abstractive and intra-literary approach is further emphasised by a belief that literary anatomy is really just a form of Menippean satire.[34] True, Burton's book itself is highly intellectualised. But Frye's notion of the term 'anatomy' as an axiomatic synonym for intellectual rigour is woefully anachronistic. Numerous instances of anatomical rhetoric in the period were violent or visceral, anxious or derisive.[35] Even those which seem largely abstract to us must have had a potent charge of corporeal immediacy for early-modern readers. All in all, Frye's explanation of Burton's title is rather like someone 'explaining' the rhetoric of computing or the internet without any reference to the social influence and novelty of these phenomena in recent history.

Frye obviously had particular reasons for excluding untidy extra-literary realities from his definition. In other cases, the approach to literary anatomy

[32] While this must remain an open question, it should be emphasised that the physicians, who tended to prize textual authority over empirical investigation or evidence, would be especially prone to textual influence.

[33] For a list of English literary anatomies see Sugg, *Murder after Death*, 213–16.

[34] *Anatomy of Criticism: Four Essays* (Princeton University Press, 1957; repr. 1973), 309–311.

[35] See for example: Thomas Achelley, *The Tragicall Historie of Didaco and Violenta* (1576), ll.1713–1828; *Volpone*, 2.5, 69–72 (*Jonson: Four Comedies*, ed. Helen Ostovich (London: Longman, 1997). For details of the work's transmission, see Arthur Freeman, 'The Writings of Thomas Achelley', *The Library* 5.25 (1970), 40–42, 41.

displays a similar lack of interest in historical context, and compounds this with a lack of relevant data. In his introduction to the Clarendon edition of Burton's *Anatomy*, J.B. Bamborough argues that anatomies were 'an attempt to get to the bottom of things and reveal everything fully and methodically'. He also rightly notes the explicitly anatomical advertisement of Burton's title-page (which 'promises ... that Melancholy will be "*Philosophically, Medicinally, Historically, opened and cut up*".) But he then goes on to observe that '"Anatomies" were something of a vogue in the late sixteenth century'.[36] This statement seems to imply only the more famous anatomies of Lyly, Philip Stubbes, Robert Greene and Thomas Nashe (and perhaps John Harington). In fact, just 13 anatomies were published in English prior to 1600, as opposed to the 26 which appeared between 1600 and 1620 (inclusive) – shortly after which the first edition of Burton's *Anatomy* appeared in 1621.

Electronic databases and catalogues mean that we now have a far better statistical overview of the rhetoric of titles and texts. Meanwhile, books such as Sawday's *The Body Emblazoned* and Andrea Carlino's *Books of the Body* have helped to shift the intra-literary bias of older scholarship back toward concrete social events and phenomena.[37] But neither of those points quite explains why Bamborough or Frye choose to ignore a clue served up to them by Democritus Junior himself: 'if the title or inscription offend your gravitie, were it a sufficient justification to accuse others, I could produce many sober treatises, even sermons themselves, which in their fronts carry more phantasticall names'. It is, he adds 'a kind of policy in these dayes to prefix a phantasticall title to a booke which is to be sold' because 'many vain readers will tarry and stand gaping' at such arresting tags.[38] This admission hardly seems to correspond with the 'intellectualised approach' of Burton's chosen form.

But Burton himself is a minor culprit when it comes to commercial (or rhetorical) opportunism. Perhaps most notably, Robert Filles' 1577 translation of a French devotional work as *Godly Prayers and Meditations* was reprinted in 1590

---

36 *The Anatomy of Melancholy*, ed. Thomas C. Faulkner, Nicolas K. Kiessling, Rhonda L. Blair, 3 vols (Oxford: Clarendon Press, 1994), xxv.

37 For a similar approach to the later growth of anatomical culture in North America, see Michael Sappol, *A Traffic of Dead Bodies: Anatomy and Embodied Social Identity in Nineteenth-Century America* (Princeton: Princeton University Press, 2002).

38 *The Anatomy of Melancholy* (Oxford, 1621), 5. By way of example Burton cites a Latin anatomy (Antonius Zara, Bp., *Anatomia Ingeniorum et Scientia* (Venice, 1615), and two other works in his margin ('Anatomy of poperie' and 'Anatomie of immortalitie'). The nearest surviving matches prior to 1621 are: Thomas Bell, *The Anatomie of Popish Tyrannie* (1603), and George Strode, *The Anatomie of Mortalitie* (1618). Burton fails to mention a work which he in fact owned – John Harington's *An Anatomie of the Metamorphosed Ajax* (1596) (Nicolas K. Kiessling, *The Library of Robert Burton* (Oxford: Oxford Bibliographical Society, 1988), no. 750). For further discussion of Zara's book, see T.J. Arthur, 'Anatomies and the Anatomy Metaphor in Renaissance England' (University of Wisconsin-Madison, PhD. diss., 1978), 298.

as *The Anatomie of the Soul*. While the high profile anatomies of Lyly, Stubbes, Greene, and Nashe may have been responsible, it seems unwise to rule out the physicians' new public anatomical demonstration, begun in 1584, as a possible factor. Whatever the reasons, it is useful to ask: was Filles' book (whose text itself was probably unchanged) in fact a *different* one in 1590?[39] Again, having published his *Comfortable Treatise for the reliefe of such as are afflicted in conscience* in 1595, 1601, and 1607, it was only in the edition of 1610 that Robert Linaker was moved to speculate in his preface: 'I may therefore well call this treatise the anatomie of the contrite and broken heart'.[40] Conversely, Roger Gostwike's *The Anatomie of Ananias* (1616) shows how opportunistically 'anatomy' tags could be stuck onto the outside of a work (rather than being stylistically or methodically integral in the way suggested by Frye) when it reappears in 1618 as *The Truth of Tithes Discovered.*

A slightly different kind of opportunism appears in those writers who hedge their bets between more traditional catchwords and the highly modish 'anatomy'. So we find the streetwise Anthony Munday offering his 1588 translation of the romance *Palmerin D'Oliva* with the subtitle: *The Mirrour of Nobilitie, Mappe of Honor, Anotamie of Rare Fortunes*. A little later, an anonymous work of 1595 advertises itself as *A Myrrour for English Soldiers; or, an Anatomy of Accomplished Man at Armes*. In such cases, 'mirror', 'map' and 'anatomy' all implicitly promise a certain totalising overview.[41] These authors do not, however, trouble themselves about the differences between a 'mirror' and an 'anatomy'. The former in particular suggests a faithfully accurate reflection of a subject, and an implicit sense of impartiality: the writer has simply 'held up the mirror' and offered the resulting picture to his readers. A 'map', meanwhile, probably implied to many readers a commendable detachment, emphasising a common alliance between sight and understanding, at the expense of immediate physical contact.[42]

By contrast an anatomy offers an in-depth portrait, and a potentially greater impression of impartiality. The literary anatomist is ruthlessly unflinching in his attempt to reveal the final truth, however difficult and distasteful it might be. As already noted, the anatomist is also either tacitly or overtly active. They engage

39 The 1590 edition has since been lost. A manuscript note before the title page of *Godly Prayers...* states that 'This book was reprinted by Richard Watkins in 1590, and entitled *The anatomie of the soule*'. The assumption of an unaltered text is based on the evidence of other, re-titled but otherwise identical, publications.

40 A6v–A7r. I owe this reference to Mary Morrissey's valuable article, 'Narrative Authority in Spiritual Life –Writing: The Example of Dionys Fitzherbert (fl. 1608–14) ', *The Seventeenth Century* 15:1 (2000), 1–17.

41 On the impact of superior glass mirrors after the early 1500s, see Herbert Grabes, *The Mutable Glass: Mirror-imagery in Titles and Texts of the Middle Ages and English Renaissance*, trans. Gordon Collier (Cambridge: Cambridge University Press, 1982), 4–5. Certain writers appear to deliberately emphasise the special clarity of new glass mirrors by reference to a 'crystal mirror' (see, for example, title page of: Robert Greene, *Penelope's Web* (1587)).

42 Cf. for example André du Laurens, *A Discourse of the Preservation of the Sight* (1597), 10–16.

with their subject in detail, and sometimes in a conspicuously violent way. Here the individual action of the author potentially conflicts with his supposed neutrality – a failing perhaps registered by those authors who self-consciously promised the 'true anatomy' of their subjects.[43] While Munday and the anonymous author of 1595 rather loosely synonymise different catchwords, others might prefer to 'anatomise' what should seem a natural candidate for 'mapping'. Hence we find Sir Walter Raleigh, in 1596, claiming to have 'anatomized the rest of the sea towns as well of *Nicaragna, Jucata, Nueva Espanna,* and the ilands'.[44]

To some extent we can identify a division between writers who are genuinely interested in the comprehensive rigour, depth and detail of anatomy, and those who more or less unthinkingly paste the word on to the outside of the work as an eye-catching label. These latter cases broadly resemble certain more obviously pragmatic and performative sales techniques: a merchant, for example, might put the word 'luxury' on boxes of tea which are otherwise identical to those previously sold under more mundane descriptions. Having posited this division, it should be added that authors may be at once modish *and* genuinely captivated by the spell of anatomy.

When using anatomical rhetoric in more precisely deliberate ways (usually within works, rather than as titles), various authors do consciously register peculiarly dissective qualities. By 1579 Lyly had already signalled the opposition between 'superficial' description and anatomical scrutiny: 'whereas I had thought to shew the cunning of a chirurgian, by mine anatomy with a knife, I must play the taylor at the shoppe board, with a paire of sheeres'.[45] In the same year Stephen Gosson asks, 'how is it possible, sir, for you, with the sight of your eye, which reacheth no farther than her face, to take an anatomie of her conceite?'.[46] Probably writing in 1582, Philip Sidney describes how, 'in piercing phrases late,/ Th'anatomy of all my woes I wrate'.[47]

Along with these evocations of depth and penetration, writers also allude to the particular skills of the anatomist's craft. Lyly, again, admits that 'if the butcher should take upon him to cut the anatomy of a man, bicause he hath skil in opening an oxe, he would prove himself a calf'.[48] Later, Donne states in a sermon that

[43] See, for example: John Davies, *The Holy Roode* (1609), F2r; *The Whole Works of William Browne*, ed. W. Carew Hazlitt, 2 vols ([London,] 1868), 1:79.

[44] Walter Raleigh, *The Discoverie of ... Guiana* (1596), A5r.

[45] 'To ... Edward de Vere', in *Euphues and his England* (1580). In keeping with my general attempt to ascertain earliest dates of composition, I am following the work's entry date of 24 July 1579.

[46] Stephen Gosson, *The Ephemerides of Phialo* (1579), fol. 63r. Cf. also: John Taylor, 'A sad, Joyfull... Elegy... upon the Supposed Death of ... Mr Thomas Coriat... ', ll.43–4, in *All the Workes* (1630), 60. On the poem's origin and date, see Bernard Capp, *The World of John Taylor the Water-poet 1578–1653* (Oxford: Clarendon Press, 1994), 13–14.

[47] 'Astrophil and Stella', *The Poems of Sir Philip Sidney*, ed. William A. Ringler, Jr. (Oxford: Clarendon Press, 1962), 194, no.38, ll.9–10; on date see Ringler, xliv.

[48] *Euphues: The Anatomy of Wit*, in *The Complete Works of John Lyly*, ed. R.W. Bond, 2 vols (Oxford: Clarendon Press, 1942), 2:180.

'You may as well call him an anatomist, that knowes how to pare a naile, or cut a corne, or him a surgeon, that knowes how to cut, and curle haire, as allow him understanding, that knowes how to gather riches'.[49]

A particularly dense and rigorous use of anatomy occurs in Robert Southwell's poem, *St. Peter's Complaint* (1595):

> This fawning viper, dumme till it had wounded,
> With many mouthes doth now upbraid my harmes:
> My sight was vaild till I my selfe confounded,
> Then did I see the dissenchanted charmes.
> Then could I cut th'anotomy of sinne,
> And search with *linxes* eyes what lay within.[50]

Connoting the grim but relentlessly clear 'twenty-twenty vision' of a 'dissenchanted' eye previously 'vaild', Southwell emphasises with unusual explicitness anatomy's crucially active, interventionist stance: 'Then could I *cut* th'anotomy of sinne'. This stance, and the implicit detachment of one who can see so comprehensively and accurately, are both consistent with the fact that the speaker is presented as having escaped, and detached himself from sin. The peculiarly demanding rigour of anatomy matches the speaker's implicitly painstaking, unsparing ability to all but wrench himself from himself. For a sufficiently pious Christian, one's shadowy and deceitful interior cannot be too thoroughly probed and purged: seemingly virtuous thoughts could easily be sinful ones in disguise. In this sense, Southwell's anatomy is a violently alienating process, intensely distrustful of what might seem to be one's familiar and natural self.[51]

Compounding this impression of unflinchingly accurate vision, the dissector proposes to focus 'linxes eyes' on the sinful interior.[52] The metaphor conveys an aggressively piercing gaze, and aptly chooses an animal which seems to see so clearly because it does so without *feeling*, its eye displaying the cold, steady,

---

[49] *Sermons*, 9:385.

[50] Robert Southwell, *St. Peter's Complaint* (1595), 24. F.W. Brownlow gives 1592 as latest possible date of composition (*Robert Southwell* (New York: Twayne Publishers, 1996), 73).

[51] Such a tactic would in many ways have been typical of Protestant interiority; it is therefore interesting to note that, while the poem was reproduced in a collection belonging to the poet Elizabeth Grymeston (or Grimston), who is thought to have had lingering Roman Catholic sympathies, a later re-use was that of Sir William Mure, who appears to have been devoutly Protestant, and actively anti-Catholic (see, respectively: Grymeston, *Miscelanea* (1604), D4v, E2v; 'A Counter-Buff to Lysimachus Nicanor; Calling himself a Jesuite, By PHILOPATRIS', in *The Works of Sir William Mure of Rowallan*, ed. W. Tough, 2 vols (Edinburgh: Scottish Text Society, 1898), 2:6. On Grymeston's recusant background, see Betty S. Travitsky in DNB. Travitsky argues that Grymeston died in 1601. Evidence on Nicanor (the pseudonym of John Corbet (1603–1641)) suggests that the poem was written between 1639 and 1641. For more on Mure, see S.M. Dunnigan in DNB.)

[52] For a comic twist on this unsparing rigour, see George Chapman, *Bussy D'Ambois*, ed. Maurice Evans (London: Ernest Benn, 1965), 3.2, 334–75.

inhuman air associated with the negative extremes of the analytic mentality. In that sense, Southwell broadly echoes the icily dispassionate behaviour of Castiglione's 'ungrate woman'.

Southwell's metaphor is atypical in its precision, and may well have been inspired by his continental contacts. At this early stage in the rhetoric of anatomy, dissection was largely monopolised by writers such as Lyly, Greene, Nashe, Sidney, and Donne – figures known for their modish astuteness or for their delight in the concrete detail of London life. Matters seem to have changed when we come to a work such as Charles Pierse's book, *Vertues Anatomie*, in 1618. Subtitled *a compendious description of that late right honorable ... the Lady Cheany ...*, this book implies that the new metaphor has now been sufficiently abstracted to avoid causing offence to the dead woman's friends or relatives. Around five years later we find the term used in speech without any need for the kind of explanatory gloss employed by Mainardi's translator or the surgeon John Hall. At a Virginia Company meeting of 5 February 1622/3, Sir Edward Sackville remarked that 'he would not nowe stand to anatomize the carriage of Mr. Wrote seeinge the Lord Cavendish had so fully donn it'.[53]

The appearance of Crooke's two striking textbooks and Harvey's ongoing work as Lumleian dissector may well have played some part in this easier familiarity. Yet not all writers were quite so comfortable with dissective rhetoric at this stage. In 1622, Thomas Robinson still felt obliged to qualify his *Anatomy of the English Nunnery at Lisbon in Portugal*: 'if the title of this book … do make thee expect some chirurgical mysteries, or profound lecture upon a dissected body, let me satisfy thee, and save thee a labour of reading it' (A4r). But intriguingly, alongside this explanation we find Robinson also insisting that 'what he promiseth by the title, he hath performed in the treatise, and hath truly anatomized this handmaid of the Whore of Babylon; laying open her principal veins and sinews in such sort, that he is bold to challenge the proudest Doctor of her [the nunnery's] acquaintance to traduce his work' (A4v). In part this usage shows that Robinson finds anatomy attractive for its polemical violence. What is especially interesting, though, is that for all the acknowledged novelty of his title, the author now feels that literature (and presumably speech) has advanced its own extra-medical rhetoric far enough for his second claim to be justified. That is: he has 'truly anatomized' because he has done what preceding literary dissectors have done, and it is in this sense that he expects his promise to be judged.

I have indicated that the quaintly intra-literary stance of Frye is an impoverished approach to the whole early-modern culture of anatomy. Yet that kind of stance does have some limited use. If an intelligent Martian came to England in (say) 1623, and spent a good deal of time reading, he or she would quite soon be able to make convincing rhetorical use of anatomy, without actually knowing what a medical dissection was. The fullest awareness of much literary dissection does require familiarity with the period's medical dissection and associated

[53] *The Records of the Virginia Company of London*, ed. Susan Myra Kingsbury, 4 vols (Washington, 1906–1935), 2:257.

publications. But at the same time, much of the 'meaning' of anatomical rhetoric was dispersed across a web of literary uses, of titles, and of related terms. It should be added, however, that even if confining him- or herself to books and speech alone, our Martian might have been more confused about the meaning of anatomy in 1623 than he or she would in 1923. As we have seen, the word could be used to connote rigour, violence, precision, depth, and skill. It was often used in the sense of 'epitome', and yet at the same time was also very likely to imply a kind of essential reduction, one which was somehow both compressive and exhaustive.[54] Such seemingly contradictory claims were in one way little different from those writers offering the essential 'pith' or 'marrow' of a topic. In another, they had a special advantage. As Mary Douglas has pointed out, the human body is an attractive metaphor for almost any bounded system.[55] In early anatomy rhetoric, writers seem to covertly transpose the limits of real bodies onto the potentially unlimited subject matter they address. By this rhetorical sleight of hand, they can claim to have comprehensively probed all the recesses, joints, and cavities of that particular topic.

One other peculiar feature of early modern rhetorical dissection is its ability to balance between spatial and dynamic registers. Although it is difficult to pin down our own sense of this elusive term, we are probably likely to think (consciously or otherwise) of 'the anatomy' of melancholy or abuses as a kind of static container. But early-modern titles or individual uses almost certainly connoted the *process* of anatomising for many readers and authors. 'Anatomy' sounded liked 'anatomising' in a way that it would not in later centuries. My contention here is not that the dynamic and active resonance of literary dissection should be preferred to its spatial aspect, but that the two were able, at this point, to co-exist in a privileged, if short-lived, way.[56]

### *Related Terms*

Between 1581 and 1650 at least 125 English titles claimed to 'lay open' their subjects.[57] The same period also saw a large number of books which offered to 'open' their chosen topics. Both of these terms were common synonyms for dissection or autopsy, and both clearly had important spatial implications.[58]

---

54 See for example William Folkingham, *Feudigraphia: The synopsis or epitome of surveying methodized. Anatomizing the whole corps of the facultie* (1610).

55 *Purity and Danger* (London: Routledge and Kegan Paul, 1969), 115.

56 Burton himself often uses 'anatomy' in an explicitly active way (see *Anatomy* (1621), 1:162, 169; see also: 110, 112, 113, 115).

57 Seven of these works were translations. In the 1648 translation, *Satans Stratagems*, the translator appears to have added the phrase (for the original, see Jacobus Acontius (d. 1566), *Stratagematum Satanae libri octo...* (1565)).

58 See for example: Anon., *The Frogges of Egypt ... truly dissected and laid open*; Richard Ward, *The Character of the Warre or the Miseries Thereof Dissected and Laid Open* (1643). Thomas Rogers, Robert Greene, Robert Pricket, John Andrewes, Thomas Heywood, and Richard Bernard all wrote at least one 'anatomy' and one 'laying open'.

Interestingly, we have now so thoroughly absorbed that spatialising of ideas as to risk forgetting how common it is. On one hand, 'lay open' has itself been flattened into the phrase 'lay bare'. On the other, we routinely talk about 'the opening page' of a book or 'opening scene' of a play without consciously registering the spatial qualities of such language. In early-modern usage, 'lay open' seems to have been more closely synonymous with dissection than was 'opened'. In some cases titles quite clearly refer to the opening of a box (or even a pack of cards). But we must bear in mind that, in more ambiguous cases, readers could easily make an anatomical link which writers had not intended or overtly signalled.

Between 1585 and 1650 twenty seven 'analyses' were published in English.[59] The spatialising tendency of such works, and their associations with the controversial logic of Peter Ramus, have been emphasised by Walter J. Ong, who has also briefly noted how anatomy contributed to this spatialising mentality.[60] But it has not been appreciated how closely the two terms could be associated. In 1599, in his preface to *Greene's Arcadia*, the exuberantly visceral Nashe derides literary hacks who 'vaunt the pride of contraction', likening them to those starving Scythians who 'tooke in their girdles shorter' to reduce the sensation of hunger, and showing contempt for their ability to 'bound their base humours in the beggerly straights of a hungry analysis'.[61] Besides Nashe's own pronounced fondness for anatomy and anatomically-derived imagery there are two reasons why this appears to indicate an association with dissection, actual or rhetorical.[62] One is that 'hungry analysis' seems suspiciously interchangeable with 'hungry anatomy'. As a noun referring to an entity, either a skeleton or partially-dissected body, 'anatomy'

A large number of 'openings' were also published in the sixteenth and seventeenth centuries, most of them from the 1580s on. Although 'opening' and its cognates often meant 'anatomy' or post-mortem (see, for example, *Annals*, 30 May 1632, 3.2:341) the term, used rhetorically, clearly shaded into a more general spatial sense which was not necessarily corporeal. For just a few examples, see John Mayo, *The Popes Parliament* (1591); Paul Baynes, *The Diocesans Tryall* ([Amsterdam], 1621); Baynes, *A Commentarie upon ... Colossians* (1634); Simpson Sidrach, *Reformation's Preservation* (1643); Sidrach, *The Anatomist Anatomis'd* (1644).

59 Five of these titles use the verb form, and two are adjectival. Three are translations. Burton's 1621 *Anatomy* also has an 'analysis of the third partition' (489).

60 *Ramus, Method, and the Decay of Dialogue* (Camb., MA.: Harvard University Press, 1958; repr. 1983), 315.

61 While the authors of the 'barren compendiums' remain obscure, the words 'No Cunning in Logicke or Dialogue Latine' may imply that their field ideally requires logical competence (*Greene's Arcadia* (1590), B1r).

62 In addition to Nashe's *The Anatomie of Absurditie* (1589), see also *Pierce Penilesse*, 1:196, 213; and *Strange News*, 1:260, 306, for direct uses. For a language of viscerality which may have more indirect anatomical inspiration, see also: *Pierce Penilesse*, 1:180; *Strange News*, 1:272; *The Unfortunate Traveller*, 2:225, 235 (*The Works of Thomas Nashe*, ed. Ronald B. McKerrow, 5 vols (A.H. Bullen, 1904; repr. London: Sidgwick and Jackson, 1910).

was an extremely popular tag for the description of a living but emaciated body.[63] Here Nashe evidently means the latter, as a skeleton could not strictly 'bound the base humours of the body', in the way that his analysis punningly does. As with Nashe's phrase, such uses were frequently derisive or contemptuous ones. Equally, as a title, or a description of a body of text, 'anatomy' very frequently meant something like 'abridgement' or 'summary'. Playing on these two senses, Nashe would have expected his readers to hear an echo of 'anatomy' in his phrase.

The fourth and perhaps most easily overlooked term is 'rip'.[64] True, we have Donne's self-dissection in 'The Legacy': 'When I had ripped me/And searched where hearts did lie'. There is also Macduff, 'untimely ripped' from his mother's womb.[65] But the first of these is not a professional anatomy, and the second implies a certain violence through its sense of rude premature excavation. Yet, whereas 'rip' now tends very frequently to denote the rapid, often aggressive or impatient tearing of a purely two-dimensional entity (for example, paper or cloth), in the time of Shakespeare and Donne it was readily used to mean a calmly professional incision, and one which, either literally or metaphorically, involved a three dimensional interior.

In medical terms, we find that the autopsied horse of 1587 was 'ripped, to see the cause of his death'.[66] In 1635 one Laurence Price warned the Christian reader against swearing by example of 'the miserable death of Thomas Miles, who did forsweare himselfe, and wished that God might shew some heavie example upon him, and so it came to passe for as hee sate at his meate hee choked himselfe, and died in short space after'. Upon 'being ript up by the chirurgions of S. Bartholomewes Hospitall' Miles 'was found to have a gub of meate sticking fast in his throat'.[67]

In literary instances the word could certainly have violent overtones. This is perhaps especially notable in certain of the four titles which employed the term between 1581 and 1613. In that first year, one John Keltridge published *Two Godlie and Learned Sermons...preached before the Jesuites... in the Tower of London. In which...al such articles as they defend ... were layed open and ripped up unto*

---

63 See for example: Joshua Sylvester, *DuBartas Divine Weeks* (1605), ll. 99–100, and 1273–74; Samuel Rowlands, 'The Life & Death of John Leyden' in *Hell's Broke Loose* (1605), ll.569–70; Philip Massinger, *The Picture* (1630), 3.1, 1–17.

64 One other word which may have also have been caught up in the rhetorical net of anatomy is 'articulate'. Various forms of this were often used to refer to a jointed body. Used verbally, in the sense of 'article', the word appears to have become common only in the later sixteenth century (whereas the noun 'article' is recorded by the *OED* from as early as c.1450). In this sense it could mean 'particularise' – something which would obviously have encouraged association with the rigorous division and subdivision of anatomy. The two earliest users recorded by the *OED* – John Foxe (1562) and Thomas Nashe (1589) – were notable for exploiting anatomy with (respectively) great promptitude and great frequency. (I am very grateful to Elizabeth Heale for suggesting this link to me).

65 *Macbeth*, ed. A.R. Braunmuller (Cambridge: Cambridge University Press, 1997), 5.8, 15–16.

66 Stowe, *Annales* (1594), 17 March 1586/7, 719.

67 Reference is from title-page to: Laurence Price, *A Wonderfull Wonder*, which dates the incident 8 Aug. 1635. Price's title is therefore thought to belong to that year.

*them*. If anything, the hostility of that work is exceeded in the year of the Armada, when an anonymous author exposes *A Packe of Spanish Lyes, sent abroad in the world ... Now ripped up, unfolded, and ... condemned* (1588). In 1613, Richard Johnson's *Looke on me London: I am an honest Englishman, ripping up the bowels of mischief* is clearly less violent, but still broadly aggressive. Meanwhile, when Thomas Newton tellingly retitles his translation of a devotional work as *The True Tryall and Examination of a Mans Owne Selfe: a worke plainly ripping up each corner of a mans conscience* (1602) we can assume the same kind of unsparing rigour displayed by Southwell.[68]

But the crucial point is that such rhetoric is not *merely* violent, any more than are the numerous pieces of aggressive dissection themselves. Indeed, when considered in detail, literary ripping peculiarly complicates the whole question of violent polemic. For such rhetoric is often considered more successfully aggressive just *because* it is so painstaking and so thorough, rather than savagely uncontrolled. Part of this thoroughness involves the three dimensions implied in the titles of 1588, 1602 and 1613 ('unfolded', 'each corner', 'bowels'). Meanwhile, in Dekker's Caroline drama, *The Noble Spanish Soldier*, the whole point is that the invasion of one's victim will be thoroughly imperceptible. The Duke of Medina, proposing to question the King ('my self in person will sound the King's breast'), claims:

> I'le venture it ... and rip up
> His very entrailes, cut in two his heart,
> And search each corner in't, yet shall not he
> Know who it is cuts up th'anatomy'
> (4.1, 91–95).[69]

Along with their relatively controlled nature, the peculiarly spatial quality of early-modern rippings is attested by numerous examples. Keltridge indeed performs the kind of analytic dissection which we see in the bracketed contents tables of Burton's *Anatomy*. Interestingly, Keltridge employs this spatial bracketing throughout the text. While for the most part this takes the form of points grouped merely within single brackets (see for example B1v–B2r), the division is also found occasionally double, or three- or four-fold (B3r). In discussing the Lord's Supper, the format takes on the complexity and scale of Robert Burton's tables, dominating two facing sides.[70] Moreover, the decision to use this method *within* the text (rather than as a prefatory frame) could well imply a desire to keep returning to the body of doctrine Keltridge opposes, and to engage with it immediately and precisely.

---

[68] The original work was by Gerardus Hyperius. Newton's earlier English versions of 1586 and 1587 both lacked the 'ripping' metaphor. Cf. also (slightly outside my general chronology): John Lanseter, *Lanseter's lance, for Edwards'es gangrene: or, A ripping up, and laying open some rotten, putrified, corrupt, stinking matter ...* (1646).

[69] The play was entered 16 May 1631, and published in 1634. For other violent uses, see *The Returne from Pernassus* (1606), F1r; Thomas Dekker, *The Wonderfull Yeare* (1603), C3r.

[70] Following the book's dual pagination, the reference is either 32–3, or fol.165v–166r.

A number of other occurrences suggest something like 'unfold', 'explore', 'unearth', or 'dwell on'. In 1573 George Gascoigne talks of 'ripping up many old griefes'.[71] In 1579, Stephen Gosson wonders if he 'might ripp up that controversie of the academikes'.[72] In the second part of his *Zelavto*, Anthony Munday has the Soldane remark to the eponymous hero, that 'to rip up the whole estate of your talk it were needless'.[73] William Warner talks of 'the ripping up of many daungers, distresses, and shipwrackes', of 'ye ripping up of al circumstances', and of 'the ripping up of Thetis her inconstancie'.[74] If the synonym of 'anatomise' (and therefore of a three dimensional body) was not recognised in such cases, the reader could be forgiven for understanding something like 'disposing of' (ripping up paper and casting it away) or 'forgetting'; whereas in fact the reverse is evidently intended. The subjects in question are often being brought *back* to light ('ripping up many old griefes'; 'I might ripp up that controversie of the academikes'). Once alerted to such a register, we find that previously unnoticed details are foregrounded: note for example the spatial qualities of 'the whole estate'.

Similiarly, when Burton states of the causes of melancholy that, 'I will adventure to guess as neere as I can, and rippe them all up, from the first to the last, generall and particular to every species', he appears thorough, but not obviously in a spatial sense. Yet he effectively rewrites this sentence later on: 'As a purly hunter, I have hitherto beaten about the circuit of the forrest of this microcosme [of the body], and followed onely those outward adventitious causes; I will now break into the inner roomes, and rip up the antecedent immediate causes which are there to be found'.[75] In this latter version the context is, firstly, that of the body; and, secondly, of a conspicuously spatialised body, expanded *via* the analogy with a building.

In terms of actual titles which rip subjects or opponents, we seem to find a particularly strong example of the transient modishness of anatomical rhetoric, with the four extant cases (prior to 1642) appearing only between 1581 and 1613. But as a whole the anatomical web was far more enduring than this. Arguably its greatest legacy is the term 'analysis'. In the present day this is very possibly the most popular intellectual catchword in existence. It has considerable rhetorical power, although users are rarely likely to be challenged as to their analytical rigour. It frequently implies a kind of piercing, unsentimental examination, somehow more authoritative than mere subjective opinion or description. In all of these ways it is remarkably like early-modern literary anatomising.

---

[71] *The Adventures of Master Ferdinando Jeronimi*, 265. On Gascoigne's pragmatic re-invention of this work as a translation, see Ronald C. Johnson, *George Gascoigne* (New York: Twayne Publishers, 1972), 119–20.

[72] *The Ephemerides of Phialo*, Br.

[73] *Zelavto* (1580), 85.

[74] *Pan His Syrinx* (1584), F4v, T3v, Ev.

[75] *Anatomy* (1621), 55, 220.

In the case of 'open' and 'lay open' it is finally quite difficult to know if certain instances are anatomical or general. What we can say is that the anatomical web of the era also includes certain isolated works, such as two titles published under the name of Paul Baynes. His *The Diocesans Tryall* (Amsterdam, 1618) has 'all the sinnews of D. Downams Defence … brought unto three heads, and orderly dissolved' (title-page), while the 1643 *Commentary* on Ephesians promises that its chosen text will be 'learnedly and fruitfully opened, with a logicall analysis' (title page). Still more strikingly, we have William Pemble's *Vindiciae Gratiae. A Plea for Grace ... wherein ... the maine sinews of Arminius doctrine are cut asunder* (1627).[76] In 1621, the preacher Richard Preston published *The Doctrine of the Lords Supper Handled. And plainely layd open out of the 1. Cor. 11.23.24 ... with ... the words of consecration emboweled....* Not only does '[dis]embowelled' defamiliarise the by then relatively common act of literary anatomy; but the date of Preston's dedicatory epistle (19 March 1621) falls squarely within Lent of that year, and thus implies the influence of the new 'anatomy season' of the post-Lumleian era. The fifth anatomically-related term of the period is one which is now almost always used in a bloodless, relatively abstract way; but which seems to have been unavoidably concrete and surgical in England until at least the 1570s.

## Dividing the Body of Knowledge: Anatomical and Literary Sections

In the present day, people habitually 'section' up their writing without any awareness of implicitly wielding a scalpel. In the eras of Vesalius or Harvey, to 'section' very frequently meant to dis-sect, or to cut into a living body in the process of surgery. The *OED*'s first instance for any sense of the word is indeed an overtly anatomical one. Geminus's Vesalian epitome of 1559 makes a cross-species comparison: 'Neyther in man only … but in the anatomie or section of any other beast'. This itself is in fact preceded by a translation of Erasmus, which in 1534 talks of 'an Anothomye or section … made of the deed body'; and by the physician Christopher Langton, who refers in 1545 to 'the elementes, the temperatures, the section of the body'.[77] In Italy, we find a character in Francesco Negri's 1546 *Tragedia del Libero Arbitrio* lamenting the contemporary fragmentation of Christianity: 'here are hundredes of sectes, whiche do not only divide Christ, but make even the smallest anatomie of him that may be'. In this post-Veslian usage, there is a conscious link between those divisive sects, and the anatomy into which they cut the body of Christ.[78] Later, in 1600, the *OED* has a reference to surgery from Philemon Holland ('killed him out of hand in the very section'), and in 1611

[76] These titles may have been the work of editors, as Baynes and Pemble died in 1617 and 1623 respectively.

[77] [Ye dyaloge called Funus] (1534), [5v]. This book lacks a title page or pagination. *An Introduction into Physicke* (1545), vi verso.

[78] I am quoting here from an English translation, sometimes attributed to Henry Cheke in 1561. But Leicester Bradner argues that the work was in fact translated by Richard

Randle Cotgrave's French/English *Dictionarie* defines 'Anatomie' as 'a section of, and looking into, all parts of the bodie'. In the conclusion to the 1621 edition of his own *Anatomy*, Burton casts a sly double glance at the numerous 'sections' of his long book, and their anatomical derivation: 'The last section shall be mine, to cut the strings of Democritus' visor, to unmaske and shew him as he is'.[79]

English literary sections seem to have arisen at almost the exact same time as the literary anatomy. The *OED* has 'section' as denoting 'a subdivision of a written or printed work' only in 1576; and its first instance of the word in the sense of 'the action of … cutting or dividing' comes in 1577. In fact John Knox had used the word in its formal, literary sense as far back as 1560. But he seemed to be in a distinct minority at this time, and may well have been influenced by continental authors.[80] As that case indicates, it would be wrong to ignore other possible influences besides anatomy. Evidence shows that 'section' as a noun or verb was also used in the contexts of architecture or geometry.[81] (Arguably, these parallels could be seen to reinforce the status of anatomical sectioning, given the emphasis on skilled and meticulous division in all three cases.) Many writers would probably also have been far quicker, in this heavily Latinate period, to make links at the level of etymology rather than in terms of concrete phenomena such as public anatomies. Nevertheless, the chronology of English-language data, its context, and its authors, all strongly suggest that anatomy was the dominant factor in promoting the new vogue for the use of 'sections'.

At least 36 English-language titles which explicitly refer to a 'section' or 'sections' were published in Britain between 1577 and 1650.[82] None appear before this, and the word itself is also very rare before that time in English.[83] Evidence from early-modern dictionaries confirms the novelty of the term. In the 1598 edition of his *Worlde of Wordes*, the often up-to-date John Florio has only the verb form: 'secare', meaning 'to sawe in sunder'. In 1611, Florio goes on to define 'settione' as: 'a section, a cutting, a desection, a dividing, a parting. Also the forfeite or confiscation of one's goods in penaltie'.[84] The progress between the two editions seems tellingly to reveal a shift from a *merely* physical act to a term

Jugge, and published shortly after 1572 (see 'Henry Cheke's *Freewyl*', *PMLA*, 49.4 (1934), 1036–1040, 1036.)

79 *Anatomy* (1621), Dddr.

80 *An Answer to a Great Nomber of Blasphemous Cavillations* (1560), 2.

81 See for example: Leonard Digges, *A Geometrical Practise* (1571), H4v; Edward Wright, *Errors in Navigation* (1599), D1r–v; and (again) Dee in *Elementes* (1570), 23r. For architecture see Henry Adamson (d.1637), *The Muses Threnodie* (Edinburgh, 1638), 35, 61. For details on Adamson and his poem see Katherine A. Craik, *DNB*.

82 The first of these is Heinrich Bullinger, *Fiftie godlie and learned sermons … written in three severall tomes or sections*, trans. H.I. (1577). Bullinger's original (*Sermonum decades quinque*, (Tiguri: Christoph. Froschaueri, 1552), has just 'in three tomes'.

83 When not used in obviously surgical or anatomical contexts, early references are usually to the 'sections' of continental Latin works.

84 *Queen Anna's New World of Words*.

which shares this originary sense with more abstract synonyms. As late as 1637, John Cockeram's *English Dictionarie* has only the verbal sense of the word ('A cutting off').

A survey of context and authorship is also revealing. In general, we see a certain fluidity at the level of literary division. Initially there is no clear hierarchy of chapters over sections, and writers often refer to 'parts' or 'sections'. More precisely, we find that the *OED*'s 1576 citation comes from Abraham Fleming's translation, *Caius' Englishe Dogges* (1576). Unlike Caius' original, Fleming's version is divided into five 'sections', to which he frequently refers by this name. In his preface Fleming stresses how Caius' original treatise on dogs '*rippeth up* so apparantly their manners'.[85] Some time before 1612, Sir John Harington, author of the 1596 *Anatomie of the Metamorphosed Ajax*, is prompted to the pun 'Ile say thy sect is of a double section' while whimsically debating the religious affiliation of Leda.[86]

Rare in vernacular use at this point, 'section' was rarer still in the form of simile or metaphor. Given this, it seems significant that Phineas Fletcher (1582–1650), perhaps best known for his long anatomical poem, *The Purple Island*, appears to have had a relative monopoly on metaphoric incidences of the word in the earlier seventeenth century. In 1615 he features it in his translation of Boethius: 'First let him view the heav'ns wide-stretched section'.[87] Here, while the sense might be seen as broadly geometrical, it seems probable that Fletcher's interest in anatomy needs to be taken into account. Neither Boethius' original Latin, nor the virtually contemporary, 1609 translation (*Five Bookes of Philosophicall Comfort*) give any hint of Fletcher's 'section'. The Latin is 'Late patentes aetheris cernat plagas', and the version of the otherwise anonymous 'I.T.' is, 'Let him behold the largenesse of the skies'.[88] In *The Purple Island* itself, Fletcher describes an angel whose

---

[85] A3v, italics mine. Fleming's later work, *The Diamond of Devotion: Cut and squared into six severall points* (1581), shows, again, that such literary cutting could also operate beyond the medium of the body. Similarly, when one 'T. Tyro' describes his book *Tyros Roring Megge* (1598), as 'cut into two decads' his inspiration seems to be logical rather anatomical (cf, also, his reference to Ramus: Decad. 1, Epig. 2, A4v).

[86] *Most Elegant and Witty Epigrams* (1618), E2r. The work was published posthumously, Harington having died in 1612. The same piece refers to 'The Families of Love' (ibid.). E.K. Chambers thinks that Middleton's *The Famely of Love* was first produced between 1604 and 1607, but also notes that references to this sect were fairly common from at least 1603 (*The Elizabethan Stage*, 4 vols (Oxford: Clarendon Press, 1923), 3:440–1).

[87] 'A translation of Boëthius', book 2 verse 7, *Poetical Works of Giles and Phineas Fletcher*, 2 vols, ed. F.S. Boas, (Cambridge, Cambridge University Press, 1908), 2:245.

[88] *Five Bookes*, 47v. Latin from: Boethius, *The Theological Tractates*, trans. H.F. Stewart and E.K. Rand (London: Heinemann, 1918), 218. The translation is signed 'I.T.' after the 'Epistle Dedicatorie' (A4r). The impression that Fletcher's interest in anatomy more or less obliquely prompted his 'sectioned' heaven is supported also by Henry Vaughan's version of the poem, which has 'expansed skies' (Henry Vaughan, *The Complete Poems*, ed. Alan Rudrum (Harmondsworth: Penguin, 1976; repr. 1995), 120.

> arms with flaming tongues all sparkled bright,
> Bright flaming tongues, in divers sections parted.[89]

Titles bearing 'section' and variants show various associations with anatomy or the interior body. John Searle, author of a 1609 'sectioning' (*An Ephemeris for Nine Yeeres*) is styled as 'Master in Chyrurgery'. In 1630, Anthony Cade's *A Justification of the Church of England* offers the 'pith and marrow of the principall bookes written by both sides', and in 1647 Thomas Collier sections up his corporeal title, *The Marrow of Christianity*. The prolific Richard Brathwait made considerable use of anatomical rhetoric, and in 1621 published both *Times Curtain Drawne, or the Anatomie of Vanitie*, and *Nature's Embassie: or, the wilde-man's measures: danced by twelve satyres, with sundry others contained in the next section*. The Dean of Peterborough, Thomas Jackson (d.1640), explicitly sectioned his *The Knowledg of Christ Jesus* and *The Humiliation of the Sonne of God* in 1634 and 1635 respectively. Back in 1615 Jackson's *Justifying Faith* was also internally sectioned, and this earlier work contains a striking vivisective analogy which indicates that Jackson had read Realdus Columbus' *De Re Anatomica* (Venice, 1559).[90]

Considering works internally sectioned without titular advertisement, we find that one of these was William Folkingham's *Feudigraphia: The Synopsis or Epitome of Surveying Methodized. Anatomizing the whole corps of the facultie* (1610). Another was Robert Anton's *The Philosopher's Satyrs (1616). This work – possibly influenced by one or both of Crooke's new anatomy books – opportunistically restyled itself as Vice's Anotomy in the following year.*[91] *The Bishop of Galloway, William Cowper, internally sectioned his book A Holy Alphabet,* and was also the author of *The Anatomie of a Christian Man* (1611). Additionally, Cowper's 'Heaven Opened' features a Ramistic chart which describes itself as an 'analysis'.[92]

As so often, the most famous instance of literary sectioning occurs in Burton's *Anatomy* – a work obsessively particularised at the skeletal level of organisation, despite its tendency to swell almost unstoppably at the fleshly level of the text. But for all Burton's knowing play with the verbal and noun forms of 'section', he is not quite so fiercely aggressive as certain of his contemporary authors. I will look here at three of these, using order of interest rather than chronology.

---

89 *The Purple Island, or the Isle of Man*, in *Poetical Works*, ed. F.S. Boas, 120. While *The Purple Island* was published only in 1633, it is thought to have been written some years before, with parts of it completed by 1610. (I am very grateful to Peter Mitchell for this information.)

90 For the analogy, see Sugg, *Murder after Death*, 167–8.

91 There are no entry dates for the 1615 or 1616 editions of *Microcosmographia*; Anton's first version was entered on 23 Jan 1616.

92 *The Workes of Mr. William Cowper* (1623), 12. (The 'analysis' does not appear in the original, single edition of this title, and was probably an editorial addition, as Cowper had died in 1619. Cf also: Cowper, *A Holy Alphabet for Sion's scholars* (1613), 5.

The reforming minister Richard Bernard (1568–1641) is significant for the way in which he exploits a range of anatomical terms. Bernard is officially credited with at least three relevant titles: *Christian See to thy Conscience, or a treatise of the nature ... of conscience ... fully laid open* (1630); *The Article of Christ's Descension into Hell, fully in the true sense thereof layd open* (1641); and *A Short View of the Praelaticall Church of England ... layd open in ten sections by way of quaere and petition to the high and honourable court of Parliament* (1641).[93] There is good reason to think that Bernard implies a mingled sense of both verb and noun in that last title: he is actively dissecting this vexed and highly-charged topic. To some extent we can infer such precision and active engagement from his other publication of 1641, carefully implying its genuine use of potentially opportunistic anatomical rhetoric ('*in the true sense* thereof layd open').

In addition, we find that Bernard is also one of two possible candidates for the authorship of *The Anatomy of the Service-book, dedicated to the High Court of Parliament*. Again published in 1641, under the pseudonym 'Dwalphintramis', this title has been attributed, alternatively, to one John Bernard. That writer is in fact thought to have died in 1567. The recurrence of the phrase 'the high court of Parliament' in the two titles offers us some clue. Moreover, in 1661 the *Short View* was reprinted, with the text of Dwalphintramis's *Anatomy* appended to it, the latter now going under the title *An Anatomy of the Common Prayer*.[94] In terms of its actual text, Bernard's *Short View* is arguably the work which has the strongest claim to the pretensions for rigour associated with literary sectioning. Its 39 pages are divided into ten sections, and each section subdivided numerically. At times these roman numeral headings are further split into separate points under arabic numerals; and occasionally single sentences are themselves broken up into numbered points.

In 1604 there appeared a work attributed to the anti-Catholic polemicist Matthew Sutcliffe: *The Supplication of Certaine Masse-Priests falsely called Catholikes ... Published with a marginall gloss ... and by sections applied to the severall parts of the supplicatory declamation.* Three versions of this were published in 1604, two carrying the phrase 'by sections applied' (STC 14430 and 14430.5). All three versions differ to varying extents, and the corresponding sense of polemical urgency is compounded by the fact that the work Sutcliffe answers, John Colleton's *A Supplication to the Kinges most Excellent Majesty,* had itself only been published in the same year. We can reasonably assume that this urgency was in part spurred by Sutcliffe's uncertainty about the anti-Catholic vigour of a new, partly unknown monarch. I will also argue that the changes to the rapidly updated text offer us some intriguing anatomical parallels.

---

93 As Richard L. Greaves notes (*DNB*) Bernard is traditionally seen as the author of *A Short View*, though here the ascription is slightly less certain than with other of his works.

94 There is also an edition of the same year (again appended to the *Short View*), with the title *The Anatomy of the Common-Prayer.*

A few points of context help us to frame this examination. In 1604, 'sectioning' was still relatively novel. Only five titles had advertised the term at this stage. Similarly, those authors using the term often tended to be ones already attracted to dissective language, or to be modishly alert in their literary habits. Harington of course provides examples of either case. We should also recall, secondly, that aside from these still rare figurative transpositions, readers were generally likely to encounter the term 'section' in straightforwardly anatomical or surgical contexts at this time. As we saw, Holland talked in 1600 of a prince killed 'in the very section'. More broadly, we find that the whole practice of cutting for the (all too common) bladder stone was itself highly novel just around the turn of the Elizabethan and Jacobean eras. In February 1602 the young lawyer John Manningham notes that 'this cure by cutting' is 'a new invention'. It seems indeed to have been notorious as well as novel, given that 'one Burneham of London' had recently died after a failed operation.[95] Thirdly, we need to bear in mind that within living memory a number of Catholics had been all but anatomised alive, with the most recent case occurring after the Babington conspiracy in late 1586.

What of the texts themselves? The difference between the unsectioned STC 14429.5, and its two successors involves far more than the mere pasting on of a new rhetorical label. The first edition of Sutcliffe's response was composed of a continuous reprinting of Colleton's original text, annotated by a typically pugnacious marginal gloss. Sutcliffe's reply to the supplication was then appended in eight chapters. In the following two versions, however, Colleton's supplication is not allowed to stand alone. Sutcliffe's fuller, chaptered rebuttal now interrupts after Colleton's first section, running for a full five chapters before the appearance of the second section, which is itself immediately answered by chapter six. Although, after section four Sutcliffe's 'Answers' are no longer referred to as 'chapters', the alternation of sections and responses continues throughout.[96]

To understand this altered mode of attack, we need to understand both the psychology of religious antagonism at this time, and the recent and ongoing changes in the practice of anatomy and surgery. It should also be stated at once that Sutcliffe's books do not make explicit use of dissective language. His polemic is anatomical in its methods rather than in its overt or particular rhetoric. First, then, Sutcliffe's psychology: a ferocious hatred of his opponent is evident in the very first of Sutcliffe's responses. Even the marginal gloss seems to form a kind of literary scalpel, continually, violently, and obsessively puncturing the defenceless body of Colleton's text. The sense that Sutcliffe is thus anatomical in implicitly recognising anatomy's potential for shame rather than for instruction matches the frequently childish (and at times outrightly comic) quality of his marginal interjections ('Catholike Masse-monger'; 'Avaunt Masse-mongers with your

---

[95] *The Diary of John Manningham of the Middle Temple 1602–1603*, ed. Robert Parker Sorlien (New Hampshire: University Press of New England, 1976), February, 1601/2, 54.

[96] The sequence described is essentially the same in both later versions. I will be referring to STC 14430.

Churches'; 'He that cometh to such dogboult Masse-mongers is well served').[97] It is not merely a flippant point to say that these are the kind of hecklings which would be suppressed by a reasonably impersonal chair in a debating chamber: Sutcliffe often comes across as pathologically antagonistic, rather than as rationally convinced of his own case. Thus the gloss can be seen (in its more reasonable moments) as effectively combining the legitimate labelling procedures of anatomy, and the common tendency of anatomical polemic to more or less obviously foreground the violence and invasiveness implicit in medical dissection. This latter aspect is, importantly, not quite the same as repeatedly stabbing a body, because it slyly blurs itself into the more legitimate, objective strategy of labelling.[98]

In psychological terms, Sutcliffe genuinely *is* piercing and re-piercing a body effectively composed of both Colleton and his argument. And in these terms his behaviour has a certain logic to it. Unconsciously, Sutcliffe sees Catholicism as a 'live threat' – with some reason, as history would soon confirm. To put this another way: along with its real physical dangers to state and monarch, Catholicism offers such a radical assault on reality itself, for an English Protestant, that it will never quite die. It is always a dangerously mobile, excessive mental presence, which must be compulsively attacked for so long as these cerebral powers persist, even in the form of seemingly inert and marginal literary texts.

Yet this view is necessarily an anachronistic one. To those involved in religious controversy at the time, their position was consciously seen as absolutely right and true.[99] Sutcliffe must have been convinced that his attack was just and rational. What I want to suggest is that he indeed came to view his marginal comments as too mild and too disengaged.

In terms of the period's anatomical rhetoric, Sutcliffe's changing versions of his response match two different literary habits. The first printing of the book is a slightly intensified version of those literary anatomies which 'lay open' false arguments with a certain triumphant flourish. In that instance Sutcliffe is unconsciously violent and invasive; yet he comes to see his tactics as merely demonstrative. He simply sets out the allegedly diseased body of argument, and his greatest intervention is to offer the pathological diagnosis provided by his title. In the second versions, he is actively and far more precisely sectioning in the way that Bernard and the author of *Moro-mastix* will later do.

---

97 D4v, Gr, H4r.

98 For a similar case of sectional polemic, see Anon., Moro-mastix: Mr. John Goodwin whipt with his own rod. Or dis-secting of the sixteenth section of his book ... Hagio-Mastix (1647). The author was evidently Catholic (see L.H. Kendall, 'Notes on Some Works Attributed to George Wither', *RES* 20.5 (1954), 390–94, 392. Kendall is rightly baffled to find the book attributed (by the British Library catalogue) to the stationer Thomas Underhill.)

99 Cf. Alexandra Walsham, *Charitable Hatred: Tolerance and Intolerance in England, 1500–1700* (Manchester: Manchester University Press, 2006), 1–5.

Turning to medical dissection itself, we need first to recall the existing method of anatomy lecturing at early-sixteenth-century universities. The procedure was tripartite. A lecturer read from a venerable textbook – something which we would see as hopelessly outdated, but then generally regarded as an established and unchallengeable authority. A *sector* or cutter (usually a humble surgeon) sought to find these organs or structures as best he could; while an *ostensor* pointed them out for the benefit of those looking on. This seemingly perverse hierarchy of theory over observation was attacked vigorously by Vesalius in a number of ways.[100] But the tendency of physicians to shun such degrading engagement with the viscera was still pronounced in England in the late sixteenth century. In terms of autopsies, we find surgeons overseen by physicians well into the Caroline era.[101]

Seen in this context, Sutcliffe appears at first to behave rather like the lecturer or (at most) the ostensor. He is aloof and distant, and does not deign to soil his hands in the putrid recesses of the *Supplication* itself. This stance very quickly alters. This could have been because Sutcliffe heard rumours that the uninterrupted reprinting of Colleton was gaining unwanted sympathy in some quarters, or simply because he himself grew nervous about allowing Colleton even the potential for such sympathy. But perhaps most of all, the newly sective method of the later versions seems to imply that potent unconscious fear of a text left 'alive' in its holistic, original state. In this sense we can imagine Sutcliffe doing far more than merely launching a rational, highly analytic attack. More intriguingly, he can be seen to reduce Colleton's text to a collection of fragments which are crucially far more *impersonal* than the complete original *Supplication*. We can perceive this approach itself in at least three ways. One: Colleton comes across without the kind of human engagement that a person would command. Two: he loses the continuity of his original literary voice – something which enjoyed an implicit power long before it was scrutinised by Jacques Derrida and his disciples. And three: he and his text are objectified in a remarkably similar way to those corpses which became purely anonymous vehicles for the transmission of general truths about human organic structure.

Sutcliffe provides an intriguing variation on the rhetorical sleight of hand common to so many literary anatomies. The gesture of neutrally 'laying open' the body of argument was especially attractive to those authors claiming a gravely exhaustive – rather than satirically vicious – approach to their subjects. Having tried this tactic and become nervous about it, Sutcliffe more actively and precisely plunges in the knife. At the same time, he still retains Colleton's entire text. By doing this, and then thoroughly dismembering it (a procedure which was presumably *more* time-consuming than simply removing it, and printing only his own eight chapters), Sutcliffe may have been attempting to compromise between

---

[100] See, for example: Roberts and Tomlinson, 133; and *Andreas Vesalius' First Public Anatomy at Bologna: an eyewitness account by Baldasar Heseler*, ed. and trans. Ruben Eriksson (Lychnos Bibliotek, 18 Almquist & Wiksells, 1959), 285.

[101] See Sugg, *Murder after Death*, 137.

the desire to 'anatomise' an immediately *present* body, and a fear that this presence was in fact too dangerously intrusive and vocal. To put it another way: not all laypeople could be trusted to read the specimen correctly. Hence the industrious professional intervention of a skilled anatomist, merging the role of sector and lecturer in the way that Vesalius was to do in the frontispiece to his *De Fabrica* in 1543. At the same time, we are probably right to suspect that Sutcliffe's laboured and repeated dissection offered the author a certain primitive satisfaction: an unconscious version of those magically destructive ceremonies of corporeal invasion and annihilation performed on the bodies of various Catholics throughout Elizabeth's reign, and very soon to be witnessed once more in Jacobean London.

Finally, it is necessary to recognise that anatomical rhetoric was one feature of a large, flexible and varied textual culture. Many writers ignored it; some readers may have been baffled, faintly irritated, or merely uninterested. As early as 1587, the title of Nashe's 1587 *Anatomy of Absurdity* may imply a certain mockery of the new fashion, and not very long after, Shakespeare's sly use of 'anatomy' as an unflinching truth-claim in the mouth of the clearly biassed and villainous Oliver, in *As You Like It*, gives us an early example of how early-modern thinkers could be sceptical of dissective strategies.[102] Again, those authors who carefully advertised the 'true anatomy' of their subject may have been guarding against the general misuse or inflationary tendency of anatomical habits as the seventeenth century progressed.[103]

If we include related terms, the rhetoric of anatomy was sizeable in quantity. But what is most significant about the efflorescence of dissective titles and language is, first, its relative suddenness and rapidity of diffusion; and, second, its early flexibility, range, and complexity of meaning. Seen more broadly, this new rhetorical habit sits on a line which runs down through the epistemic shifts of scientific medicine, and whose later descendant, 'analysis', has immense intellectual cachet at the present moment.

[102] 1.1, 155–58. For further details, see Sugg, *Murder After Death*, 61–2.

[103] Bacon's 1605 criticism of those who pretended to methodical division without justification may also include rhetorical anatomists to some degree (*Novum Organon*, in *The Works of Francis Bacon*, ed. James Spedding, Robert Leslie Ellis and Douglas Denon Heath, 14 vols (London, 1858) 4:85.)

Chapter 4

# Medical Humanism, Rhetoric, and Anatomy at Padua, circa 1540[1]

Andrea Carlino[2]

In 1945, the linguist Emile Benveniste published a short paper in the *Revue de l'histoire des religions* devoted to what he called the medical doctrine of Indo-Europeans. In this paper, Benveniste advances a precise definition of the word "medicine" that he dates at "a highly prehistoric era": medicine applies "a well-conceived plan to a troubled condition," that is, it intervenes not only empirically but with "reflection, competence and authority." This definition brings Benveniste to trace the outlines of a general doctrine that structures medical activity within the vast domain of Indo-European culture and civilization. From the comparative analysis of three texts—the Avesta (tenth to sixth centuries B.C.E.), the third Pythic of Pindarus (fifth century B.C.E.) and a hymn from the tenth Mandala of the Ṛg-Veda (second half of the second millennium B.C.E)—there emerges a tripartite typology of diseases, treatments, and therapeutic functions common to this civilization. Hence, according to Benveniste, we can perceive, already at a very early era, an articulation of medicine into three types of care and therapeutic practices: the medicine of the knife, the medicine of herbs, and the medicine of speech. Benveniste's argument demonstrates consistency with the tripartite patterning which, according to Georges Dumezil, structures Indo-European society in its entirety (Dumezil 1958)[3] and which is reflected in the orders-based organization of feudal society (Duby 1978).

This classification of therapeutic functions is hierarchically ordered, following the associations of cleric / speech, warrior / knife and farmer / herbs. In fact, this tripartition structures the organization, the attribution of competencics, and thus the hierarchy of therapeutic activities during classical antiquity, the Middle Ages and modernity: the doctor (word), the surgeon (knife), and the apothecary (herbs) are indeed the three figures (and the three instruments) that dominate the history of western medicine over several centuries, including the social organization

---

1 With Andrea Carlino's kind permission, this article has been translated by Vincent Halford and Stephen Pender. It first appeared as "Les fondements humanistes de la médicine: rhétorique et anatomie à Padoue vers 1540," in *Littérature et médicine: approches et perspectives (XVI-XIX siècle)*, ed. Andrea Carlino and Alexandre Wenger (Geneva: Droz, 2007), 19–47.

2 To Joseph, for his 80th.

3 Dumezil takes up the essay on Beneviste's medical doctrine on 21–2.

of health professions into guilds. In this context, ancestral associations emerge between medicine and speech, intimate and stable links that span centuries: on professional, social, and cultural levels, these associations display one of the features characterizing the activity of physicians in earlier times; moreover, they fix the demarcation distinguishing doctors from other healers and practitioners who operate with their hands. Physicians were masters of words. Over several centuries, their profession was built on texts, their intellectual profile and their social status were in fact comparable to that of philosophers, scholars, and philologists.

By recognizing the foundational value of speech in medicine, Beneviste's article occasions consideration of the multiple relationships between medical and literary fields, relationships that could constitute challenging areas of research and reflection for historians: the role of ancient textual authorities; philological and exegetical exercises (reading, commentary, interpretation, translation, epitomizing) that characterize the intellectual practices of medical culture in the Middle Ages and modernity; physicians' nominalist passions and lexicographical enterprises; the intimate relationship between care, persuasion, and healing, and thus the conscious use of rhetorical techniques as tools at the heart of therapeutics; the issue of style in medical writing; treatments accomplished by words, charms and incantations in healing practices; critical and satirical debate about the perversion of "philological doctors" into "logophile doctors" (for example, in Ferrand 1610, f. aVr).

With a view to bringing to light this essential relationship between medicine and speech, often forgotten by a historiography ensnared in the separation between disciplines and fields of knowledge, in this article I shall limit myself to exploring this question in relation to the category of medical humanism, a category dear to medical historians investigating the Renaissance: . More particularly, I will develop this discussion proposing the inscription of a medical text—the *De humani corporis fabrica libri septem* (1543) of Andreas Vesalius—within the production of humanist culture. Re-assessing Vesalius as part of the learned milieu active in Padua during the late 1530s and early 1540s will allow some new, unexpected, but nevertheless intimate relationships between anatomy and rhetoric to emerge.

Studying the period from about the mid-fifteenth through the sixteenth centuries, historians of medicine employ the historiographical category "medical humanism" when they are confronted with the imposing mass of documents that attest to the abstruse, almost obsessive work by a number of physicians in order to recover, restore, and annotate classical sources of medical knowledge, particularly Hippocrates, Galen, and Dioscorides. The intellectual profile of these humanist doctors is thus characterized primarily by the deployment of philological competency, by an encyclopaedic vocation, by a distinct will to restore the pristine bases of the ancient medicine, after the hazardous transmission of this knowledge in the Middle-Ages and, especially, after textual and interpretive corruption by Arab authors.

Principally active at Ferrara, the physician, philosopher and philologist Niccolò Leoniceno (1428–1524) is an emblematic figure with respect to the humanist attitude towards the ancient medical texts. He devoted a good portion of his activity to editing, translating, and publishing Greek texts, above all Galen, but also Hippocrates and Aristotle. According to Leoniceno, the works of these authors had been misread and misinterpreted—in short, corrupted—by Arab doctors (Avicenna, in particular) and by certain Latin authors. The *De Plinii et aliorum in medicina erroribus* (1492),[4] in which Leoniceno corrects the errors of Latin commentators that "polluted" Greek medicine, has become, for his contemporaries and in the recent historiography, the text that exemplifies the humanistic critical and intellectual posture in medicine (French, 84–6).

Leoniceno's critical activity centres on reconstituting the textual foundations of medical knowledge through philological expertise. His work has been recognized by modern historiography as a typical humanist contribution to the medicine of the period, itself characterised by a return to the past in order to enable future developments in medical scholarship. To my knowledge, the first time the category "medical humanism" appears in the title of a scholarly work was Walter Pagel's 1977 article "Medical Humanism: A Historical Necessity in the Era of the Renaissance." In this essay, Pagel justifies the notion—on its own rather suspect—of "historical necessity" by explaining that the reconstruction of ancient knowledge (Greek, of course, but also Latin) undertaken by humanists during the fifteenth and early sixteenth centuries furnished the bases on which a new medicine might be built and affirmed. About the central figures of the renewal of medicine in the Renaissance, Pagel writes: "the soil from which the Vesalian as well as the Paracelsian reform emerged was humanism" (Pagel 1977, 379). This is how he summarizes the impact of humanism on Paracelsian medicine:

> If it is not the quest for new and pure manuscript sources, or the yearning for beauty, the contempt for scholasticism and Arabism, for logic and rhetoric was surely the ground which Paracelsus had in common with the humanists. (1977, 383)

This passage is problematic, not with respect to Paracelsus—Pagel is an authority on the subject (Pagel 1958)—but rather concerning the supposed disdain of humanists for logic and for rhetoric. Actually, Pagel's interpretation seems biased by a reductive and simplifying designation of humanism, explained as a return to classical sources of medical knowledge and, all in all, little more than an exercise in critical philology applied to texts.

---

[4] This text was first published at Ferrara, *de Rubeis et de Grassis*, 1492. Following the success and polemics it instigated, it was republished with the title *De Plinii, et aliorum medicorum in medicina erroribus opus primum ... Eiusdem Nicolai Epistola ad Hermolaum Barbarum in primi operis defensionem. Eiusdem Nicolai De Plinii ... novum opus ...*, Ferrara, per Ioannem Maciochium, 1509. On Leoniceno and humanism see Nutton 1997 and, more generally, Nauert 1979 and Mugnai Carrara 1991 (in particular for the polemic on Pliny, 25–31).

To correct this interpretation, it will be necessary to widen the historical panorama and to question literary and intellectual history in order to find a more appropriate definition of the humanist movement and, in turn, to evaluate more precisely its contribution to the medical culture of the sixteenth century.

Among the most lucid contributions, Francisco Rico's *Le rêve de l'humanisme* holds a special place. In its first pages, Rico offers the following proposition:

> We can designate humanism a perfectly delimited historical tradition, a continuous succession of men of letters who transmitted learning one to another, who felt themselves to be trustees of the same heritage and who considered themselves mutually linked. (13)

He then details the cultural values that inspired this community:

> Humanism's most illustrious family of minds, the richest in ideas, has always held the tenet that one must seek the foundation of all culture in the arts of language, deeply assimilated owing to the relentless reading, commentary and imitation of the Rome and Greece's great authors; that classical languages and literatures, models of clarity and beauty, should be the entry to any doctrine or work worthy of esteem, and that the correctness and elegance of style [...] constitute a sine qua non condition for any intellectual enterprise; and finally, that the studia humanitatis thusly conceived, in reviving antiquity, should end up producing a new civilization. (Rico, 2002, 19)

From this definition, I retain three elements: the idea of a community interlocked by shared values; the conviction that the foundation for all intellectual enterprise resides in the arts of language; the identification of a stereoscopic intellectual approach, peculiar to the *studia humanitatis*: the gaze fixed on the past, yet directed toward a radical recasting of learning.

Rico's definition rests on a solid historiographical tradition and, in particular, on the synthesis furnished by P.O. Kristeller on the figure of the humanist in the Italian Renaissance: the humanist is a scholar—often a teacher—engaged in the *studia humanitatis*; these are a specific set of disciplines (grammar, rhetoric, poetics, history, and moral philosophy) based on the study of the classics and considered as the foundation of all intellectual, scientific, and artistic enterprise.[5] As Lorenzo

---

[5] "The term *humanista*, coined at the height of the Renaissance period, was in turn derived from an older term, that is, from the 'humanities' or *studia humanitatis*. ... By the first half of the fifteenth century, the *studia humanitatis* came to stand for a clearly defined cycle of scholarly disciplines, namely grammar, rhetoric, poetry, history, and moral philosophy, and the study of each of these subjects was understood to include the reading and interpretation of its standard ancient writers in Latin and, to a lesser extent, in Greek. This meaning of the *studia humanitatis* remained in general use through the sixteenth century and later, and we may still find an echo of it in our use of the term *humanities*" (Kristeller 1979, 22). This essay was presented by Kristeller in 1954 in the Charles Beebe Classical Lectures at Oberlin College (Ohio) and was published in Kristeller 1995. On this subject, see also Kristeller 1960 and the bibliographic discussion in Kristeller 1962.

Valla clarifies, in one of the reference texts of humanist culture, the *Elegantiae Linguae Latinae* (1440), without the humanities (*sine studia humanitatis*), it is impossible to seriously know any discipline: eloquence is as necessary to those who study civil law as canon law, medicine as philosophy, theology as the Holy Scripture (Rico, 20–21).[6]

So, *pace* Pagel, the arts of language, and among them rhetoric, are at the very heart of humanist culture, a culture that, though originally defined by a circumscribed range of knowledge, unfurls itself on a much wider set of disciplines, deploying an encyclopaedic vocation that is justified and legitimized, on the one hand, by the study of ancient sources and, on the other, precisely by the mastery of language, of language and discourse in its technical, even professional aspects.

This specific definition of "humanism" is not necessarily in contradiction with the more generic version that historians of medicine have usually adopted when they speak of "medical humanism." Yet, , it allows reassessing, in a significant historical moment, the intense relationship among medicine and language evoked by Beneviste, a relationship which a superficial reading of the history of medicine, boringly progressive and obtusely specialized, had made us forget.

These general discussions about medical humanism, leads me to consider the *De humani corporis fabrica* of Andreas Vesalius from an unusual perspective.[7] In medical hagiography, this work is rightly considered the founding text of modern anatomy, a text that, via observation on the cadaver and direct experience, allowed its author to break free from the unwieldy heritage of the ancients, in particular Galen. Moreover, the knowledge of anatomy is here presented as the condition that establishes a rational, verifiable, in a word scientific medicine. Hence the challenge to assign this work to its humanist context and to focus on Vesalius and his role in the scholarly circles active in Padua around 1540, in order to attempt to erase borders historically erected to circumscribe a separate, autonomous field of activity and reflection specific to anatomy, and at a stroke, to medical knowledge. Accordingly, this approach implies resituating Vesalius among his fellow humanists. This is a move already initiated by Ludwig Edelstein in an article published over half a century ago, "Vesalius, the Humanist" (1943).[8] In a prudent, almost circumspect tone, Edelstein summarises his proposition towards the end of his essay as follows: "not only was [Vesalius]a classical scholar, not only did he wear the robe of the humanist, but he also professed the main articles of the humanistic faith." His proof rests essentially on three arguments: first, Vesalius

---

6 I consulted the *Elegantiae Linguae Latinae* in the Laurentius Valla edition, *Opera*, Basileae, apud Henricum Petrum, 1540 (facs. ed. in Laurentius Valla, *Opera omnia*, Torino 1962, t.1). The passages referenced are in the introduction to Book 4 and in Book 6 at Chapter 34.

7 On Vesalius, I refer to the standard biographies of Roth 1892, Cushing 1962, O'Malley 1964. On the contribution of Vesalius to the rise of modern anatomy, see also, for example: Cunningham 1997 (88–142) and Carlino 1994.

8 On the contribution of L. Edelstein to the history of medicine, see Rütten 2006.

manifests the awareness of founding modern anatomy from the resurrection of, not in opposition to, classical anatomy; next, an ethical spirit governs the conception of the *De humani corporis fabrica*, a spirit comparable to the humanist project that associates the quest for knowledge with the discourse on the dignity of man as encouraged by, among others, Pico de la Mirandola; finally, in his writing, Vesalius consciously adopted a style borrowed directly from the works of Cicero.

In the footsteps of Edelstein, here I wish to reinforce those arguments by showing Vesalius' cultural and personal engagement in the humanist movement. I shall consider, first, the significance of the word *fabrica* in Vesalius' work; next, I will explore the cultural context in which he operated in Padua; and, finally, I shall examine the heuristic value that the humanists close to Vesalius recognized in the anatomical method with respect to the arts of language.

Vesalius' term *fabrica* has been the object of several discussions, interpretations, and translations among historians: they hesitated amongst "structure," "fabric," "composition," "œuvre."[9] As some have noted (e.g., Bylebyl 1979, 358–9), this term had already been employed in the title of the Latin translation of a Byzantine anatomical text by Theophilus Protospartarius. Published at Venice in 1537, this translation was the work of Giunio Paolo Crasso, philosopher, physician, and philologist,[10] who after having occupied a chair in moral philosophy, was one of Vesalius' teachers at the University of Padua and one of the *promotores* for his doctorate (Bylebyl 1979, 359 and Papadopoli 1726, t.1, 322–3).[11] In the dedicatory epistle, although Crasso shows a precise consciousness of the literary stakes and contemporary debates concerning the ethics of translation, he eschews the term *fabrica* in the text and prefers to adopt other synonyms such as *apparatus, structura, artificium.*[12]

---

9 Charles O'Malley, the latest biographer of Vesalius, chose for example the word *structure*, "as best representing Vesalius' concern with the underlying bony structure of the body" (139).

10 With respect to Crasso, Scardeone writes: "Inter omnes docos pollet nunc Paulus Crassus philosophus et medicus clarissimus, et tam Graecae quam Latinae linguae disertissimus, et publice in scholis eruditissimus medicinae professor, et privatim in curandis aegris magister peritissimus …" (s.v.).

11 The full title of Crasso's translation is: *Theophili Protospartari de corporis humani fabrica libri quinque a Iunio Puolo Crasso Patavino in Latinam orationem conversi. Hippocratis preterea de purgatoriis medicamentis Libellus ...*, Venetiis, [Ottaviano Scoto], MDXXXVI. This text was then published in a compilation edited by Johannes Guinterius, , , Vesalius' teacher while he was a student in Paris (Winther, 1539).

12 In the epistle, he writes about the practice of translating: "Ergo mirari desinant Grammatistae, si, quod graeci faciunt, nobis etiam concedendum petimus, ut nova rerum latinis novarum nomina fabricemur, ut aiebat. M. Tullius, aut ex aliis transferamus, semperque illius Galeni, Platonisque dicti mihi veniebat in mentem, verba iis esse negligenda, quibus multarum magnarumque rerum contemplatio esset proposita, laudandamque magis orationem, quae verbis apertioribus, (modo ne forent prorsus barbara) quam quae limationibus uteretur" (Crasso, *De corporis humani fabrica* 1536, 5–6).

By following Edelstein's indications, and by examining Vesalius closely, we can indeed ascertain that Vesalius chose the word *fabrica*, not in homage to one of his university masters (namely Crasso), but rather in reference to his literary model, Cicero. As Jackie Pigeaud demonstrated, "Vesalius takes *fabrica* in the sense that he reads it in the *De natura deorum*" (155–61). In book two of Cicero's text, the word *fabrica* appears twice, precisely in passages where anatomical issues are discussed. If in the first passage Cicero uses the locution "admirabilis fabrica membrorum" in relation to the animal body (*De natura deorum*, 2.47.121), the second occurrence is even more significant:

> Illa potius explicetur incredibilis fabrica naturae: nam quae spiritu in pulmones anima ducitur, ea calescit primum ipso ab spiritu, deinde contagione pulmonum, ex eaque pars redditur respirando, pars concipitur cordis parte quadam, quam ventriculum cordis appellant, cui similis alter adiunctus est, in quem sanguinis a iecore per venam illam cavam influit. Eoque modo ex is partibus et sanguis per venas in omne corpus diffunditur et spiritus per arterias; utraque autem crebrae multaeque toto corpore intextae vim quondam incredibilem artificiosi operas divinique testantur. (Cicero, *De natura deorum,* 2, LV, 138)

The use of the term *fabrica* arises in a passage that provides an anatomical description; more cogently, it occurs in a section of the *De natura deorum* devoted to the celebration of Providence and of Nature's intelligence ("naturae ratio intelligentis") where the wonder generated by the enterprise of the *Faber* (the gods, Nature) is asserted.[13]

Beyond the stylistic argument and beyond some citations from Cicero that we find sprinkled throughout the *Fabrica*, we have the proof that Vesalius knew very well these crucial passages of the *De natura deorum*. When he discusses the names that must be attributed to the different parts of the intestine, he writes: "Cicero autem in tertio de Natura Deorum intestinum aliquod ita vocari arbitratus medium intestinum ucertit … ." Actually, it is not a quotation of the third book, but of the second. In any case, this passage precedes by only a few lines in Cicero's text the occurrence of the term *fabrica* in relation to human anatomy (Vesalius 1543, 504).[14] Further, the expressions *fabrica naturae* and *fabrica membrorum* are recurrent not only in Vesalius' text, but also in the dedicatory epistle to Charles V, for example, where the term is used with the same philosophical and ethical connotations as in the *De natura deorum*.

*Fabrica* also belongs to another semantic and disciplinary field, architecture. In sixteenth century architectural theory, it defines the process of material construction enacted on the base of a detailed project previously conceived by a coherent

13 "Facilius intellegitur a diis inmortalibus hominibus esse provisum si erit tota hominis fabricatio perspecta omnisque humanae naturae figura atque perfectio" (Cicero, *De natura. deorum*, 2, LIV, 133).

14 The passage dealt with is *De natura deorum*, 2, LV, 137. On this subject see Pigeaud 1995, 156–7.

theoretical abstraction. This disciplinary context allows us to move from the word *fabrica* to the milieu in which this term was used. The Italian architect Sebastiano Serlio is the author the *Sette libri d'Architettura*, one of the most important treatises on architecture of the Renaissance, as well as one of the greatest illustrated editorial enterprises of the sixteenth century. The seven books were published between 1537 and 1575, with the exception of the sixth, which remained a manuscript until 1966 (Dinsmoor 1942, Bury 1989, Deswarte-Rosa 2004).[15] As scholars have shown, this treatise, in particular its structure and the conceptt that underpins it, is closely aligned with the encyclopaedic project of a "theatre of omniscience" elaborated by the humanist and master of rhetoric Giulio Camillo.[16] Over the course of several years in Italy and France, Camillo was occupied with producing a system and a machine, at once theoretical and architectonic, that would be able to contain and allow the control of terrene knowledge as well as of the eternal ideas that govern it. It was founded on the application of the "divisive method," which had its roots and its chosen terrain in the arts of language (mostly rhetoric, grammar, and the topics) and which consisted of a "retrogradation of the sensible to the intelligible" measured in seven levels.[17] Although it was virtually applicable to all domains of knowledge, Camillo employs this method, comparatively, for architecture, while Serlio exploits it to organise his intellectual programme in the seven books of his treatise (Carpo, 78–80).[18]

---

[15] In chronological order, the books published by Sebastiano Serlio (1475–1554) during his lifetime were: *Regole generali di architettura* (Quarto Libro), Venetia, F. Marcolini, 1537; *Il terzo libro ... nel quale si figurano e si descrivono le antiquità di Roma*, Venetia, Marcolini, 1540; *Il primo libro d'architettura*, Paris (Jean Barbé, 1545); *Il secondo libro di perspettia* [sic], Paris, Jean Barbé, 1545; *Quinto libro d'architettura*, Paris, Michel de Vascosan, 1547. *Le Livre extraordinaire de Architecture*, Lyon, G. de Tourne, 1551, which was not originally part of the work, was published as the missing sixth book in several editions of the "complete" treatise of Serlio after 1566 (in Venetia, appresso Francesco [de Franceschi] Senese, et Zuane Krügher Alemanno).

[16] The definition "theatre of omniscience"—as opposed to "theatre of memory"—was correctly given by Deswarte-Rosa 2004, 31–66. On the question of the Serlio–Camillo relationship, see: Olivato 1971; Olivato 1979; Carpo 1997, in part pp. 47–137; Deswarte-Rosa 2004, in part pp. 38–46. Carpo proposes the idea of an influence of Camillo's "pedagogic method" on the conception of Serlio's *Sette libri*; on the other hand, Deswarte-Rosa insists on the contribution of Serlio's architecture on Camillo's philosophical thought. With the state of proof available today, I will content myself with the established fact, well documented by such researchers, of the close collaboration and the personal relationship of Camillo e Serlio.

[17] Here is not the place to enter into the details of Camillo's complex project. On this matter, see the works of Yates 1966; Bolzoni 1983; Bolzoni 1984; Carpo 1993.

[18] The complete project of the treatise is presented by Serlio in 1537 in the preface to the first volume published, the *Regole generali di Architettura o Libro Quarto cit.*, "L'autore alli lettori," f.5. Camillo's passage on the seven degrees of architecture is in the *Idea dell'eloquenza*, a text that remained manuscript and was published by Bolzoni 1984, 121–2.

We can observe several similarities in form and approach between the *De humani corporis fabrica* and the *Sette libri di architettura*: the organisation in seven books, the attitude toward classical sources, the place devoted to the communication of knowledge by illustration, the importance accorded to the rapprochement between theory and practice, the relationship between scholarly inquiry and experience, the articulation between parts, structures, and functions. A personal rapport between Vesalius and Serlio is highly probable, since the two are present between Venice, Padua, and Bologna around 1540, and since they frequented the same scholarly milieux: around Pietro Arctino, Jacopo and Francesco Sansovino, Tiziano Vecellio and his workshop, the Venetian printing houses of Bernardino de Vitalis and Francesco Marcolini, the networks of Spanish patrons in Italy, in particular around the governor Alfonso d'Avalos and the ambassador Don Diego Hurtado de Mendoza.

One trace of this Serlio–Vesalius relationship can be seen in the frontispiece of the *Fabrica*: the dissection scene takes place in the middle of a temporary wooden theatre, built inside a courtyard surrounded by seven columns, above which is a frieze decorated by triglyphs, metopes, and bucranes. The same decoration of the frieze is described, analyzed, and represented in Serlio's *Quarto Libro* (Serlio 1537).[19] Further, in the same period Serlio built a temporary wooden theatre in the courtyard of the Palazzo da Porto at Vicenza, analogous to the one represented in the frontispiece of the *Fabrica*.[20]

The cultural and contextual proximity of Vesalius and Serlio leads me to advance the hypothesis of another significant connection: that of Vesalius and Camillo, who both share the aim to reveal the interactions between science and the arts of language under the aegis of humanist culture. If it is true that Camillo, great friend of Serlio,[21] frequented the same cultural milieu and the same networks of clientele as Vesalius, we also know—and I will return to this point below—that Camillo manifested in his writings a remarkable interest in anatomy as knowledge of the body, but also as an intellectual approach, as a method. In Camillo's eyes, anatomy is, as it were, the "divisive method" in action, the tangible and practical version of the course of "retrogradation of the sensible to the intelligible."[22] Some clues of his

---

19 I consulted Serlio's edition of 1600. La frieze is reproduced on p. 117r., in the third book, illustrating the details of the Porta dei Leoni at Verona, and on p. 140v., in the fourth book, describing the doric order.

20 Serlio recounts this and describes the wooden theatre in the *Trattato sopra le scene* contained in Serlio 1545, ff. 63r.–66v.

21 Camillo came to be the universal heir in the will that Serlio drew up in 1528. This testament was found and published by Olivato 1971.

22 The Venetian numismatist and polymath Sebastiano Erizzo, who also studied medicine at Padua with Bassiano Landi, defines the "via divisiva" as the master path to investigate into the essence and the very nature of everything. To this method, which Erizzo said he learned by following Bassiano's anatomy lessons, he devoted a treatise that today one would define as epistemology applicable to all disciplines indiscriminately (Erizzo 1554).

anatomical engagement are given, for example, when Camillo recounts assisting at a dissection in Bologna (was it the one carried out by Vesalius in 1540?[23]) or when he writes, in his *Sopra Hermogene,* about the conceptual relationship between eloquence and architecture, where he regularly uses the term *fabrica* to designate a construction and a system achieved by means of a theoretically founded project:

> Si come l'Architetto, non con sanamente si condurrebbe à fabbricare alcuno edificio con le pietre, et altri semplici, se prima nella mente non avesse con belli, et dotti pensieri fatta una mental fabrica, ad imitation di cui, di fuori essercitasse le mani. Cosi di niuno consiglio è da giudicare quello componitore, il quale à caso si dà a mettere insieme le parole, et altri ornamenti, senza regger lo stile, secondo alcuna forma prima collocatasi nella mente. (Camillo 1579, t. 2, 77)

Moreover, in the *Della imitazione*, a polemic text written against the *Cicerionanus* of Erasmus, Camillo offers a comparison between eloquence and anatomy that emphasises the similarity of these two disciplines proceeding from the notion that their very objects (the body and discourse) are both invariably organised by complex but stable structures (grammar and the bone structure, respectively):

> Ricordomi già in Bologna, che uno eccellente anatomista chiuse un corpo humano in una cassa tutta pertugiata, e poi la espose ad un corrente d'un fiume, il qual per que' pertugi nello spazio di pochi giorni consumò e portò via tutta la carne di quel corpo, che poi di sè mostrava maravigliosi secreti della natura negli ossi soli, e i nervi rimasi. Così fatto corpo dalle ossa sostenuto io assomiglio al modello della eloquentia dalla materia e dal disegno solo sostenuto. E così come quel corpo potrebbe essere stato ripieno di carne d'un giovane o d'un vecchio, così il modello della eloquenzia può essere vestito di parole che nel buon secolo fiorirono o che già nel caduto languide erano. (Camillo 1544)[24]

This set of arguments, as well as the few biographical elements available, make the hypothesis of an intellectual complicity between Vesalius, Serlio, and Camillo very plausible. To firmly prove it, we would need, as it were, *the* letter in which their personal relationships are clearly attested.

As for the notion of *fabrica*, the move from word to context will also prove useful for notions such as *studia humanitatis* and, above all, *humanista.* Again, this brings us back to Padua. If, on the one hand, the notion of *studia humanitatis* started to circulate in Italy towards the middle of the fifteenth century, on the other hand the term *humanista*, and especially its vernacular version *umanista*, after a couple of sporadic occurrences at the end of the fifteenth century, seems mostly

---

[23] I here allude to the dissections documented by the notes taken by Balthasar Heseler in 1540 at Bologna during the anatomy lessons of Matteo Corti and Vesalius, now published in Heseler 1959.

[24] I consulted the edition of this text in Giulio Camillo Delminio, *L'idea del teatro e altri scritti di retorica*, San Mauro (To), Res, 1990. (The quotation is on 192.)

to have circulated towards the end of the 1520s,[25] in particular in Northern Italy (Bologna, Venice, Padua, Florence). Several significant occurrences had been used to designate as humanists scholars such as Cola Bruno, Benedetto Varchi, Lazzaro Bonamico, Francesco Sansovino, but also Romolo Amaseo, Paolo Manuzio, and Lodovico Domenichi, all in more or less direct relation with the *Accademia degli Infiammati*, an academy founded at Padua in June 1540. I would even say that this Paduan coterie could be considered the humanist academy *par excellence*; in many respects, despite its brief existence (1540–1542),[26] it served as model for the foundation of several scholarly academies to come, for example the *Accademia Fiorentina* and the *Accademia della Fama* at Venice.

The *Accademia degli Infiammati* was founded by a group of enthusiastic scholars, engaged in the *studia humanitatis* and, at the same time, in cultural innovation founded on a deep knowledge of ancient learning. It is rather difficult to quickly summarize the cultural program of the *Infiammati*, animated as they were by the notable presence of numerous, charismatic polymaths. Among the clear objectives of the *Accademia*, we find the reading and discussion of literary works (Petrarch, for example), as well as the commentary and translation of philosophical works, foremost Aristotle's texts and in particular *Ethics*, *Poetics*, and *Rhetoric*, all works immediately pertinent to the *studia humanitatis*. More cogently, the study of the *bonae litterae* and the debate about language and its use were central to its concerns. This implied the study of Latin and Greek classics, but also the vernacular was taken into account as a scholarly language in any disciplinary field, including philosophy and the sciences.

More generally, what emerges here—and what constitutes the essence itself of the *Infiammati*'s cultural project—is the fabrication and the promotion of the professional figure of the *literatus*. This ambitious and decisive project in European intellectual history is configured as a professionalization of literary practices and techniques, whether in Latin or in the vernacular, in poetry or poetics, in moral or natural philosophy, in history or law, in botany or medicine (Bruni 1967; Mazzacurati 1961; Vianello 1988). For the *Infiammati*, the *literatus*, whom we

---

[25] For the reconstruction of the history of the term "humanista", see: Campana 1946; Avesani 1970; and Lanza 1991. The *loci classici* indicated in the Renaissance tradition are Cicero, *De re publica*, I, xvii, 28–9 and Aulus-Gellius, *Noctes Atticae*, XIII, xvii, 1–4.

[26] On the *Accademia degli Infiammati* the principal source of information is the book of Tomitano [1545]. The critical literature is, surprisingly, rather limited; see Bruni 1967; Samuels 1976; Vianello 1988; and Mikkeli 1999. On the model role of the *Accademia degli Infiammati* for the academic movement of the sixteenth century, it suffices to recall the passage of a lesson given at Florence in the *Accademia Fiorentina* by Benedetto Varchi – one of the inspirers of the *Infiammati* and, later, eminent figure of the *Accademia Fiorentina* – in which he proclaims the Padua Academy as the prototype of the scholarly academies: "dalla quale e questa nostra, chente ella si sia, e tutte l'altre che si sono create di poi per tutta l'Italia, si può dire, con verità, per quanto stimo io, che siano procedute ed abbiano non pur l'origine avuto da lei, ma buona parte ancora delle leggi ed orientamenti loro" (Varchi 1858–59, v. 2, 379).

can also call here the humanist, is a scholar who has transformed the pursuit of knowledge into a profession,, a scholar who is in command of specific skills and competencies in the arts of language, and who is driven by an encyclopaedic vocation. In this precise context, the *literatus*' intellectual activity is consistent with the conviction that a profound relationship links different domains of knowledge and that a transdisciplinary approach is essential to any humanist enterprise. This was possible, of course, in the context of an institution which presents itself explicitly as a space of intellectual liberty, as an alternative to that offered by the university, limited by its traditions, its disciplinary constraints, its *curricula*, its rituals.[27]

From these premises, the *Accademia degli Infiammati* gathered over the course of two years a considerable party of scholars: artists, philosophers, aristocrats, humanists, secretaries, writers, teachers, and students of the university, as well as expatriate Florentines, Venetian nobles, and young *Germani* students, all engaged, as amateurs or professionals, in the most diverse domains of arts and learning. Among them, we find, for example, philosophers and *literati* engaged in the front line of the debate on the use of the vernacular, such as Benedetto Varchi and Sperone Speroni; commentators on Aristotle such as Vincenzo Maggi and Marcantonio Passeri; writers, poets, and polymaths such as Pietro Aretino, Luigi Alamanni, Ludovico Dolce, and Francesco Sansovino; jurists such as Leone Orsini, Mariano Sozzini and Giovanni Andrea dell'Anguillara; the *magister ciceronianus* Lazzaro Bonamico, the scholar Pierio Valeriano, as well as professionally elusive and intellectually versatile figures such as Daniele Barbaro—translator of the Vitruvius' *Architecture* into Italian, commentator on Cicero's *Academica* and Aristotle's

[27] L'Accademia degli Infiammati – writes Mario Pozzi – is the "espressione di una cultura alternativa a quella dello Studio e manifestazione del nuovo prestigio raggiunto dal volgare" (Pozzi, *Sperone Speroni.* Nota introduttiva, in Pozzi 1978, 476). Benedetto Varchi, one of the founders of the Accademia degli Infiammati, regarding the different objectives that animated the University and the Academy and, in taking some distance from the methods used at the Studium, underlines that it is desirable "ab eis dissentire non modo possumus, sed debemus, cum alia eorum, alia sit nobis ratio Academiae nostrae." In his *Lezione sopra la generazione de' Mostri,* pronounced at the Accademia Fiorentina in July 1548, Varchi in the Proemio insists on the advantages of undertaking philosophical activity preferably at the academy (Varchi 1590, 89). Similar arguments that include grammar in the field of philosophy - thus pertinent to the activities specific to the academy's cultural space—are also developed in the *Lezione ... dei tempi dei verbi,* of December 1551 at the Accademia Fiorentina: "Perciocché se bene l'insegnare i tempi è ufizio del gramatico, il dichiarare il tempo, senza il quale i tempi intendere non si possono, a colui solo appartiene, a cui tutte l'altre cose s'aspettano, cioè al Filosofo. Onde non posso fare che non mi rida alcuna volta tra me medesimo della semplicità di certi, i quali non intendendo, per quanto stimo, quello che dicono, e il contrario a punto chiedendo di quello che disiderano, non vorrebbero che nell'Accademia cose filosofiche filosoficamente si dichiarassero, come se propriamente cosa alcuna trovare si potesse in verun luogo, la quale sotto la Filosofia non caggia, e di cui non dico non possa, ma non debba favellare il Filosofo." This lesson was published in Varchi 1810. The quotation is on pp. 43–4.

*Rhetoric*, author of an important dialogue on eloquence—who figures among the creators and promoters of the first botanical garden in Europe.[28] Remarkably, among the *Infiammati* we also find several eminent figures in the histories of science and medicine: not only Alessandro Piccolomini, author of a text on the sphere and of the first general treatise on natural philosophy in the vernacular, but also Luca Ghini, Girolamo Fracastoro, and Giovan Battista Montanus (or da Monte), physicians and philosophers, each one engaged in projects of reform in their own field of expertise (botany, contagion theory, clinical medicine) (Vianello 1988, 47–70).

And Vesalius? There is no doubt that Vesalius frequented the *Accademia degli Infiammati* as a spectator; maybe he also was formally affiliated with the academy and he participated in the same project of cultural renewal promoted by its members. In the *Fabrica*, Vesalius rarely names his contemporaries. When he does, it is with the precise intention of indicating their excellence and, at the same time, the familiarity he enjoyed with them. Hence, we find an eulogy of the "infiammato" Giovan Battista Montanus ("divini ingenii vir, ob singularem illam tum Medicinae, tum caeterarum scientiarum cognitionem, nulli aetatis nostrae medicorum secundus." [Vesalius, 309]). Similarly, Marcantonio Passeri, one of the leading figures of the academy and of Paduan aristotelianism, is described as "non modo musicorum absolutissimus verum nostrae aetatis philosophorum eximium decus" (Vesalius, 35).

Better attested is Vesalius' close link with Benedetto Varchi, the Florentine *literatus* who had elaborated the *Infiammati*'s program and occupied a pre-eminent place in this coterie. Beyond the multiple attestations of esteem and of friendship towards Vesalius diffused in Varchi's writings,[29] we have five autographed letters

[28] Here is not the place to enumerate the considerable bibliography devoted to these humanists; for Benedetto Varchi, Pirotti 1971 and Firpo 1997 (in particular 218–290 on Varchi, *il letterato*); for Sperone Speroni, Pozzi 1978, 471–509 and the special issue devoted to Sperone Speroni of *Filologia veneta: lingua, letteratura, tradizioni*, Padova 1989; for Daniele Barbaro, Laven 1957 and Angelini 1999. For bio-bibliographies of other members of the Infiammati, see Vianello 1988.

[29] I will limit myself here to recalling the sonnet Varchi wrote in Vesalius' honor in 1543, to encourage him to accept the anatomy chair which Cosimo 1 had offered him at the University of Pisa (Varchi 1555); the laudatory passage in the *Questione sull'alchimia* (1544) (Varchi 1827, 54) and the passage on the third lesson on the soul, delivered in 1544 at the Accademia Fiorentina: "il dottissimo et mio amicissimo esser Andrea Vesalio, huomo singolarissimo et che non solo aggiugne a gl'antichi in quella professione, ma gli passa." This lesson belongs to the "lezioni sul canto XXV del Purgatorio" published, in part, in *La prima parte delle lezioni di M. Benedetto Varchi, nella quale si tratta della Natura, della generazione del corpo humano e de' mostri*, Firenze, Giunti, 1560. The third lesson, which remained manuscript, (Biblioteca Laurenziana Firenze, ms. Med. Pal. 113), was recently published in Andreoni 2004. The quotation is on p. 211.

of Vesalius addressed to Ser Benedetto, written between 1543 and 1546.[30] In these letters, we find the attestation of the intimate relationship between these two scholars, of their intellectual collaboration, and of shared projects that go back to the years spent together in Padua at the precise moment when the *Accademia degli Infiammati* was active.

In a letter addressed to Varchi, dated 26 March 1544, Vesalius alerts his friend, at the time settled back in Florence, to the publication of Daniele Barabo's commentary on Aristotle's *Rhetoric*. He insists on the opportunity to offer this work to Pietro Vettori, a central figure in the period's scholarly community and the intellectual and moral guide to numerous Italian humanists, including Varchi. In effect, Vettori had built his reputation as a great philologist by working on editions, translations, and commentaries of several Greek and Latin texts, in particular the works of Aristotle and Cicero. Several times, he edited the *Rhetorica ad Herennium,* at the time attributed to Cicero. In 1544, Vettori already envisioned Latin editions of and commentaries on Aristotle's *Poetics* and *Rhetoric.*[31] The brief notation in Vesalius' letter shows, on the one hand, a first-hand insight into Florentine and Venetian humanist networks and concerns and, on the other, provides a clue to Vesalius' specific curiosity about questions germane to the *studia humanitatis*, especially about domains of study, namely rhetoric, central to both the *Infiammati*'s discussions and the European humanist milieu of the period.

Barbaro's commentary on Aristotle's *Rhetoric* appeared in 1544 in Venice and Lyon (Barbaro 1544a, Barbaro 1544b) and it echoes issues relevant to medical learning.[32] Barbaro proposes a comparison between medicine and rhetoric which, after the textual and contextual exploration thus far, sends us back to another level of the intersection between medicine and language, this time of a philosophical, methodological and epistemological order:

> Omnis dicendi facultas, ita mentes humanas deducit, et flectit, ut medicina partes, et membra corporum nostrorum: qua ratione fit, ut recte admoneat nos Plato eundem haberi medicinae, ac Rhetorices modum, quoniam in utraque facultate subjectae rei vis, et natura dividenda est, in altera quidem corporis, in altera vero animae, ut non usu quodam rationi esperti, nec levi cura, sed arte, et ratione corpori sanitatem medicamentis, animae rectum sensum dicendo inducete studeamus [...]. (Barbaro 1544a, f.1r.)

30 Two letters are held at the Biblioteca Apostolica Vaticana (Fondo Chigiano, L, III, 60, cc. 90–91 and cc. 95–6 ; and three letters at the Biblioteca Nazionale di Firenze (Aut. Pal., II, 116, 117 and 118), now published in Ongaro 1968 (116 and 117) and in Ciliberto 1972.

31 The bilingual edition of the *Rhetoric* dates from 1548 (Vettori 1548). I note that this text was re-edited at Basel in 1549 by Johannes Oporinus, editor of both editions of Vesalius' *Fabrica* (1543 and 1555). Another edition appeared in 1549 at Paris by Michel Vascosan. For the erroneous attribution of *Ad C. Herennium de ratione dicendi* to Cicero, see Harry Caplan's introduction in the Loeb Classical Library edition of this text.

32 Another edition appeared in 1545 at Basel, ex officina Bartholomaei Westhermeri.

This comparison is taken up frequently, and demonstrates well, here as in other works he subsequently edited (in his translation and commentary of the *Architectura* by Vitruvius, for example [Barbaro 1556][33]), that Barbaro searches constantly for internal and intimate relationships between different domains of knowledge, akin to the encyclopaedic impulse we have seen animating the *Infiammati*. Further, in the dedicatory epistle to Cardinal Benedetto Accolti, dated February 1542, that opens his paraphrase of Cicero's *Academica*, Barbaro indicated that he adopted, in philology, an anatomical approach. Like an expert anatomist, he sectioned, analyzed, and reconstructed Cicero's text like a human body:

> Habebis autem in Academicarum Quaestionum dialogos sectiones quasdam meas eorum medicorum similitudine, qui humana membratim corpora dissectant, ut quibus quaeque partibus constent, inspiciant; quod, si parum perspicax et cautus in ea dissectione fuerim et aliquod membrum praetervolando omiserim, tu optime Ciceroniane id minutius concisum et in minima quaeque dispartitum considerato meque innitentem atque adeo tentantem adiuva, quoniam non cadaverum sectores, sed vivorum inspectores sumus.[34]

The fundamental convergence of anatomy, philology, and textual analysis, three disciplines founded on the exercise of the "divisive method", is explicit. In this passage, Barbaro exemplifies the relentless quest for a philosophical *instrumentum* common to all disciplines, a quest that was critical to the transdisciplinary approach envisioned by this humanist circle (Angelini 1999, VIII et passim). In the same context, in fact, the humanist physician Giovanni Battista Montanus, friend and colleague of Vesalius, offers a generic comparison between element of

---

[33] A second edition, reviewed and expanded, and a Latin translation, for the European market, came out in Venice in 1567 from the press of Francesco de Franceschi and Giovanni Chrieger, (Barbaro 1567). It is worthy noting that in this work Barbaro takes up and analyses the notion of *fabrica* in a manner entirely compatible with that of Vesalius, Camillo, and Serlio: "[Vitruvius' text] *Architettura è Scienza ornata di molte dottrine, et varie eruditioni. Essa nasce da fabrica, et da discorso. Fabrica è continuo, et essercitato pensamento dell'uso, che di qualunque materia, che per dar forma all'opera proposta si richiede, con le mani si compie. Discorso è quello, che le cose fabricate prontamente, et con ragionevole proporzione puo dimostrando manifestare.* [Barbaro's commentary] Divino è veramente il desiderio di quegli, che levando la mente alla consideratione delle cose, cercano la cagione di esse, et riguardando come dal disopra, et da lunge la verità s'accendono alle fatiche ... . Sono anche molti, che avenga dio che del certo sappiano esser bisogno per l'acquisto d'una scienza particolare di molte altre. [Vitr.] *Fabrica è continuato, et essercitato pensiero dell'uso.* [Barb.] Ogni artificioso componimento ha l'esser suo dalla notizia del fine, come dice Galeno. Volendo adunque fabricare, fa di mestieri havere conoscimento del fine. ... Volendo adunque fabricare, bisogna conoscere il fine, come quello che al mezzo impone forza e necessità. Ma per la cognitione del fine è necessario lo studio, et il pensamento" (Barbaro 1556, 8).

[34] Barbaro's text is found in ms. Biblioteca Nazionale di Firenze, Magl. VIII. 1492, fasc. 7. (The quotation is at c. 1v.). It was published in Schmitt 1972, Appendix B.

natural philosophy and grammar (Siraisi 1987, 100; Maclean 2002, 330). Above all, Montanus suggests that anatomical discourse is a reservoir of metaphors and a method, which humanists might borrow and apply to other domains of the *studia humanitatis*, in particular to grammar and to rhetoric.[35]

We have already seen the significant recurrence of the term *fabrica* in Giulo Camillo's work on the rhetoric of Hermogenes of Tarsus (*Sopra Hermogene*), and how in his *Della imitazione* he compares structures of anatomy and eloquence. But the rapprochement goes even further. In a letter addressed to his friend Marcantonio Flaminio, in which Camillo explains his method in relation to both Latin and vernacular texts "of the most lauded scholars" on the arts of language (namely grammar, rhetoric, and topics), he elects "the marvellous *fabrica* of the human body" as his heuristic model, as well as an organizing principle of the discursive matter:

> E' il vero che da una parte avevamo la maniera in alcuno edificio da Cicerone principalmente tenuta; dall'altra quella di Metrodoro ne' dodici segni del cielo, dove trecento sessanta luoghi secondo il numero de' gradi gli erano famigliarissimi. Ma veggendo ne l'una poca dignità, ne l'altra molta difficultà, et ambedue forse più alla recitazione che alla composizione acconcie, rivolgemmo tutto l' pensiero alla meravigliosa fabrica del corpo humano. Avvisando, se questa è stata chiamata picciol mondo per avere in sè parti che con tutte le cose del mondo si confacciono, potersi a qualunque di quelle accomodare secondo la sua natura alcuna cosa del mondo, e conseguentemente le parole quella significanti.[36]

Further, aligned with his project of constructing a theatre of omniscience, he concludes by proposing the human body as the "measure" of all knowledge:

> Potete omai [...] aver in parte compreso con quanta facilità e con quanta bellezza per le membra dell'umano corpo noi apparecchiamo l'una e l'altra lingua. Così potessi dimostrarvi con qual ordine l'agricoltura, la cosmografia e l'altre facultà, perciò che in questa medesima fabrica potrò in brevissimo tempo e con poca fatica, non solamente le parole, ma anche le cose insieme allogare, e così rendere una imagine di quel vincolo della sapienza et eloquenza da Socrate a gran torto disciolto. (Camillo 1990, 9)

The anatomical body becomes for Camillo the "figure" of the link between *sapientia* and eloquence, a link which is also the explicit epistemological approach shared by other *Infiammati* humanists.[37]

---

35 On the relationships between medicine and rhetoric, see also Pender 2005.

36 To my knowledge the first edition of this letter is in Camillo 1579. It was also published in Camillo 1990. The quotation is on p. 6.

37 Giovanni Battista Goineo, an *Infiammato* student of Romolo Amaseo, writes: "nemo est qui istud ignoret, eloquentiam sine scientia esse verborum volubilitatem inanem, scientiam sine eloquentia mutae et infanti statuae similem prope videri" (1537, [5–6]); and,

Even if Sperone Speroni—the key figure of the *Infiammati*, "prince" of this academy from October 1541 until its crisis and extinction, and great defender of the vernacular against Latin—was a critic of this postulate, in his dialogues the reference to the anatomy / rhetoric intersection remains nevertheless constant: the anatomic metaphor still works effectively to designate the practices proper to the arts of language. In a crucial passage of his *Dialogo della retorica* (written between 1538 and 1540) that aims to define the technical characteristics of rhetoric in order to confine it specifically to the writing practices in the literary field,(designated as "discourse of delectation"), Speroni makes Brocardo, one of thc protagonists, say:

> [...] io vi prego che, non guardando alla fama degli scrittori della retorica, poniate mente alla verità, la quale, da ragione aiutato, io mi apparecchio a palesarvi. Perciò che altra cosa è il parlar di questa arte, le vene sue, i membri, l'ossa, i nervi e la carne sua annoverando e partendo, la qual guisa d'anatomia lei insegnando con le ragioni operiamo; e altra cosa è il parlar oratoriamente al vulgo, a' giudici, a' senatori quelli allettando e muovendo. (Pozzi 1978, t.1, pp. 637–82)

In distancing his position from the dominant humanist tradition and its *auctoritates* who extolled the possibility of an encyclopaedic knowledge via the professional management of the arts of discourse (above all, Aristotle and Cicero), Speroni again uses a comparison with anatomy to propose a new configuration of rhetoric, distinctly more circumscribed as a set of rules, forms, and relationships structuring discourse, comparable to those which organize parts of a generic disincarnate body deprived of subjective features.

This configuration points at the use of these rules and forms as specific competencies of the *literatus*. It constitutes, as Giancarlo Mazzacurati writes, a decisive step, consciously accomplished by Speroni, towards constituting a literary field established *juxta sua principia* (Mazzacurati 1985).[38] In the *Dialogo della retorica*, Speroni adumbrates a straight forward definition of literary and discursive practices, finally purified, as it were, of their traditional and instrumental use in the political or juridical arena or even in the utopian fabrication of theatres of omniscience. We are here confronted with a pragmatic 'rough copy' of the figure of the *literatus* as a profession of literary writing. What matters most, is that, despite the polemics concerning the function of rhetoric among the *Infiammati* - for or against the instrumental use of writing, the

in this same tone, Benedetto Varchi in one of his academic lessons: "conciosia che nessuno possa essere né veramente eloquente senza dottrina, né veramente dotto senza eloquenza" (Varchi 1590, 90). On these two quotations, see Vianello 1990, 110 and 147.

[38] This essay by Mazzacurati was also published under the title *Sulla funzione della retorica nel '500: dal governo del sapere all'esercizio della letteratura, in Letteratura e Società. Scritti di italianistica e critica letteraria per ... Giuseppe Petronio,* Palermo, 1980, I, 97–113). On this subject see Bruni 1967 and Vianello 1988, in particular Chapter. VII "L'esigenza della litterarietà", 39–170.

comparison between the *fabrica* of the body and the *fabrica* of discourse survives and remains epistemologically meaningful.

Exploring the intersection of medicine and rhetoric in the *Infiammati*'s milieu, as well as registering Vesalius' activity in the context of this academy and the issues that dominated it, allows us to draw some conclusions. By following Benveniste's guidance with respect to the profound and ancestral link between medicine and speech and, concurrently, in bringing the notion of humanism to its original connotation in specific relation to the *studia humanitatis*, I have attempted to propose another context for understanding medical humanism, constituted by institutional configurations, cultural interests, and personal interactions. I particularly focused on Andreas Vesalius' cultural milieu in Padua, as well as the conception and impact of his anatomic œuvre, a context of eminently humanist character, dominated above all by discussions concerning the use and function of the arts of language. This has allowed me to investigate the effects of discussions concerning language and discourse in the elaboration of an intellectual project like the *Fabrica*, as well as to emphasise the adoption of the anatomical body as a model that structures different areas of inquiry. Anatomy is, in this milieu, an epistemology applicable to diverse domains of knowledge—above all to rhetoric, the master discipline of humanist cultural practice.

Moreover, in pushing forward Edelstein's insights on Vesalius as a humanist, I propose to consider the conception and publication of the *Fabrica*, designated by historians as a founding text in modern anatomy, under a radically different light: it consists of a foundation which can be explained as part of a more general humanist project of reforming knowledge, and which includes a reconsideration of the professional and cultural profiles of the actors involved—a project that, as we have seen, is rooted in the critical evaluation of classical antiquity, fashioned and pursued thanks to a professional usage of the arts of language, governed by a scholarly approach that is essentially transdisciplinary.

If we consider the operation of defining the competencies specific to the *literatus* through, say, Speroni's anatomical comparison, and if we take into account the coexistence, in the same humanist cultural space, of the will to found a literature *juxta sua principia* and of a similar will, explicit for Vesalius, to found modern anatomy by dissection, the rapprochements between medicine and literature take on quite a distinct significance in the context of the more general debate about the relationships between humanist and scientific culture. This brings me to contemplate an idea that, perhaps, goes beyond the cultural history of the Renaissance. The separation of the subjective from the objective, of the *verba* and the *res*, postulated as a condition for the establishment of a truly scientific endeavour—in medicine as in the study of nature—thus appears in all its fragility and in its historical inconsistency. The experience of the *Infiammati*, as well as the actors, texts, and contexts of medical humanism, constitutes one of the multiple areas in which—I believe—the practice of history can fruitfully intervene in order to dispel the illusion of the autonomy and separateness of medical and scientific learning.

# Chapter 5
# Political Pathology

Daniel M. Gross

Although one would not know it reading Georges Gusdorf, Michel Foucault, Donald Kelley, Roger Smith, or for that matter most of the recent scholarship in the leading journal *History of the Human Sciences*,[1] we should credit the German Reformation theologian Philipp Melanchthon for practically grounding the modern human sciences as he reformulates the classical homology between rhetoric and medicine. Melanchthon's innovation lies in his practical treatment of a human being forged at the intersection of two theological principles. First, since God works through a living human being, human nature can be studied in terms of natural philosophy and not just Scripture. Second, since human nature is essentially wanting—*Infirma natura hominum*—we are subject to the practical arts of rhetoric and medicine. Considering Melanchthon's influence in schools and universities across Europe,[2] it is worth reconsidering these humanistic origins of the modern human sciences designed to *reshape* humankind instead of merely describing it or subjecting it to experimental science. Psychology and pedagogy are two human sciences I have elsewhere approached from this humanistic and more specifically rhetorical perspective, with passions as the focal point.[3] In this essay,

---

1 Georges Gusdorf, *Introduction aux sciences humaines; essai critique sur leurs origines et leur développement* (Paris: Les Belles Lettres, 1960); Michel Foucault, *The Order of Things: An Archaeology of the Human Sciences*, trans. Alan Sheridan (New York: Vintage, 1970); Donald R. Kelley, *History, Law, and the Human Sciences* (London: Variorum, 1984); "*Altera natura*: The Idea of Custom in Historical Perspective," in *New Perspectives on Renaissance Thought: Essays in the History of Science, Education and Philosophy*, eds. John Henry and Sarah Hutton (London: Duckworth, 1990); Roger Smith, *The Norton History of the Human Sciences* (New York: Norton, 1997).

2 Sachiko Kusukawa, *The Transformation of Natural Philosophy: The Case of Philipp Melanchthon* (Cambridge: Cambridge University Press, 1995); Heinz Scheible, *Melanchthon: Eine Biographie* (Munich: Beck, 1997); Karl Hartfelder, *Philipp Melanchthon als Praeceptor Germaniae* (Nieuwkoop: Graaf, 1964); Theodor Muther, *Die Wittenberger Universitäts- und Facultäts-Statuten vom Jahre 1508* (Halle: Buchhandlung des Waisenhauses, 1867); Christoph Scheurl, *Briefbuch, ein Beitrag zur Geschichte der Reformation und ihrer Zeit*, eds. Franz von Soden and Joachim K.F. Knaake, 2 vols. (Aalen: Zeller, 1962).

3 Daniel M. Gross, *The Secret History of Emotion: From Aristotle's* Rhetoric *to Modern Brain Science* (Chicago: The University of Chicago Press, 2006); a few passages in the following section on Melanchthon's physics originally appeared in Daniel M. Gross, "Melanchthon's Rhetoric and the Practical Origins of Reformation Human Science," *History of the Human Sciences* 13.3 (2000): 5–22.

I similarly reconsider the origins of modern political science from Melanchthon through the German Baroque.

***

> Certainty [in human affairs] cannot be achieved because the souls of men are mutable. Wherefore the poet says all that is surely changed is changed by love. And Plato says that with love, animal nature can be transformed.
>
> —Philipp Melanchthon, *Liber de anima*

In asking "What is the end and use of physics?" Melanchthon reveals his profound pragmatism alien to our experimental and descriptive sensibilities: "From this doctrine comes the art of medicine through which we discern elements, natural properties, properties of action, contraries, human parts, the causes of change in pure and mixed elements, the various humors in the body, temperaments or combinations, and the correlative spirits, inclinations, and passions of man. To a certain degree, [a doctrine of physics] actually leads to the investigation of ourselves as human beings, the maintenance of our health, and the mastery of our inclinations."[4] So what we immediately encounter is neither a primitive form of biophysics nor sociobiology. Rather it is a therapeutic physics of human nature, a curative medicine of the soul.[5] For Melanchthon suggests not that we try to reduce human behavior or inner experience to material and function, but rather that we increase our competence in that properly human domain marked out in Holy Scripture under headings of nature and grace, and designated in the world of fallen humankind under the categories of privation, contingency, free will, mutability, and second causes. Physics and Scripture are intimately bound, and both are indispensable.[6] Moreover the consistency with which these two domains of knowledge are integrated into a program for soulful therapy distinguishes Melanchthon's work from his contemporaries and creates space for modern social studies as protreptic arts rather than human sciences in the narrow, late-modern

---

4 "Ex hae doctrina extruitur ars medica, quia hic discernuntur elementa, qualitates, qualitatum actiones, cognatio, dissidia, causae alterationum in elementis et mixtis, naturae dissimiles humorum in corpore humano, temperamenta seu crases, et his congruentes spiritus, inclinationes et adfectus in hominibus. Haec aliquantulum et vel obiter aspicere in nobis multum conducit, et ad valetudinem tuendam, et ad mores regendos." Philipp Melanchthon, *Initia doctrinae physicae* (1549), in *Corpus reformatorum* Philippi Melanthonis opera quae supersunt omnia (hereafter, CR), vol. 13, eds. Karl B. Bretschneider and Heinrich E. Bindseil (Halle: Schwetschke, 1846), 190.

5 See Nancy S. Struever, "Rhetoric and Medicine in Descartes' *Passions de l'âme*: The Issue of Intervention," *Renaissance-Rhetorik/Renaissance Rhetoric*, ed. Heinrich F. Plett (Berlin: Gruyter, 1993).

6 "multa sunt in doctrina Ecclessiae, quae sine physicis explicari non possunt." Melanchthon, *Initia*, 190–191.

sense. And when it comes to therapies of human nature, rhetoric and medicine are the two leading arts.

No doubt the homology between rhetoric and medicine was commonplace in Plato's early modern wake. In the case of both rhetoric and medicine, we read in the *Phaedrus*, "there is a nature that we have to determine, the nature of the body in the one, and of the soul in the other, if we mean to be scientific and not content with mere empirical routine when we apply medicine and diet to induce health and strength, or words and rules of conduct to implant such convictions and virtues as we desire" (*Phaedrus* 270b).[7] More than mere artifice, rhetoric has long been considered an invasive art with curative, as well as destructive, powers. Typical of this perspective is doctor of medicine Johannes Placotomus's "Oration on Correct Speech, or Precepts of Medicine" collected, significantly, in a 1552 Leipzig volume along with humanists Erasmus, Sabino, Curtius, and Melanchthon's biographer, Joachim Camerarius. In a fashion resonant with the psychoanalytic methods of our era, Placotomus argues that young doctors must be trained to recognize the ways in which everyday language can be a site for curative, psychosomatic intervention.[8] Doctor and "philippist" Paracelsus gives this homology between rhetoric and medicine a decidedly theological spin, emphasizing the dual function of art in contrary states of nature and grace: "Disciplines of the New Creature are not administered in the old manner—that is, from the stars down through reason—but as Paul revealed, according to the will and graces of God. Thus we have a rhetoric and eloquence different from that of heathens: our eloquence is true talk and the speech of tongues on fire. The same is true for other disciplines, such as medicine."[9] Along with a new rhetoric, then, new creatures are subject to "new medicine" that would channel God's will.[10] Melanchthon himself discusses rhetoric and medicine in his declamation "Contra empiricos Medicos" (1534), warning that, if overdrawn, the homology between the two can lead to bad science. Both disciplines treat the passions and both are grounded in physics, but their modes of intervention are, and should remain, different. Rhetoric moves and

---

7 See also Aristotle, *Topics* 1.3: "We shall be in perfect possession of the way to proceed when we are in a position like that which we occupy in regard to rhetoric and medicine and faculties of that kind: this means the doing of that which we choose with the materials that are available. For it is not every method that the rhetorician will employ to persuade, or the doctor to heal; still, if he omits none of the available means, we shall say that his grasp of the science is adequate."

8 Johannes Placotomus, *Oratorio de ratione discendi, ac praecipue medicinam* (Leipzig: V. Papae, 1552).

9 "Also in nova creatura ist kein austeilung der officia nach alter art, das ist; aus dem gestirn und unser vernunft, sondern nach dem willen und gaben gottes, wies Paulus ausleitet. also haben wir aliam rhetoricam et eloquentiam quam ethnici. verum dicere et igneis linguis loqui est nostra eloquentia. so mit andern officiis, als mit medicina." Paracelsus, "De eclesiis veteris et novi testamenti," *Sämtliche Werke* 1.2 (supplement), eds. Kurt Goldhammer and Franz Steiner (Wiesbaden: Steiner, 1973), 35.

10 "De officiis, beneficiis, et stipendiis." Paracelsus, 45.

cures by way of speech, and medicine by way of material intervention including pharmacology. When it strays too far from experience and draws its art from rhetoric alone, medicine becomes the theoretical quackery that warrants divining from a urine sample not only the subject's illness, but also a narrative in which the subject's age and life accomplishments are magically revealed.[11] But ultimately both are messy, "interventionist" disciplines, resisting assimilation to a familiar story in which Descartes's epistemological solipsism is the founding gesture of modernity.[12]

The question is one of pragmatics: to what extent is human nature mutable? At what stratum is medicine of the heart and soul effective: the individual? the political body? humankind? Certainly not the latter, since in the end it is only by way of Christ's second intervention in historical time that human nature can be restored to its original state of grace. But in the meantime, how can we best ready our depraved nature for salvation? In answering these questions, Melanchthon defines the scope of Reformation human science.

The proper object of human science, it turns out, is not exhausted by reference to collections of individuals. Corporate bodies also have to be considered and treated on their own terms. As Melanchthon modestly attests, though God may govern change in civil society, "human art is an additional factor."[13] Thus, for instance, the medical doctor must not only consider the humors, temperaments and stellar forces that affect a single body (*in singulis corporibus*), but he must also calculate how they effect the health and habit of communal life (*in communi vita*).[14] Meanwhile the rhetorician's job is not just to indoctrinate in children the verbal habits of a static society, but also to train students to competence in the mechanics of a society constantly in motion. Rhetoric was critical for public administration, courts, and the political arena. It was needed "to persuade to law and dissuade from vice, to establish the rules of war and peace, in short to determine in proper fashion all civic issues."[15] Literary science would exemplify ethical behavior in this domain proper to humankind: reading pagan authors such as Aristotle, Cicero,

---

11 Melanchthon, "Contra empiricos Medicos," CR vol. 11, 203–204. On the relationship between Melanchthon's rhetoric and natural philosophy see also Olaf Berwald, *Philipp Melanchthons Sicht der Rhetorik* (Wiesbaden: Harrassowitz, 1994).

12 In this essay a decidedly rhetorical *Staatsmedicine* will complicate Nancy Struever's succinct summary: medicine in the early modern period is obliged to therapy—cure of the body, and rhetoric is obliged to therapy—cure of the body politic. Struever, "Rhetoric and Medicine in Descartes' *Passions de l'âme*," 207.

13 "aut civitatum mutationes gubernare inquit, placidius tamen est conce dere, comitem his adiungendam esse artem." Melanchthon, *Initia*, 330.

14 Melanchthon, *Liber de anima* (1552), CR vol. 13, 87.

15 "Rhetorica, dicendi artificium usui sane magno veteribus fuit, non ad paedeian solum industria quadam tractandam, sed omnino etiam ad rei publicae administrationem, forum, consilia, suadendas leges, dissuadenda vicia, sancienda belli pacisque iura, denique ad omnia civitatis recta constituendae munera." Philipp Melanchthon, *De rhetorica* (Wittenberg: Grunenberg, 1519), Aiiij/r.

Quintilian, Ovid, Livy, Sallust, Seneca, Pliny, and Horace would provide the data from which flawed humans could infer behavioral rules of thumb then put into practice by way of rhetoric.[16]

Finally, in his physics Melanchthon analyzes the basic principle of persuasion: motion, or *kinesis*. "Motion is action or agitation—the acquisition of form or proper end; or it is the capacity for form in a subject, because that which is potential in the subject is able to take form, and tends towards that form."[17] Admitting the obscurity of this crucial Aristotelian definition, Melanchthon then turns to an example. But surprisingly, the example he gives is not a growing plant or a locomoting animal, as anyone familiar with Aristotle and Galen might expect. Instead Melanchthon turns immediately to moving speech: that is, to rhetoric. Motion literally takes shape in the heart as a physical organ. And motion incited by speech includes anger, for instance, described in the following terms:

> Anger is vibration emanating from the heart to an object *revealed as* bad which the heart attempts to expel, and in defense against which the spirits of the heart pours forth into the blood causing its agitation and rise in temperature and inflaming red bile so that the blood is dispersed with tremendous force. These agitations, which are the nature of the heart, occur in order to produce spirits. In turn it is the nature of the spirits to disperse throughout the entire body, exciting motion and heat in the heart, and propagating into the extremities so that arms and legs are readied to repel the offending object [my italics].[18]

In Melanchthon's materialism there are no inherently good or bad objects. Instead we find only objects *revealed* as good or bad—*ostenditur ut mala*—a formulation that hovers elegantly between secular and sacred rhetoric: *ex verbo Dei ostenditur*. How then does this new materialism extend to the civic realm?

---

16 "Ideo in arte admonendi sunt studiosi, ut quaerant eos in causis, ac proferant in lucem, et dicendo illustrent, ut si quis de studiis literarum dicet, non tantum ostendet, quam sint honesta, quamque utilia, sed si recte considerabit res humanas, inveniet etiam necessariam esse literarum scientiam, quia sine doctrina religionis et legum, non possunt teneri respublicae, neque haec civilis societas coli." Melanchthon, *Elementorum rhetorices libri duo* (1531), CR vol. 13, 446.

17 "Motus est actus, id est agitatio, id est acquisitio formae vel termini, vel abiectio formae in subiecto, quod est in potentia, id est, quod formam recipere potest, et ad eam tendit." Melanchthon, *Initia*, 356.

18 "Sed illustrior esset oratio, si de specie aliqua motus diceretur, et causae efficientes, finales et instrumenta recitarentur, ut si describeretur Ira. Ira est verberatio cordis orta a re, quae ostenditur ut mala, et quam depellere cor nititur, in qua depulsione spiritus cordis effunditur in sanguinem, et agitatione ipsa accenditur, et sanguinem calefacit, et bilem rubram inflat, ut depulsionis causa sanguis in exteriora spargatur, fiuntque hae agitationes, quia talis est cordis natura, ut gignat spiritus, et spirituum natura talis est, ut spargantur in totum corpus, et motu et calore cordis incalescant, et properent in extrema membra, ut ea arment ad depulsionem obiecti, quod offendit." Melanchthon, *Initia*, 357.

In a fascinating but not entirely successful passage of *Liber de anima* designed as an antidote to stoic apathy, Melanchthon proclaims that there are two ways to rule, and therefore syllogistically speaking, two ways to rule the passions: either despotically or politically. "Despotic rule is when inferiors obviously obey under duress, and those who disturb the peace are imprisoned so as to squelch rebellion. The other, called political, is when the civic soul is altered by way of persuasion so that wills comply—moved by the good, or out of fear of the bad, not to oppose the law."[19] The despotic is manifest in the force of both mind and will that stays Achilles's hand in battle despite his extreme anger, or is exemplified in the cogent locomotion that keeps us from spilling a drink even when emotionally distressed. Political rule, on the other hand, is motion "persuaded" by harmony of heart, right reason, and honest will. It is exemplified when Theseus's son Hippolytus controls his external member because he knows in his heart that incest with step-mother Phaedra would be an atrocious crime punishable by the gods. Without the heart, even right behavior falls short of virtue.

When Melanchthon published this passage in 1552, mind, will, and body were typically considered necessary media for virtuous activity. The mechanics of mind and body were discussed at length in Renaissance neostoic ethics, for instance, and free will parsed in the famous Erasmus-Luther debate. But with the Reformation also came a revival of Augustinian thought that secured the heart firmly in the centre of a life that was properly human.[20] Contrary to both Stoic and Scholastic thought, Melanchthon insisted that God judges the heart first, and not the intellect. He is thus compelled to conclude in the influential *Loci Communes* of 1521 that the will is actually synonymous with the heart, and that "the heart and its passions must be the greatest and most potent part of man."[21] It was, moreover, a sentiment that found sympathy in the work of both Luther and Calvin. "The assent which we give to the divine Word," observed Calvin in characteristic fashion, "is more of the heart than the brain, and more of the affections than the understanding … faith is

[19] "…despotikè, id est, herilis, cum videlicet coacti obediunt inferiores, ut cum homo inquietus impeditur carcere, ne tumultuetur. Altera, quae nominatur politikè, est, cum suadendo flectuntur animi civium, ut volentes obtemperent, quia videlicet bono aliquo aut metu mali moventur, ut legi non repugnent…". Melanchthon, *Liber de anima*, 129–130. Melanchthon calls the doctrine of Stoic apathy "ridiculous": "Ridicula est et apatheia Stoicorum, qui misericordiam et plerosque similes affectus bonos vituperant." See "Scholia in Epistolam Pauli ad Colossenses" (1527) in *Melanchthons Werke in Auswahl: Studienausgabe*, ed. Robert Stupperich (Gütersloh: Bertelsmann, 1963), vol. 4, 230–243; also *Liber de anima*, 133.

[20] See William J. Bouwsma's classic essay "The Two Faces of Humanism: Stoicism and Augustinianism in Renaissance Thought," *Itinerarium Italicum: The Profile of the Italian Renaissance in the Mirror of its European Transformations*, eds. Heiko A. Oberman and Thomas A. Brady, Jr. (Leiden: Brill, 1975), 3–60.

[21] "Nam cum corda deus iudicet, necesse est cor cum suis affectibus summam ac potissimam hominis partem esse." Melanchthon, *Loci Communes 1521* (Gütersloh: Mohn, 1993), I.57.

absolutely inseparable from a devout affection."[22] However, this shift from mind to heart has an importance that reaches far beyond religious doctrine, providing, in fact, a key to the new way of life reflected at the theoretical level in Reformation human and specifically political science.

As Melanchthon suggests in his uncanny metaphor, the body is best ruled despotically, which is to say it is best treated as an unreflexive mechanical device. Its proper disciplines would be physics in the narrow sense, and perhaps gymnastics. Mind would be the despotic ruler, and its first discipline dialectic: a method of sound argumentation designed to move in law-like fashion from given premises to certain conclusions (we might think of logic or mathematics). The heart, on the other hand, resides in that ambiguous domain where nothing is certain—where mechanics and logic might at times impinge, but never dominate. Natural and spiritual passions can dissemble as they do battle in the soul: hubris, for instance, may be clad in the guise of charity. And even when the good or the bad should be self-evident, they can remain obscure to a mind clouded by Satan's dust: remember the centrality of objective revelation. Virtuous action is not spontaneous. For the passions that move us must first be treated in what Melanchthon calls "political" fashion: the civic soul must be persuaded to things good or bad by way of vivid speech. If the civic soul is to behave virtuously, then, it must be subject to rhetoric.

Passions of the heart respond to the technologies of human science in a way that mind and reflexive body do not. It is therefore no surprise that a Reformation culture that puts the heart at the centre of its human science might see Scholastic logic give way in its universities to Aristotelian–Hellenistic ethics, rhetoric, the study of classical literature, and other ostensibly character building protreptic arts. Indeed it is no exaggeration when Dilthey claims that the very function of sixteenth- and seventeenth-century anthropology was to ground the human sciences in the theory of passions.[23] And if that is the case, as I believe it is, then a genealogy of the human sciences in the Reformation requires that we differentiate the passions according to their scientific consequences.

Shifting the operative metaphor, passions are, for Melanchthon, hard currency in an economy of the soul. Considered a desiring faculty of the will (*adpetitus voluntarius*), passions provide a soul with the means to interact with an external world, to evaluate situations and dispose body and mind appropriately, creating distance or intimacy as the case might demand. Anger, as we have seen, is vibration emanating from the heart to an object revealed as bad, and which the

---

22 Quoted in Bouwsma, 39.

23 Wilhelm Dilthey, "Die Funktion der Anthropologie in der Kultur des 16. und 17. Jahrhunderts," *Weltanschauung und Analyse des Menschen Seit Renaissance und Reformation. Wilhelm Diltheys Gesammelte Schriften*, vol. 2 (Leipzig: Teubner, 1914), 479; see also "Auffassung un Analyse des Menschen im 15. und 16. Jahrhundert," and "Das natürliche System der Geisteswissenschaften im 17. Jahrhundert," *Aufsätze zur Philosophie*, ed. Marion Marquardt (Berlin: Dausien, 1986).

heart then attempts to expel. Hatred is inveterate anger. Happiness is motion that soothes in anticipation of the good, a pleasant dilation that disposes the heart to accept the good object;[24] fear a constricting motion of the heart averse to future evil;[25] and so on to sadness, hope, love, shame, modesty, compassion, envy, and zeal—all passionate means to measure and negotiate a complex world. We should notice first that Melanchthon relentlessly expresses his theory of passions as a hard moral science, if that is not an oxymoron. Neither simply embracing the social psychology of Aristotle's *Rhetoric*, nor forshadowing the pathology of emotional expression made popular in the late seventeenth and eighteenth century by Le Brun and Lavater, Melanchthon instead binds every single passion to a situation that is at the same time ethical, and physical. Though Nietzschean talk of man's "interiorization" now reads as little more than a figure of speech, and Luther is forced to apologize for the profane description of a heart "dilated, enhanced, and prolonged," naturalistic discourse of this sort was no problem for Melanchthon. Nor was it a problem for other natural philosophers of his time, including the anatomist Vesalius, whose famous *De humani corporis fabrica* played a crucial role in the final revision of Melanchthon's treatise on the soul.[26] Reading Melanchthon's *Liber de anima*, one gets the sense of both a spatial and dynamic principle at work, nascent elements in the early modern physics of persuasion.

But of course the rhetorical tradition, now lost to the modern human sciences, established in fine detail the mechanics of speech situations, pedagogy, and motions of the soul. If we now compare Philipp Melanchthon's final *Rhetoric* to his *Liber de anima*, we can see in dramatic terms the transfer of techniques from the discipline of rhetoric to theology, to political science and beyond.

Following classical design, Melanchthon divides the parts of an oration into the exordium, narration, proposition, confirmation, rebuttal, and peroration. The peroration materializes rational argument by way of the emotions, and it provides a model for the hermeneutics of reading Scripture. But it is the scientific implications of the exordium that are of particular interest here. According to Melanchthon, the function of the exordium is to "prepare the souls of the auditors" along three lines (*praeparandi sunt animi audientium*): auditors are rendered benevolent, attentive, and docile (*benevolos, attentos et dociles*). Benevolence is achieved when the business at hand is set up in terms of quotidian niceties, whether that be appreciation for the opportunity to speak, a self-deprecating comment, or some other device one uses as an indirect invitation to listen. It also is a strategy the speaker uses to establish his honesty, credibility, and amicability before the real issue is addressed. Melanchthon then offers an example from Paul, who begins

24 "Laeticia est motus, quo cor acquiescit in bono praesenti, et est dilatatio, qua cor velut accipit intra sese, et amplectitur obiectum." Melanchthon, *Liber de anima*, 126.

25 "Timor est motus, quo cor constringitur, tanquam fugiens futurum malum." Melanchthon, *Liber de anima*, 127.

26 Melanchthon counted a number of medicine professors and natural philosophers as friends, including Leonhart Fuchs, Jakob Milich, Veit Oertel, and Caspar Peucer. See Berwald, 15.

his letter to the Romans by praising their faith. Second, auditors are rendered attentive when the magnitude and significance of the issue at hand is underscored, as when Paul tells the Romans that he is not ashamed of the gospel because it is the power of God. Finally, auditors are rendered docile when Paul suggests what lies at the heart of the matter: the gospel reveals God's grace.[27] Here one should also notice that the examples Melanchthon draws from Scripture do not just serve as a common reference. They also expand the scope of his rhetoric from the classroom exercise and university disputation to the very structure of religious life.

Everyday language renovates the image of God that languishes in human nature. As Melanchthon remarks in his *Liber de anima*, though fallen, nevertheless there remains in humankind a vestige of God expressed by way of common sense (a Stoic *sensus communis*). The notions thus expressed are both precepts of natural law (e.g. Thou shalt not kill) and unambiguous formulae, such as the syllogism that allows us to apply natural law in any given case (I shall not kill). The image of God that produces in human nature this *lumen naturale* is no doubt weak, but it can be strengthened by way of sacred rhetoric. We invoke God in our daily prayer (*quotidiana invocatione*) and consider God's testimony inscribed in us by way of *logos*, the Word.[28] What we see, then, when we move from a treatise on good speaking to theology, is that the rhetorical techniques used to persuade remains the same, but the rhetorical situation is redoubled. First we render *ourselves* benevolent, attentive, and docile by way of daily prayer. And only after we ready our souls can the Holy Ghost act as rhetor, delivering God's message: "The Holy Ghost is rhetorized in order to illustrate the Promise" comments Martin Luther on Psalm 121.[29] Likewise Melanchthon's discussion of self-persuasion clearly harkens back to the pagan rhetoric of Quintilian. But the inner life in which it functions has reached a new level of sophistication. Where hope dilates and guilt convolutes, prayer inscribes inner life with a modicum of order.

Finally, Melanchthon's physics of persuasion bleeds from inner life into the political arena and beyond, into the entire spectrum of human activity. Analyzed in *Liber de anima* as a subcategory of the *potentia locomotiva*, the passive intellect lets things happen.

[27] Melanchthon, *Elementorum*, 431–2.

[28] Melanchthon, *Liber de anima*, 171.

[29] "Opus est igitur hortationibus, ut ista (liceat enim sic loqui) naturalis brevitas deu angustia cordis nostri dilatetur, magnificetur, et prolongetur.… Rhetoricatur igitur Spiritus sanctur iam, ut exhortatio fiat illustrior." Martin Luther, *Dr. Martin Luthers Werke, kritische Gesamtausgabe* (Weimar: Böhlau, 1883–1987), vol. 40/3, 59–60. For commentary see Klaus Dockhorn, "Rhetorica movet: Protestantischer Humanismus und karolingische Renaissance," *Rhetorik: Beiträge zu ihrer Geschichte in Deutschland vom 16.–20. Jahrhundert*, ed. Helmut Schanze (Frankfurt: Athenaion, 1974); "Luthers Glaubensbegriff und die Rhetorik," *Linguistica Biblica* 21/22 (1973): 19–39; and Klaus Dockhorn's review of Hans-Georg Gadamer's *Wahrheit und Methode*, in *Göttingische Gelehrte Anzeigen* 218 (1966): 169–206. For a bibliography on the topic see Reinhard Breymayer, "Bibliographie zum Thema 'Luther und die Rhetorik,'" in *Linguistica Biblica* 21/22 (1973): 39–44.

Following upon the activity of the inventive intellect, another faculty recognizes and accepts the resulting dictate. This faculty is called the passive intellect. Aristotle sees it in all of life: in the arts, in public and private deliberation, in military strategy, in poetics and eloquence. Certainly the passive intellect can be more or less acute and is always stronger when combined with the inventive—since the latter is the stronger of the two faculties. As politician and general Themistocles needed forethought and the creative intellect to persuade Athenians to temporarily abandon the city for strategic purposes before the second Persian invasion of Greece, invention must eventually be reconciled with the deliberative capacities of an audience and find acceptance.[30]

So even if agency overpowers patience, patience is nonetheless necessary for activity to take effect. Sebastian Franck would say that only through sheer suffering, resignation, and surrender might we be impregnated by the power from on high; Luther that the Word of God finds entrée through natural language. Here Melanchthon suggests that products of the inventive intellect need to be heard, understood, synthesized, and, if everything goes well, accepted, if they are to have any consequences. Only then, and only if circumstances are appropriately disposed, might one expect concordant behavior.

## After Melanchthon

When it came to figuring how best to articulate social institutions that embody the more useful passions, Aristotle was the acknowledged authority mobilized by Melanchthon and others in Germany and beyond. To cite only a few examples, Thomas Hobbes translates Aristotle on the passions, Hermann Conring acknowledges that both his early treatise *Of the Diseases and Mutations of Commonwealths* and his later *Civil Prudence* rely on this same work,[31] and in his treatment of motion, Scipione Chiaramonti, the Italian opponent of Galileo and Kepler, relies heavily on the first and second books of Aristotle's *Rhetoric*.[32] For those of us who approach politics with a Cartesian frame of reference, the single strangest and most important commonality among these typically Aristotelian

[30] "Alterum officium est postea inventa intelligere, agnoscere, et tanquam dictata accipere. Ab hoc officio nominatur intellectus patiens. Vidit Aristoteles in omni vita, in artibus, in consiliis publicis et privatis, in stratagematibus, in poëtica, in eloquentia, alios aliis perspicaciores esse, et inventione plus valere: Alios inventa intelligere, et suis cogitationibus anteferre, ut Themistocles suadens, ut cives relicta urbe naves ingrediantur, plus valet intellectu faciente, quam alii, sed coeteri intelligunt consilium et adprobant." Melanchthon, *Liber de anima*, 148.

[31] Hermann Conring, *Dissertatio politica de morbis ac mutationibus rerumpublicarum* (Helmstedt: Müller, 1640), B4r; *De civili prudentia liber unus* (Helmstedt, Müller, 1662), 51.

[32] Scipione Chiaramonti (Scipio Claramontius), *De coniectandis cuiusque moribus et latitantibus animi affectibus libri decem; Opus novi argumenti et incomparabile, cura H. Conringii recensitum* (Helmstedt: Müller, 1665), 5r.

projects is monist but non-reductive understanding of corporate dynamics. Nature (*physis*)—whether human or non-human—is, under Aristotle's definition, "a principle of motion and change." But the sort of motion and change typical of rocks, plants, and animals differs qualitatively from that of humans, and thus the means of "persuasion" will differ as well. In the Aristotelian tradition then, both a crass idealism or a reductive materialism are out of the question. So is any strict division between the human and natural sciences—a distinction formalized by nineteenth-century philosophers after J. S. Mill.[33] Instead what we get is the analysis of a living continuum, subject at its higher strata to arts of persuasion inoperative in the non-human world.

In the *Leviathan*, Hobbes analyzes the corporate qualities and dynamics of people in this Aristotelian mode: ethics (or "consequences from the *passions* of men") is subordinated as a discipline to the category of "Physiques," and so are both poetics ("consequences from speech in Magnifying and Vilifying") and rhetoric ("consequences from speech in persvvading").[34] Moreover Hobbes is careful to point out that the sort of "motions" typical of human nature and subject to a physics of persuasion, such as appetites of love and hateful aversions, are not in motion by metaphor alone. "For though Words may be called metaphoricall," Hobbes remarks, "Bodies, and Motions cannot."[35]

Chiaramonti similarly analyzes corporate dynamics for practical purposes in his treatise *On the Interpretation of Mores and the Hidden Affects of the Soul*. As humans, Chiaramonti observes, we are moved not only by natural phenomena such as hunger, thirst, climate, and geography, but also by those artifacts of civilization we create on the order of second nature. Therefore in addition to analyzing how changes in air quality, temperature, and humidity excite changes in the soul,[36] human scientists must also analyze how souls are changed by institutions of state.[37] Again, the key to success for the social technician is rendering second nature first. More powerful than mere cognition swayed by fleeting fantasies and fickle beliefs,[38] mores incorporate the world of cultural value. As Chiaramonti

---

[33] For the history of this distinction see Hans-Georg Gadamer, "The Significance of the Humanist Tradition for the Human Sciences," in *Truth and Method*, 2nd, revised edition, trans. Joel Weinsheimer and Donald G. Marshall (New York: Crossroad, 1989), 3–42.

[34] Thomas Hobbes, *Leviathan*, ed. Crawford B. Macpherson (Harmondsworth: Penguin Books, 1968), 149.

[35] Hobbes, *Leviathan*, 119.

[36] "Praeter mutatio iugis ventorum perpetuam quoque varietatem aëris facit, nunc caliditatem inducendo, nunc frigiditatem, nunc siccitatem, nunc humiditatem: ad mutatio animum ad excercitationem excitat." Chiaramonti, 61.

[37] Chiaramonti, 125.

[38] "cum ex disciplina dispositio appetitus immediate descendat, quae mos ipse est, plus momenti assuetudo disciplinae ad morem quam cognitio habebit." Chiaramonti, 135; "Cognitio absque phantasmate secundo debiliter movet voluntatem; ergo propensio ex temperamento plus momenti habet ad mores." Chiaramonti, 139.

succinctly puts it, mores are habits of virtue and vice (*habitus ergo virtutis aut vitii est mos*),[39] and habit long practiced is transformed into nature (*longa consuetudo imitetur naturam, dicaturque transire in naturam*).[40]

Hermann Conring's social technology is similarly structured.[41] Conring first observes in the *New Commonwealth* that mores correspond to body temperature, and from this he infers that nature must have something to do with shaping souls both individual and collective.[42] Based on this conviction that civic souls must be treated in natural terms (*civium animos*), Conring then lays out a method to diagnose and cure the ailments the civic soul might suffer—political pathology in other words. But unlike souls of a lesser order, civic souls are subject to a strange sort of cure particularly useful to the politician: that is, the talking cure. In his *Civic Prudence*, published in the same year as the *New Commonwealth* (1662), Conring begins by questioning the utility of rhetoric as a mere art of arranging and decorating speeches. And even as a method for inventing arguments, defining topics, and teaching, rhetoric is of no use for Conring when it comes to learning civic prudence.[43] However as a "method of political discourse" defined in the pseudo-Aristotelian *Rhetorica ad Alexandrum* I.1. and the pseudo-Ciceronian *Rhetorica ad Herennium* 1.2,[44] rhetoric is deemed by Conring indispensible. "What is truly magnificent about prudence is its ability to alter the momentum of human actions, reason, and guiding principles—inciting it, deflecting it, distancing it, and when necessary, even driving it out."[45] A Stoic purging of the passions might be

39 Chiaramonti, 132.

40 Chiaramonti, 135.

41 Conring was, appropriately, an early champion of German customary law over the abstract *Systema iuris romani*. On Conring as law theorist and apologist for the German territorial state system see Klaus Luig, "Conring, das Deutsche Recht Und Die Rechtsgeschichte," in *Hermann Conring (1606–1681): Beiträge zu Leben und Werk*, ed. Michael Stolleis (Berlin: Duncker and Humblot, 1983), esp. 377–95.

42 "Mores enim animi si sequuntur temperaturam corporis … consequens est, naturae magnam esse vim flectendi animos hominem, adeoque rerumpublicum etiam formas et status commutandi." Hermann Conring, *Disputatio politica de civitate nova* (Helmstedt, Müller, 1662), Br.

43 Hermann Conring, *De civili prudentia liber unus* (Helmstedt, Müller, 1662), 50.

44 Conring, *Civili prudentia*, 53. The *Rhetorica ad Alexandrum* definition is *methodos ton politikon logon*, and the offices of the orator are according to the *Rhetorica ad Herennium*: "Oratoris officium est de iis rebus posse dicere quae res ad usum civilem moribus et legibus constitutae sunt, cum adsensione auditorum quoad eius fieri poterit"; "The task of the public speaker is to discuss capably those matters which law and custom have fixed for the uses of citizenship, and to secure as far as possible the agreement of his hearers." It is a definition drawn from Hermagoras. See [Cicero] *Ad C. Herennium. De ratione dicendi (Rhetorica ad Herennium)*, trans. Harry Caplan (Cambridge, MA.: Harvard University Press, 1989), I.i.2; Caplan footnote b.

45 "magnum vero prudentiae momentum est humanarum actionum rationem et principia exacte novisse, quum sic demum liceat aut impellere eas, aut declinare, aut removari, prout usus exigit." Conring, *Civili prudentia*, 51.

necessary in the extreme case, but under normal circumstances most important is the ability to treat the more subtle machinations of the soul analyzed with such rigor in Aristotle's *Rhetoric*.[46]

Chiaramonti and Conring also share the view that moral philosophy functions like medicine. As medicine is divided by the Greeks into five sub-disciplines—physiology, hygiene, pathology, semiotics, and therapeutics—so, according to Chiaramonti, should moral philosophy be divided.[47] Though Conring asserts in his *Universal Introduction to the Art of Medicine* that, strictly speaking, medical doctors do not treat the soul (*Medico, qua Medicus, ignota est Anima*), nevertheless in his works on political and moral philosophy, it is clear that the duty of the medical doctor to "conserve integral health" seems to apply equally well to doctors of any sort.[48] Conring's career advancement is indicative of this disciplinary seepage. In 1632 he occupied chairs in rhetoric and physics at Helmstedt, in 1637 a chair in medicine, then finally in 1650 he is named Helmstedt *professor politices sive civilis philosophiae*.[49] As Michael Stolleis observes in his introduction to a useful collection of essays on Conring, just as this polymath combined his medical practice with political engagements both in his own region and beyond (he was a member of the Braunschweig-Wolfenbüttel government), Conring also combined medical and political theory. That is, Conring understood the art of politics as applied *Staatsmedicine* in the fashion of others before him such as Henning Arnisaeus and Gabriel Naudé.[50] Moreover Conring's teaching responsibilities as listed in the *designationes laborum* indicate a fluid movement between natural philosophy and politics. For instance, in 1644 Conring is listed

46 In his *Polyhistor literarius philosophicus*, Daniel Georg Morhof treats the art of civic prudence in much the same terms: it requires attention to ways of speech (conversational virtues and axioms; 155), mores and affects (151), as well as temperaments (rhetorical invention is a matter of—among other things—nutrition, education, place of birth, and good air; 322). Its subsidiary disciplines include a moral philosophy that urges the reform of character by right training of the dynamic soul (338). Daniel Georg Morhof, *Polyhistor literarius philosophicus*, revised edition (Lubeck: Bockmann, 1714).

47 "Quinque partes Medicina continet, quae Graecis vocibus dicuntur, Physiologia, Hygiina, Pathologia, Simiotica, Therapeutica. Eas omnes Moralis quoque includit." Chiaramonti, 5.

48 "scopum Medicinae esse vel sanitatem integram conservare vel eandem collapsam restituere in integrum." Hermann Conring, *Introductio in universam artem medicam singulasque eius partes* (Helmstedt: Müller, 1654), 7. Conring's later authorities on medicine include Leonard Fuchs, Paracelsus, Thomas Erastus, Bruno Scidelius and Conrad Helvetius, and Thomas Harvey, ibid., 76; see also Edwin Rosner, "Hermann Conring als Arzt und als Gegner Hohenheims," Stolleis, 87–120.

49 Werner Kundert, "Hermann Conring als Professor der Universität Helmstedt," ed. Stolleis, 399–402. A similar figure at Schaffhausen is professor of logic, rhetoric and medicine Johann Konrad Peyer (1653–1712), whose works include *Exercitatio anatomico-medica de glandulis intestinorum, earumque usu & affectionibus* (1677).

50 Stolleis, 18.

teaching "On innate heat, on affects of the heart and their cure;" "On procuring knowledge of racial origin;" and "On the freedom of the German Republic." In 1659 listed are "Machiavelli's *The Prince*;" "On the nature of civil prudence;" "On the most grave affects of the human body;" and "On the Roman Empire according to Hopper."[51] But most significantly, it is clear that the terms Conring uses to discuss politics are regularly drawn from the disciplines of medicine and rhetoric. In his early *De morbis ac mutationibus rerumpublicarum* (1640), Conring cites Aristotle's *Rhetoric* on the affects and causes of civic mutations,[52] while proclaiming that "the origin and source of all internal motion is *persuasio*" (*Omnium igitur internorum motuum fons et origo est persuasio*).[53] The figure of the mutating political body dominates *De morbis ac mutationibus oligarchiarum* (1661), and finally in his work on *Civil Prudence*, Conring asserts outright that the art of medicine is directly relevant to sciences both moral and political.[54]

For political thinkers throughout seventeenth-century Europe, pathos was not just considered a problem to be fixed, and pathology not just the science of nature gone awry. But no matter what one's assessment of human nature and the passions, when it came to practical ethics, opposing arguments could be proleptically acknowledged at very little cost. If human nature was essentially reasonable and whole, training the passions that persisted seemed nonetheless a good idea. If human nature was essentially passionate, one could simply give a theoretical nod to some prior state of greater perfection, and then get on with the very same business of rendering the passions useful. Oddly, one's practical pathology could thus be both Cartesian and Aristotelian, both philosophical and rhetorical, both purgative and progressive. The real difference came with the function of time. For Stoic-Cartesian pathology returned naturally to a norm, and norms are most weighty when derived from atemporal, universal, and static principles. Aristotle's political pathology, on the other hand, induced norms only from the habits that constitute particular states of being. Instead of stasis, Aristotle emphasized the passions that motivate incessant cultural mutation.

Let us remember that constitutions were defined by Aristotle relative to diverse habits and ends. One is advised for instance not to employ the value of freedom as the major premise in an argument justifying the acts of tyranny, or the value of wealth in an argument to a democratic assembly (*Rhetoric* 1366a1–6). Generally

---

[51] 1644: "De calido innato, de affectibus cordis eorumque curatione. De paranda stirpium notitia. Privatim de republica Germanica." 1659: "Machiavelli, Princeps (Abschluß). De natura civilis prudentiae. De gravissimis corporis humani affectibus. De republica Imperii Romani secundum Hopperum." Kundert, in Stolleis, 406–407.

[52] Conring, *De morbis ac mutationibus rerumpublicarum,* B4r.

[53] Conring, *De morbis ac mutationibus rerumpublicarum,* A3v.

[54] "Quoniam scilicet ad artem medicam pertinet illud omne quod ad sanitatem humani corporis sive conservandam sive restituendam facit, quidni pari ratione et civilis scientiae fuerit omnia illa novisse quae emolumenti aliquid queunt parere?" Conring, *Civili prudentia* 62.

Aristotle advises in his *Rhetoric* not to structure one's persuasive efforts on the basis of all opinions, but rather on those held "by an identified group" (1395b31–34). In the fifth book of the *Politics*, Aristotle provides this constitutional relativism with a dynamic principle: "All constitutions are overthrown either from within or from without," and it is the role of a treatise on politics to explain how—how a state becomes weak and thus subject to attack from without, as well as how dissension and political revolution arises from within the political body. It turns out that revolutions and dissent from within arise as a result of passions both legitimate and illegitimate, including fear of dishonor and loss, anger, insolence and avarice, hatred and contempt, and most importantly, the desire for equality (of course not a passion strictly speaking, but rather an instigator of passion). Constitutions then move incessantly from one form to another as passions characteristic of the political culture emerge and dissipate—a fluctuation based on the political structure and its various imbalances. Thus in a famous reconstruction of political *ur*history, Aristotle conjectures that:

> The first governments were kingships, probably for this reason, because of old, when cities were small, men of eminent virtue were few. Further, they were made kings because they were benefactors, and benefits can only be bestowed by good men. But when many persons equal in merit arose, no longer enduring the pre-eminence of one, they desired to have a commonwealth, and set up a constitution. The ruling class soon deteriorated and enriched themselves out of the public treasury; riches became the path to honour, and so oligarchies naturally grew up. These passed into tyrannies and tyrannies into democracies; for love of gain in the ruling classes was always tending to diminish their number, and so to strengthen the masses, who in the end set upon their masters and established democracies (*Politics* 1286b8–22).

Thus the constitution, Aristotle concludes, "is in a figure the life of the city" (1295a40–1295b1). The role, then, of the political theorist is to analyze which passions give this political figure what we might call its tropological swerve—that is, to devise a rhetoric of the political body considering both its institutional stability, and its motivating passions. Or so thought interpreters of Aristotle in the seventeenth century.

In this light we can conclude by considering Arnold Wesenfeld, a long forgotten late-century figure of Frankfurt/O. public life, who represents doggedly this Aristotelian political pathology common in the German Baroque and beyond.[55] As an aside, it is also worth noting how Wesenfeld represents that nascent sensitivity to human dynamics that would soon show up in the new historical science of human nature.

---

[55] Arnold Wesenfeld was a professor of logic, ethics, and metaphysics at Frankfurt/O. His books include *Dissertatio de natura definitionis* (1692); *Georgica animi et vitae* (1696); *Passiones animi* (1713); and *Versuch einer Verbesserung der Moral unter den Christen* (1726). For a note on Wesenfeld's eclecticism, see Donald R. Kelly, "Eclecticism and the History of Ideas," *Journal of the History of Ideas* 62.4 (2001): 577–92.

In his 1696 *Georgica animi et vitae, seu pathologia practica, moralis nempe et civilis, ex physicis ubique fontibus* [*Georgics of Soul and Life, or Practical Pathology of Life Both Moral and Civil, in Each Case from the Wellspring of Physics*],[56] Wesenfeld attempts a high wire act balanced between a range of contrary forces, including traditional theology and new science, philosophical reason and practical pathology. He begins by contrasting the rational philosophy of Gassendi and Descartes to the civil pathology of Aristotle's Rhetoric, and then sets out to integrate the two in a scheme compatible with the Genesis story of man's creation.[57] Wesenfeld does acknowledge the natural integrity of humankind first bestowed to Adam by God—an integrity still manifest in man's *divinae gratiae lumen* and inhabited by Descartes's clear and distinct ideas.[58] But after Adam's fall, according to Wesenfeld's conventional understanding, the soul was divided into elements of a rational supernature and an irrational nature, the latter subject primarily to the passions. Wesenfeld's postlapsarian human thus populates a *status primaevi corruptique* in which we can read Christian, Hobbesian, Cartesian, and Lockean connotations: mind and body do battle, and bad habits after the fall set the association of ideas against their natural order.[59] The function of civil society, according to Wesenfeld, is to tap those mental faculties that allow us by the Grace of God to "repair the natural order" and "rule the passions"—thereby transforming our corrupt nature by better habit to a state more reasonable.[60] But not reasonable to a fault. For besides those "inordinate" passions that perturb our actions from their natural course, there are also "spiritual" passions without which God's plan would fail in us. These spiritual passions include for Wesenfeld those that help us weigh perception and judge the right course of action—the very same passions without which Aristotle thought ethical behaviour impossible, and Hobbes the life of the mind.[61] In other words, Wesenfeld's pathology would be indispensible, no matter what the state of humanity.

Wesenfeld asserts that pathology is applicable in practical and moral theology, ecclesiastical oratory, medicine, physics, military strategy, and philosophy.[62] But it must function as something more than a descriptive adjunct. Pathology must actually prepare the way for practical intervention. "Thus it is not enough simply to note those motions of the soul," one learns from the preface to Wesenfeld's

---

56 Arnold Wesenfeld, *Georgica animi et vitae, seu pathologia practica, moralis nempe et civilis, ex physicis ubique fontibus...* (Frankfurt: Volckeri, 1696).

57 Wesenfeld, unpaginated introduction.

58 Wesenfeld, 53–4.

59 Wesenfeld, 55, 4.

60 "Gratiam addimenti, ut reparetur ordo naturae institutus, sicut in ceteris mentis facultatibus, ita et in imperio passionum." Wesenfeld, 55–6; "supposito, nos in statu corrupto quidem versari, sed cuius tamen aliqualis reparatio (quantum ad usum vitae civilis necessarium est) in nostra manu posita." Wesenfeld, 56.

61 Wesenfeld, 69.

62 Wesenfeld, unpaginated introduction.

work. The pathologist must also analyze "the origins of these motions, how they are intertwined, and the ways in which they compel."[63] The uses of pathology are then threefold: first, to direct "the more perfect passions in us and others—a project felicitous in both public and private life, natural and civil."[64] This is achieved, Wesenfeld elaborates, by controlling as far as possible the circumstantial factors that effect the quality and quantity of passions, which includes everything from climate and geography to sensory input and imaginary projection into the future.[65] Second, pathology is useful for "the possible abolition of those inordinate passions both ubiquitous and tenacious, or for total suppression of those that are truly inordinate and perturb both our actions and the actions of others." Finally, one can employ pathology for "access to the perfection of instituted states in the regime of reason, and to their motions," that is, to the extent reason remains in the nature of humankind.[66] Though these two final uses are clearly Stoic in sentiment, Wesenfeld ultimately draws out the implications of Aristotle's dynamic political analysis and defines pathology as a universal science of motion pulsing through the life both moral and civil.[67]

***

Nancy Struever once remarked in conversation that epistemological determinism distorts Foucault's resilient approach to the human sciences in *The Order of Things*. This constraint explains why Foucault puts the invention of human nature that marks modernity at the end of the eighteenth century, whereas I put it two centuries earlier. For Foucault, human nature is first a product of the human sciences; no more, no less. Perhaps it was "directly presented to discourse" in the natural sciences of the Classical age, given a definitive status and accorded a good deal of attention, but it had no independent epistemological status before the nineteenth century, and thus no ontological import. On these grounds, Foucault can then polemicize the concept of human nature did not properly exist in the Renaissance, nor the "man" so addressed. I too argue that human nature is a product of the human sciences, but I define the human sciences differently. Not just the disciplines that take as their

---

63 "Neque tantum ipsos illos motus adnotare animus est, verum et motuum horum origines, nexus, modumque impellendi…". Wesenfeld, unpaginated preface.

64 "perfectior passionem directio in nobis et aliis, quod ad vitae privatae et publicae, naturalis et civilis felicitatem multum facit." Wesenfeld, 63.

65 Wesenfeld, 31–45.

66 "(2) Possibilis abolitio inordinationis universae passionibus adhaerentis, totalis vero sublatio eius inordinationis, quae nostra aut aliorum actiones externas perturbat. (3) Accessus ad status instituti perfectionem in rationali regimine motuum suorum, quousque per relictas naturae vires licet…". Wesenfeld, 63.

67 "…quod Pathologicis hisce principiis superstructum est, nempe theatri universalis motuum vitae civilis et militaris cum publico communicare aggrediar." Wesenfeld, unpaginated preface.

object humankind as an empirical entity (nineteenth-century economics, biology, and philology),[68] nor just the reflexive, "meta-epistemological" disciplines that try to explain what makes humankind capable of treating itself as an empirical entity (psychology, sociology, the analysis of literature and mythology),[69] human sciences must be understood instead as "meta-practical." They are interventionist disciplines that reflect practice in more or less systematic fashion. Hence the key disciplines are law, pedagogy, psychology, and political science, as well as certain sorts of theology, practical philosophy, poetics, rhetoric and medicine—the first such "human sciences" and resources for those that come after.

If one investigates human nature from the perspective of the history of philosophy, as did an earlier generation of intellectual historians such as Kristeller and Trinkaus, it makes sense to conclude that human nature was conceived differently in pre-modern and modern eras with the Italian Renaissance marking the break. If one investigates human nature from the perspective of epistemological history, as did Foucault, then the very concept can readily be seen as an eighteenth-century invention. Now needed are new investigations of human nature from the perspective of the history of the practical arts, including from the perspective of the first practical arts of rhetoric and medicine. Undoubtedly from such studies human nature will emerge renewed, once again.

68 Foucault, 344.

69 Foucault, 367.

# Chapter 6
# Responses to Vulnerability: Medicine, Politics and the Body in Descartes and Spinoza

Amy Schmitter

## Introduction: The Rhetorical Landscape of Vulnerability

That all humans are mortal is enough of a truism to serve as the major premise in the standard example of a syllogism. But truisms may well be true, as this one is on at least two counts: humans are vulnerable, and humans are finite. Less of a truism is the claim that humans are vulnerable *because* we are finite. Here we can learn from several of the most important seventeenth-century philosophers; both Descartes and Spinoza recognized our somatic fragility as extended things in a world full of other extended things, but took it as part of a more general vulnerability to which limited creatures are subject. Although they share the same insight, they model the relation between vulnerability and finitude in rather different ways, and so end up with different sets of recommendations about how to cope with our vulnerability. On the one hand, Descartes conceives of finite beings as intrinsically liable to internal breakdown; correcting such breakdown is the work of medicine and engineering. On the other hand, Spinoza pictured finite things as susceptible to being overwhelmed by external forces and calls for a broadly political strategy to buttress ourselves against incursions from outside.

As the talk of corrective strategies should suggest, both Descartes and Spinoza hoped their accounts would serve not only analytic and explanatory ends, but as tools of persuasion. They should move us to act, whether to support the advancement of medicine, to bring about the right kind of political state, or to undertake schemes of direct psychic and individual self-improvement.[1] In this

[1] I shall return to such "self-help" plans at the end of this discussion; they figure prominently in the concluding sections of each Part of Descartes's *Passions of the Soul*, and in his correspondence with Elisabeth of Bohemia between 1644 and 1645, as well as Part V of Spinoza's *Ethics*, and to some degree in his early *Treatise on the Emendation of the Intellect*. For further discussion of projects of self-improvement in Descartes, see Deborah Brown, *Descartes and the Passionate Mind* (Cambridge: Cambridge University Press, 2006), Chapters 7 and 8; Lisa Shapiro, *The Correspondence Between Princess Elisabeth of Bohemia and René Descartes* (Chicago: University of Chicago Press, 2007), "Translator's Introduction," especially pp. 29–35, 40–51, and "Descartes's Ethics" in *A Companion to Descartes*, ed. J. Broughton & J. Carriero (Malden, MA: Blackwell Publishing, 2008),

sense, Descartes and Spinoza shared broadly rhetorical aims. But I will argue that differences in their conceptions of our finitude and resulting vulnerability steered the strategies each championed, and so I will examine their rhetoric in a narrower sense, that is, in the choice of expressive vehicles through which to frame their arguments. The kinds of vulnerability they envisage—whether "internal" or "external"—can perfectly well co-exist, and the underlying conceptions of our finitude may well be logically equivalent. But Descartes and Spinoza present their views through alternate *models,* models with distinct emphases and shifting centers of gravity. The differences are subtle, but shape what appears salient about our finitude— which in turn affects the tenor of each philosopher's proposals. Their role in directing response explains why such issues of salience have been the special province of rhetoric at least since the discussion of the *pathê* in Book 2 of Aristotle's *Rhetoric*. In both the broad and specialized senses, then, how the expressive models stamp Spinoza's and Descartes's proposals for translating conception into action count as matters of their rhetoric.

Nonetheless, the rhetorical division of labor takes place against a broadly shared background: both Descartes and Spinoza make a sharp and emphatic division between what is finite and what is genuinely infinite, a division that configures their entire conceptual and rhetorical landscape. Although not the same, the division is closely related to the contrast between activity and passivity examined by many scholars,[2] for plenary activity appears the privilege of the positively Infinite, while to suffer or undergo—that is to be subject to passions—is a sign of limitation. The distinction between finitude and the Infinite is particularly obvious in Spinoza's conceptual repertoire, because of the role God plays as a basic ontological category. But Descartes anticipated this feature of Spinoza's thought in many respects, particularly in locating our vulnerability in the frailty inherent to finitude. The connection between finitude and vulnerability strikes me

---

especially pp. 453–9. The literature on Part V of Spinoza's *Ethics* is copious; examples include Donald Rutherford, "Salvation as a State of Mind: the Place of *Acquiscentia* in Spinoza's *Ethics*," *British Journal for the History of Philosophy* 7 (October 1999), pp. 447–73, Michael Lebuffe, "Spinoza's *Summum Bonum*," *Pacific Philosophical Quarterly* 86 (June 2005), pp. 243–66, and for a survey, Don Garrett, "Spinoza's Ethical Theory," in *The Cambridge Companion to Spinoza*, ed. D. Garrett (New York: Cambridge University Press, 1996), pp. 267–314). For overviews of the general seventeenth century interest in individual "remedies" for what ails us, particularly through the application of reason to the "passions," see Susan James, "Reason, the Passions and the Good Life," in *The Cambridge History of Seventeenth-Century Philosophy*, Vol. II, ed. D. Garber & M. Ayers (Cambridge: Cambridge University Press, 1998), pp. 1358–96, and my "Seventeenth and Eighteenth Century Theories of Emotions," *The Stanford Encyclopedia of Philosophy*, ed. E. Zalta, URL = <http://plato.stanford.edu/archives/fall2008/entries/emotions-17th18th/>.

2 Notable studies of the contrast between passion and action can be found in Susan James, *Passion and Action* (Oxford: Oxford University Press, 1997), and Paul Hoffman, *Essays on Descartes* (Oxford: Oxford University Press, 2009), especially pp. 4, 8–9, 105–141.

as an important insight, one where we can learn something from early modern philosophers (even God-intoxicated ones). For many contemporary thinkers give the fragility of the *body* its due without fully acknowledging other vulnerabilities of our condition.[3] Descartes and Spinoza do not themselves exhaustively catalogue all the forms of vulnerability; for one, neither gives much heed to the dependence we have on what is outside for sustenance, whether it be air, food, or water.[4] But they do recognize that finite minds are subject, just as finite bodies are, to both passions and disruptions. To make this point, I will close with a consideration of how Descartes and Spinoza address psychic vulnerability. But I readily admit that this topic is a trickier subject for both philosophers than is somatic fragility, for they often address the former through the latter.

Descartes is particularly clear about the nature and causes of somatic fragility, and deeply concerned with how it affects our lives, and with what techniques we can use to remedy its effects. I say "remedy," rather than "cure," since Descartes treats the body and its vulnerability as intrinsic to our earthly existence, for both good and ill. Noting these concerns with the body and with practical remedies may help undermine two of the more persistent stereotypes with which Descartes has been saddled: that he has only contempt for the body, and that his concerns are restricted to abstract speculation. Recent scholars such as Deborah Brown have tackled these unfounded stereotypes through an examination of the passions as perceptions that manifest our embodiment in ways central to our experience as full human beings making our way through the world.[5] I hope the discussion here will further this project by showing that in pursuing his practical concerns, Descartes

---

3 For an example, let me cite a discussion held during the NEH Summer Institute "How Background Practices Produce Intelligibility," at the University of California, Santa Cruz in summer 1997. In response to the query about why she had referred specifically to the body, rather than to material practices more generally, throughout her presentation, Judith Butler explained that she wanted to highlight the issue of vulnerability. I appreciated the direction of her discussion, even if I don't think that it is the sole avenue of approach; it is what first started me thinking about the connection between vulnerability and finitude.

4 Such dependence strikes me as distinctive in kind: we require an exchange of outside material—much like what Marx described as the *Stoffwechsel* [metabolism, material exchange] involved in all work—in order to survive. It is a *positive* dependence, despite making us susceptible to suffocation, hunger and thirst, and so does not readily fit into the analysis I give here. I owe this point to an excellent question asked by Katherine Loevy at Vanderbilt University.

5 For examples, see Amèlie Rorty, "Descartes on Thinking with the Body," in *The Cambridge Companion to Descartes*, ed. J. Cottingham (Cambridge: Cambridge University Press, 1994), pp. 371–92, and Brown 2006, especially "Introduction," and Chapter 1. I discuss the stereotypes and misreadings Brown confronts in "Descartes's Peepshow (and other Cascading Metaphors): Critical Review of Deborah Brown, *Descartes and the Passionate Mind*," *Canadian Journal of Philosophy* 40 (2010), pp. 485-508.. For a somewhat different approach to (and evaluation of) the current state of Descartes's reception, see Thomas Sorell, *Descartes Reinvented* (Cambridge: Cambridge University Press, 2005), especially "Introduction."

in no way contrasts the vulnerability of the body with any supposed mental impregnability. Descartes's substance dualism is, of course, terribly important to his ontology, but that does not mean that every feature of his thinking reduces to it. As we will see, the coping techniques Descartes proposes treat the boundaries between mind and body, and the external world more generally, as more porous than Spinoza allows. Spinoza's views are just as heterogeneous: on the one hand, he tolerates a fair diversity of means for individuating ourselves; on the other, he insists on the need for vigilant policing of the boundaries of whatever individual we do identify as ourselves. Perhaps we can find here a general lesson about the rhetoric of dualisms: they are not always monolithic.

## Vulnerability and Finitude

Although it upends the chronology, we may see how finitude begets vulnerability most clearly by using Spinoza as a lens for inspecting the basic conceptual connections. The last three Parts of his *Ethics* are largely devoted to describing the human susceptibility to passions, that is, to passive affects, the causes of which lie (partly) outside us. This susceptibility is inescapable, making humans inevitably prone to bondage. The nature of such bondage, and how it can be eased by forming a collective with powers of action greater than that of any individual is the subject of Part IV of the *Ethics*. Only in Part V does Spinoza suggest that humans can achieve a kind of freedom by developing the part of the intellect that is eternal. But even there, he does not allow that we can somehow evade our necessary passivity. The reason is utterly general: we find ourselves in the midst of external things, which can act on us, overwhelm us, and bring about our destruction. This point is spelled out as early as Proposition 3 of Part IV: "The force by which a man perseveres in existing is limited, and infinitely surpassed by the power of external causes."[6] It is quite simply a brute and brutal feature of the human condition that we are always subject to being overpowered by external forces. Eventually, we will succumb.[7]

This fate is not unique to humans. All "singular things," which are "in nature," are susceptible to external forces and partially passive. So basic is this point that it forms the first and only axiom advanced in Part IV: "There is no singular thing

---

6 All references to the *Ethics* will be cited by Part, type, number and when relevant, component (e.g., "IP4d" means Part One, Proposition Four, Demonstration). In this scheme, "P" stands for proposition, "D" stands for definition, "A" for axiom, "d" for demonstration, "l" for lemma, "s" for scholium, "c" for corollary and "Pref" for Preface. Translations are those of Edwin Curley's *Collected Works of Spinoza* Vol. I (Princeton: Princeton University Press, 1985).

7 Here Spinoza assumes that "can happen" entails "will happen sometime," which illustrates his commitment to an temporalist understanding of possibility: what is possible may not be necessary through its own essence, but is determined by the chain of causes that produce it.

in nature than which there is not another more powerful and stronger. Whatever one is given, there is another more powerful by which the first can be destroyed." (IVA1). The axiom is the only evidence cited in the demonstration of Proposition 3, which simply draws out its consequences when considering a series: "given a man, there is something else, say A, more powerful. And given A, there is something else again, say B, more powerful than A, and so on, to infinity. ..." (IVP3d). For example, any extended singular thing—that is, any body—no matter how determinately large, is always susceptible to being overpowered by some further, larger conglomeration of bodies (which insofar as it acts in tandem, could count as a "singular thing" by Spinoza's lights). There can be no larg*est* body that is less than the whole of extension, and yet the whole of extension is not, properly speaking, a singular thing in nature.[8]

The point, however, is not restricted to bodies, that is, to finite modes of extension. Any sort of finite things with a determinate existence count as singular things (IID7). Now, there is a sense in which some singular things can be found in God's infinite intellect or infinite attributes, rather than in nature; for example, what-it-is-to-be a circle of radius R is not *in* nature, and so not vulnerable to conditioned natural forces.[9] But any singular thing that "actually exists" is *ipso facto* "in nature." Actually existing singular things are embedded in an infinite chain of finite causes, which explains the fact of their existence. To be "in nature" entails being located in such causal chains—being "conditioned," as Kant would later say. As such, both bodies and modes of thinking (that is, minds) count as conditioned, singular things (see IIA5). So all existing finite things are liable to overpowering and overwhelming by external forces, whether as a matter of being open to destruction or simple passivity. Indeed, the capacity to be acted upon can be taken as the distinctive mark of finite existence. It is rooted in one of Spinoza's earliest definitions whereby "something is finite that can be limited by something else of the same nature" (ID2). Since it is impossible that there exists only one finite thing, or one most powerful finite thing, existing finite things can always be limited by other existing finite things. Only what is absolutely infinite has the kind of self-sufficiency and self-containment that would guarantee invulnerability. The Infinite[10] exists necessarily in a particularly strong sense, and as such, it constitutes an entirely different order of being and intelligibility from the finite. We are not, and cannot be infinite in this sense—although Spinoza will concede a sense in which there is something of the human mind that partakes in the eternal (see VP23).

---

[8] On some related points, see Gabbey (2008), "Spinoza, Infinite Modes and the Infinitive Mood," *Studia Spinozana* 16 (2008), pp. 41–65, p. 54.

[9] See IIP8. The passage is difficult, but for our purposes, I suggest glossing Spinoza's thought as holding that a formal essence, such as what-it-is-to-be some finite thing X, is not *in* nature as an actually existing X is.

[10] I think that this holds true not only for infinite substance, but also for infinite attributes, or modes, but for some caveats about the sense in which attributes and modes can be infinite, see Gabbey (2008).

Although he was unique in elevating it to an axiom of his system, Spinoza was not the first early modern philosopher to note the necessary vulnerability of natural things.[11] As we will see in the next section, Descartes showed an abiding concern with the fragility of the (human) body and its repair. Still, Descartes did not connect vulnerability to finitude anywhere nearly as explicitly as Spinoza did. Since he also focused on medical engineering as the most important fix for our frailties, it may seem that he assumed that only bodies are vulnerable, despite recognizing the existence both of a positively infinite substance, and of minds distinct from bodies. It is true that unlike Spinoza, Descartes did not consider even finite minds to be *naturally* destructible. But he maintained that they are receptive to passions, that is, to being acted upon, even to the extent of being acted on in ways that inhibit autonomous action. More exactly, he considered *finite* minds to be susceptible. Once we look for it, we can find plenty of evidence that Descartes understood the infinite to constitute a different order of being and intelligibility from the finite. Both his letters on the eternal truths and the Fourth Set of Replies to the *Meditations on First Philosophy* explain that we cannot, strictly speaking, *comprehend* the Infinite. But we can conceive it; indeed, we can conceive it more clearly and distinctly than anything else.[12] Our inability to comprehend the infinite stems from the disproportional relation in which we finite things stand to the positively Infinite (see the Fifth Set of Replies, AT VII: 368; CSM II: 253). Descartes identifies the positively Infinite with God (see the First Set of Replies, AT VII: 113; CSM II: 81, and the *Principles of Philosophy* §27, AT VIIIA: 15; CSM I: 202), and attributes the various Divine perfections to the positive lack of limitations that constitutes God's Infinity. It belongs to the being of the positive Infinite to be without parts and to have only attributes, not modes (*Principles of Philosophy* §56, AT VIIIA: 26; CSM I: 211), and so God has the perfections of simplicity, immutability and activity without passivity. Descartes's letter to Clerselier of 23 April 1649 is particularly telling: here he identifies the Infinite with the absolute essence of substance, as well as with being and truth (AT V: 355–6; CSMK III: 377–8). For the same reasons, Descartes insists on the conceptual and ontological priority of the positive Infinite over finitude, even in understanding our own finite natures (Fifth Set of Replies, AT VII: 365; CSM II: 252; letter to Hyperaspistes, August 1641, AT III: 427; CSMK III: 192). Nonetheless, he also maintains that none of the properties by which we dimly compare ourselves with God can be applied to both in the same sense (the Second Set of Replies,

[11] I would argue that Hobbes is another predecessor, although he may not recognize the generality of the point, since he concentrates exclusively on the vulnerability of bodies. But since there is nothing besides bodies in Hobbes's universe, the limitation follows simply by set inclusion.

[12] That we can conceive of the infinite more clearly and distinctly than anything else is the lesson of the "causal" proofs of God's existence in Meditation III; see AT VII 45–6, CSM II: 31–2, also letter to Mersenne of 21 January 1641 (AT III 284, CSMK III: 169) and the *Principles of Philosophy* §19, AT VIIIA 12, CSM I 199.

AT VII: 137; CSM II: 98–9).[13] The sharp conceptual and ontological division between finitude and the Infinite rules out treating the Infinite as vulnerable, or indeed, even as mutable. And so, like Spinoza, Descartes treats invulnerability as the privilege of the Infinite. But as we will see below, Descartes diverges from Spinoza in identifying the difference that makes a difference as a matter of the relation between part and whole.

## Descartes, Divisibility, and Doctoring

In the "Preface" to the French edition of the *Principles of Philosophy*,[14] Descartes introduces a metaphor that sketches the relations among various philosophical disciplines: "the whole of philosophy is like a tree. The roots are metaphysics, the trunk is physics, and the branches emerging from the trunk are all the other sciences, which may be reduced to three principal ones, namely medicine, mechanics and morals" (AT IXB: 14, CSM I 186). Although the *Principles* restricts itself to the roots and trunk, Descartes makes it clear that the true "fruits" of philosophy are gathered from the branches. Those fruits are largely practical, but they also spring from an understanding of the nature of matter—that is, an understanding of the nature of extended substance, its modal variations and the mechanical causes that govern them. For this reason, the branches share important similarities: mechanics is a kind of engineering directed at how and to what ends to manipulate matter—as are both medicine and morals. Medicine is largely a matter of managing the structure of the body to maintain its functionality, and ultimately its integrity. Morals has the broad aim of directing our actions towards the good, but on Descartes's view, the main practical difficulty for morals is disciplining and cultivating our passions, those perceptions of the soul that are "caused, maintained and strengthened" by bodily processes, so that they harmonize with our best-considered reasons.[15] Doing so in turn involves retooling various bodily systems.

---

[13] The extremity of the difference may be part of the loss of univocal, and even of analogous relations between God and creatures in early modern thinking; on this topic, see Tad Schmalz, "The Disappearance of Analogy in Descartes, Spinoza and Regis" *Canadian Journal of Philosophy* 30 (2000), 85–113.

[14] This "Preface" was originally titled "*Lettre de l'Autheur à celuy qui a traduit le Livre, laquelle peut icy servir de Preface*" ["Letter from the author to whoever translates this book, which may here serve as Preface"], and was added to the 1647 French edition, translated by the Abbé Claude Picot from the original Latin, published in 1644. Because Descartes hoped that the *Principles* would take on the rule of a textbook, it is natural to include some reflection on the structure of the "sciences." See "Avertissement," AT IX, iii, CSM I 177, and for the status of the *Principles*, letter to Mersenne, 31 December 1640, AT III 276, CSMK III: 167.

[15] On this issue, see my "The Passionate Intellect: Reading the (Non-)Opposition of Intellect and Emotion in Descartes," in *Persons and Passions: Essays in Honor of Annette Baier*, ed. J. Whiting, C. Williams, and J. Jenkins (South Bend, IN: Notre Dame U. Press, 2005), pp. 48–82

For this reason, Descartes's later (and last) work, *The Passions of the Soul*, can claim to consider the passions simply "*en physicien*" [as a physicist], even as it ends with a lengthy consideration of the ties between the passion of *generosité*, virtue, and happiness. The ultimate aim is to discipline—not suppress—our passions, so that we achieve a kind of *felt* autonomy, habitualized as *generosité*; we do so by manipulating our bodily configuration, so that it disposes us to feel particular passions in response to outside causes in ways that can be approved by reason. The importance of working through the body to experience habits of autonomous action explains why *generosité* is both a passion and a virtue. Although the techniques that Descartes recommends in the *Passions* use the imagination to reconfigure relevant body parts, rather than (say) surgery, they nonetheless constitute a kind of self-doctoring.[16] So, the branches of the tree of philosophy are largely devoted to the same thing: the manipulation of matter, and particularly of our own bodies, in ways that promote our good.

That Descartes conceives of our good largely in terms of health is witnessed by a number of his letters. In the spring of 1645, Descartes writes Elizabeth of Bohemia that "perfect health" is "the foundation of all the other goods of this life" (AT IV: 220; CSMK III: 250). Later in the same year, he declares "the preservation of health has always been the principal end of my studies …" (to [the Marquess of Newcastle], October 1645, AT IV: 329; CSMK III: 76). And seven years earlier, Descartes wrote to Constantijn Huygens that he was working on a "compendium of medicine" (AT I: 649; CSMK III: 76). That compendium never materialized (although the *Passions* and various physiological works, such as the unfinished *Description of the Human Body* might constitute parts), and Descartes seems to have abandoned some of his early ambition to extend human life by 100 or more years (see the letter to Huygens and *Discourse on Method*, AT 62; CSM I: 143). It seems likely that Descartes found that the roots and the trunk of the tree occupying most of his time, forcing him to leave it to the future to inch along the branches. Be that as it may, I maintain that the conceptions of physics and metaphysics not only provided the explanatory framework within which he hoped to realize his ambitions for medicine, they also motivated the turn to medicine as the proper response to the weaknesses of the human condition.

Central to Descartes's revolutionary metaphysics is a streamlined conception of matter, one freed from "the useless lumber of scholastic entities" and irrelevant causes (see *Comments on a Certain Broadsheet*, AT 366; CSM I: 309), and reduced to the fully intelligible modes and causes proper to extended substance. Extended substance is capable of taking on various modal variations, including size, shape and motion, and of transmitting motion from part to part through some form of contact. Motion is a particularly important mode, for it is the distribution of motion

---

[16] Indeed, this may be the kind of self-doctoring that Descartes (citing Tiberius) thought anybody who had survived to the age of thirty should be well equipped to practice (see letter to [the Marquess of Newcastle], AT IV: 329–30; CSMK III: 275–6, as well as the "Conversation with Burman," AT V: 179; CSMK III: 354).

throughout the continuum of extension that explains how we are able to make further modal distinctions such as those between size and shape. But divisibility is just as central to the conception of matter as is motion.[17] Any chunk of matter can be divided into smaller parts, each of which behaves as does matter in general, according to the laws of motion that govern the transfer of motion through impact or across a rigid medium. Divisibility and mobility are the conditions allowing for any modal variation to distinguish among the parts of extension. Yet of the two, divisibility seems even more basic, necessary for differentiating parts at all. The world of extension is a plenum of extended substance, and as such, the only kind of motion conceptually possible is internal, relative motion of parts. That possibility requires, in turn, the possibility of differentiating among the parts of extension, and hence requires divisibility. Part Two of the *Principles* explains:

> The matter existing in the entire universe is thus one and the same, and it is always recognized as matter simply in virtue of its being extended. All the properties which we clearly perceive in it are to be reduced to this one: which is its divisibility, and accordingly, the mobility of its parts [*ad hoc unum reducuntur, quòd sit partibilis, & mobilis secundùm partes*] and its resulting capacity to be affected in all the ways which we perceive as being derivable from the movements of the parts. (AT VIIIA: 52; translation modified from CSM I: 232; see also *The World*, AT XI: 34; CSM I 91).

So, divisibility plays a central role in Descartes's accounts of the essence of extended substance: most notably, in the Sixth Meditation, where it is used to mark "the very great difference between the mind and the body, inasmuch as the body is by its very nature always divisible ..." —a difference that alone is sufficient to show the real distinction between mind and body (AT VII: 85–6; CSM II: 59).

Moreover, the divisibility of bodies is a divisibility *ad indefinitum*, divisibility without end. Descartes insists on this point: holding against those who maintain that all series must come to an end, "on the contrary, I think that in the division of the parts of matter there really is an endless series ..." (letter to [Mesland], 2 May 1644, AT IV: 113; CSMK III: 232). But this unending divisibility is not a form of infinitude: Descartes is likewise adamant about reserving the notion of infinity for God alone, Who is extended only in the sense that Its power reaches everywhere. We understand that God possesses infinitude as a real attribute—a trait that we cannot adequately comprehend, but that can nonetheless give content to a clear and distinct idea. In contrast, "things in which we observe no limits [*nullum*

---

17 In Descartes's technical language, the determinate divisions into which a chunk of matter has actually been cut and the determinate motions of any chunks constitute modes. But because mob*ility* and divis*ibility* seem explanatorily central among modes, they may in fact be only conceptually distinct from the *attribute* of extension, which makes them rather more than mere modes; for further discussion of related points, see my "The Wax and I: Perceptibility and Modality in the Second Meditation," in *Archiv für Geschichte der Philosophie* 82 (2000), pp. 178–201.

*finem*]—such as the extension of the world, the division of the parts of matter, the number of stars, and so on—should instead be regarded as indefinite [*ut indefinita spectabimus*]" (AT VIII: 14f; CSM I: 201f). The indefinite, unlimited divisibility of bodies is not a kind of *positive* infinity and perfection, but merely shows "in a negative way that any limits which they may have cannot be discovered by us." Such indefiniteness is thus a lack, something metaphysically and conceptually downgraded from the genuinely Infinite.[18]

Such indefinite divisibility is also, I maintain, why any configuration of extension will be prone to disruption. Because it is always subject to splintering into smaller and smaller, differently sized and shaped pieces, *no* configuration can be kept fully immobilized. It can neither be quarantined from the rest of extension, nor have its parts so tightly packed as to bar incursion of alien particles. As a result, even the most stable arrangement can be disarranged.[19] That which is true of bodies in general is also true of our bodies specifically. Our bodies are typically very well-engineered for the ends of self-maintenance, and self-development. At a minimum, they are designed to maintain the amount of heat and the integrity of the whole sufficient to constitute life. The heat fuels internal systems that maintain the mass of the body, alert us to external dangers and goods, prompt us to act accordingly, and allow us to diagnose whether the systems are functioning properly. In this way, we come equipped with various "maintenance" systems that help us to preserve the sort of continuity enabling us to treat our bodies as persisting over time, and with the diagnostic systems that allow us to maintain those maintenance systems.[20] But no matter how well-engineered these systems may be, and no matter how magnificently self-maintaining our bodies might be as a whole, they cannot be made immune to breakdown. The configuration of parts that constitutes the well-engineered body can be disrupted either by the introduction of alien particles at its interstices (disease), or by the disarrangement of the very

[18] Alan Gabbey suggests that Spinoza makes a related distinction grammatically (borrowing from Scholastic logicians), depending on whether "infinitus" is used categorematically or syncategorematically: the former, but not the latter, describes the absolute and unconditioned infinity of God; see section 2 of Gabbey (2008). But see the letter to Johann Hudde, discussed by Gabbey *passim*, where Spinoza muddies the waters a bit.

[19] It is instructive to look at the order of articles in the relevant section of the *Principles* in light of these considerations: articles 26–7 insist on the mere indefiniteness of extension, which Descartes follows with article 28, which rules out the use of final causes, "the purposes which God or nature may have in view when creating," to explain the operation of extended things. Article 29 then declares that God is not the cause of our errors (see AT VIII: 15–16; CSM I: 202–203). Part of the reason *why* God cannot be considered the cause of our errors is because however well God may have engineered our bodies, it belongs to the constitution of bodies that they do not follow the order of purposes, and things can go wrong. On this topic, see further my "How to Engineer a Human Being: Passions and Functional Explanation in Descartes," *A Companion to Descartes,* ed. J. Broughton & J. Carriero, Blackwell Press, 2007, pp. 426–44.

[20] For the notion of a "maintenance system," see Amélie Rorty (1994), p. 378.

parts themselves (maiming and destruction). This is where medicine comes in, and why there will always be a business for medicine: the inherent divisibility of finite matter means that we will always be prone to breakdowns. Medicine is in the business of repairing those breakdowns, and perhaps even improving the fabric of our bodies so that they will be more resistant to the sorts of incursions that disrupt their functioning. For this reason, the capacity to doctor ourselves may be the most effective of our systems of self-maintenance. What medicine cannot do is make us invulnerable, and so it cannot put itself out of business. Vulnerability is built into our very fabric, because of its unlimited divisibility. Although later sections will examine other therapeutic models of therapy entertained by Descartes, we should now appreciate just how central medical engineering is to his vision of our capacities for self-improvement.

## Spinoza's Political Response, or Size Really Does Matter

Vulnerability is built into our very fabric for Spinoza too—at least if we understand our fabric in terms of its finitude, as a finite mode less than and dependent on the whole. Again, it is because we are "in nature" in this sense, embedded within and dependent on an unending chain of conditioned causes, that we are subject to being overpowered by external forces. Spinoza is crystal clear that both minds and bodies are singular things in nature. However, because of the parallelism he maintains between the attributes and modes of thinking and of extension, we can look simply at the vulnerability of our bodies to understand most of the shape of Spinoza's explanation.[21] In particular, we should consider how Spinoza accounts for the identity and persistence through change of a finite mode in the case of the human body. This is no easy issue, whether we are considering the human mind, or the human body; there is no deep ontological basis for differentiating a finite mode from the chain of modes in which it is embedded, no real distinction between it and everything else. The finite modes that are the human mind and the human body interact with and depend on the rest of the conditioned universe in which they are embedded. So what makes a human body a "singular [and single] thing?" Well, the parts of singular things concur in their causal efficacy, that is, they act as a single cause, and they have greater "reality" or "perfection" in proportion to their active power (see IIP13s). And so, Spinoza seems to take it as a condition for granting something enough reality to count as a singular thing with some sort of

[21] Spinoza's psycho-physical parallelism rests mostly on the famous claim that "the order and connection of ideas is the same as the order and connection of things" (IIP7), or more generally, that the causal ordering under each attribute of God or Nature is the same. So, although Spinoza prohibits any talk of causation *between* modes of different attributes, the explanatory form—given by tracing causes—will be the same for each. Of course, sometimes it may seem as if Spinoza relies heavily on explanation in one mode without properly acknowledging how difficult it may be to apply an analogous explanation to a very different mode or attribute.

identity that the thing acts to preserve its being and increase its power of action. Such concerted action is what Spinoza calls *conatus*, or the striving toward self-preservation (IIIP6–7). But making conatus the basis for individuation means that there are no privileged, or exclusive, conditions for enumerating singular things: one singular thing can be found "inside" another singular thing.

The reliance on conatus also leaves the constitution of a singular thing unexplained. The question is particularly pressing because Spinoza allows that the extended parts of which a body is composed can be replaced by other bodies, the parts can become greater or less, and the parts can change the direction of their motion as a whole, or even sometimes in relation to each other, yet the "Individual will retain its nature, as before, without any change of its form" (IIP13L4–7). To allow for such changes, Spinoza offers the following definition:

> When a number of bodies, whether of the same or of different size, are so constrained by other bodies that they lie upon one another, or if they so move, whether with the same degree or different degrees of speed, that they communicate their motions to each other in a certain fixed manner, we shall say that those bodies are united with one another and that they all together compose one body or Individual, which is distinguished from the others by this union of bodies (IIP13Def).

In this account, Spinoza hopes to capture the sense in which a human body can be considered an individual, even though it is composite, grows and changes, moves, and "to be preserved, requires a great many other bodies" (IIP13Pos.I–VI). What the various motions and transactions between interior and exterior that belong to the conatus of the body tend toward is preserving "the proportion of motion and rest" that allows the body to move in enough unison to demarcate its inside from the outside.[22] In short, the body preserves its identity by cultivating what systems theory calls a "systems-environment boundary." The identity is dynamically maintained, and as such cannot last forever. But such transience is not tantamount to a built-in expiration date; Spinoza insists that only what tends to its preservation can be counted as a singular thing, or proper part of a singular thing. Rather, the very maintenance of system boundaries requires a constant exchange with the world outside. Because the world is full of things outside of the individual's boundaries that are bigger and more powerful than it, the world contains forces capable of overwhelming any singular thing in it.

Still, that very circumstance suggests a general strategy to resist the battering that leads to destruction: to expand one's boundaries, both to incorporate more in the "interior" of the individual and to be better able to resist what is outside. Spinoza's account is perfectly capable of accommodating nested sets of "singular things," and there is nothing in the account of the dynamically achieved identity of

---

[22] This proportion itself is no easy matter, and Spinoza suggests that no simple ratio will capture it. For further discussion, see Martin Lin, "Memory and Personal Identity in Spinoza," *Canadian Journal of Philosophy*, 35 (2005) pp. 243–68.

the human body that rules out our taking on yet other identities. Indeed, Spinoza encourages us to think of the possibilities:

> ...if we should conceive of a ... kind of Individual, composed [of many individuals] ..., we shall find that it can be affected in many other ways, without any change of its form. And if we proceed in this way to infinity [*in infinitum*], we shall easily conceive that the whole of nature is one Individual, whose parts, i.e., all bodies, vary in infinite ways, without any change of the whole Individual (IIP13L7dem).

One kind of response to our vulnerability, then, would be to seek some sort of union with the whole of nature. Spinoza certainly toys with this possibility; indeed, Part V of the *Ethics* does rather more than merely toy with it. I will turn to this topic in the last section, although it must be acknowledged that whatever Spinoza has in mind is not crystal clear. But there is another strategy that works with our finitude, and looking at it may illuminate Spinoza's thinking in general. The strategy is political: it advocates that we associate ourselves with others to form a larger and more powerful individual, one better able to fend for itself, while fending off incursions from outside. This is where Spinoza borrows a trick or two from Hobbes; as in Hobbes, the aim of association is to form a genuine polity, where the body politic is understood with deadpan literalness. It is an "artificial" body that is much larger than any of the individual subject-bodies that make it up.[23] Insofar as we build this social body on the basis of what is "common" to all humans—the rational pursuit of our own "advantage"—it too can count as a singular thing seeking to preserve its own boundaries and proportions of motion and rest. Hobbes too conceives of the commonwealth as a corporate body with a life and endeavor [conatus] of its own. Because it is much better positioned to pursue its own interests than are any of its subjects individually, it ends up benefiting (or tending to benefit) those "natural" individuals who are its constituent parts. But Hobbes is almost solely concerned with our vulnerability to others of the *same* kind, with the threat posed by our (rough) "equals"—to which his solution is to build an unequal artificial body. In contrast, Spinoza seems mostly concerned with threats posed by what is *more* powerful than the individual. Such a restriction may be sensible by Spinoza's lights; since singular things are *essentially* nodes of resistance to external forces (at least insofar as they are "real"), anything that threatens them must be capable of overcoming their essential resistance, and so counts as more powerful than they. Even so, because of its finitude, no singular thing can achieve invulnerability. Forming a larger, corporate body is an effective strategy not so much because it introduces something of unequal power into a field of roughly equal powers, as simply because that body gains in power and thus "perfection." All else being equal, bodies that truly count as singular things should increase their

[23] The metaphor of the body politic is elaborated in enormous detail in the "Introduction" to Hobbes's *Leviathan*, and mentioned often in Spinoza's *Theological-Political Treatise*, most notably in Chapter XVI.

perfection by increasing their size. Moving more and more across the boundary from outside to in, both decreases the threats from outside and gives the whole increased powers to maintain the integrity of the system.[24] The increase in power is only a matter of degree: we should now see why it makes no more sense to talk of a most powerful singular thing than it does to talk about a largest finite thing. Corporate bodies are more durable than their parts, but hardly indomitable.

## Descartes v. Spinoza: Vulnerability from Within and Without

If I am right, then Descartes and Spinoza fasten on to rather different ploys for addressing our vulnerability. Since their proposals are not incompatible—except as a matter of time management—we might wonder whether each philosopher could appreciate the proposals of the other. There is some evidence that Descartes at least might be sympathetic to what we might call the "agglutinative" approach adopted by Spinoza. The *Passions of the Soul* describes how "devotion" may be directed at "our sovereign, our country, [and] our town" (AT XI: 390; CSM I: 357–8). Devotion is a species of love, the passion that moves the soul to consider ourselves as "joined with what we love in such a manner that we imagine a whole, of which we take ourselves to be only one part, and the thing loved to be the other" (AT XI: 387; CSM I: 356). Moreover, in identifying with the loved object, we consider the whole to be more perfect than we are alone (see AT XI: 432; CSM I: 377). The very possibility of appropriate political love suggests that association with others might be a way of increasing our perfection, much as Spinoza thought. Still, since Descartes hardly goes very far with any political philosophizing, it would be sheer speculation to say much more.

In contrast, Spinoza does not seem to accord medicine the same place as he does politics. Just after describing the advantages of political association, Part V of the *Ethics* declares that "it does not pertain to this investigation to show how the intellect must be perfected, or in what way the Body must be cared for, so that it can perform its function properly. The former is the concern of Logic, and the latter of Medicine" (V Pref). However, we have another work, the early *Treatise on the Emendation of the Intellect* (before 1662), which does concern itself with how the intellect can be perfected. There Spinoza lists various steps to be taken to achieve what he has laid out as the good for humans: medicine makes it onto the list of instrumentally valuable disciplines, right after moral education: "*Third*, attention must be paid to Moral Philosophy and to Instruction concerning the Education of children. Because Health is no small means to achieving this

24 Note that this really does assume that all else is equal; it is a necessary and serious constraint that the increase in size does not disrupt the stability of the whole system. For most natural bodies (plants and animals), increase past some optimal adult size will disrupt the whole system—which is why mere weight gain does not as such signal an increase in perfection.

end, *fourthly*, the whole of Medicine must be worked out."[25] The end served by the various items on the list is the same, for Spinoza insists, "I wish to direct all the sciences toward one end and goal, viz. that we should achieve, as we have said, the highest human perfection" (ibid., p. 11). That end is acquiring "a nature much stronger and more enduring than [our] own" (ibid., p. 10). But even though medicine is means for achieving human perfection, Spinoza spares little thought for it, putting it almost at the end of his list, followed only by mechanics, and then failing to consider it again. In contrast, Spinoza ranks other pursuits a bit more prominently: "it is necessary, *first* to understand as much of Nature as suffices for acquiring such a nature; *next*, to form a society of the kind that is desirable, so that as many as possible may attain it as easily and surely as possible" (ibid., p. 11). Indeed, this sort of political association is itself part of the end, that is to attain "knowledge of the union that the mind has with the whole of Nature." Elsewhere, Spinoza simply ignores medicine

Spinoza's approach shows the marginal place medicine occupies in his corpus and why he chooses a different focus for countering threats to our bodies than does Descartes. What steers their choice of practices, I suggest, is a rather different conception of how finitude brings vulnerability, which in turn may rest on a different model of the finitude in question. Spinoza gives a fairly clear indication of his conception of finitude in the already cited demonstration to Proposition 3 of Part IV: "given a man, there is something else, say A, more powerful. And given A, there is something else again, say B, more powerful than A, and so on, to infinity…." Here, to be finite is a matter of being a member of a series that is always followed by yet a greater member. Just as with the counting numbers, we can always generate another member by some successor function. Thus, the finitude of any singular thing is shown by its relation to what lies outside and following it – in particular, by its being *less than* what follows. So, the characteristic feature of finite things on this view is just what makes them vulnerable to something else.

Spinoza's "Letter on Infinity" (to L. Meyer, 20 April 1663)[26] muddies the waters a bit by distinguishing several senses of infinity: Spinoza distinguishes there between what is infinite by its nature or definition and what is infinite solely by virtue of its cause (as well as what is merely "indefinite"). The distinction between what is essentially Infinite and what is infinite only by virtue of its cause (and thus can be conceived without its infinitude) marks the special Spinozistic distinction between substance and (infinite) modes. We need not worry about this

[25] Curley (1985), p. 11. Taking "this end" to be served by health to refer to the antecedent "moral philosophy" would marginalize medicine yet further: medicine would then be merely a means to a means. But this does not seem the most plausible reading of the passage cited above. My thanks to Don Garrett, Michael Rosenthal and Erica Tucker for pressing me on this point.

[26] A translation of this letter can be found as letter 12 in Spinoza, *The Complete Works*, tr. S. Shirley (Indianapolis, IN: Hackett Publishing, 2002), especially pp. 787–8, 790, and in Curley (1985), esp. pp. 201–202, 205

distinction here, noting only that Spinoza talks of the infinitude of the latter in terms of a lack of limits [*nullos fines*]. He likewise emphasizes the unboundedness of the first sense of Infinite in his letter to Johann Hudde of 10 April 1666,[27] where he explicitly states that an infinite being cannot be conceived as determinate [*determinatum*], for the reason that any such conception would suppose bounds, outside of which the being did not exist. Although the same letter mentions various other necessary properties of infinite beings, including simplicity and indivisibility, many of Spinoza's arguments rest on the centrality of the notion of a single, unbounded being. Alan Gabbey uses these passages to argue that "the key idea" in Spinoza's conception of infinity is "indeterminateness through the absence of termini."[28] Just as in his conception of the finitude of singular things, then, what matters most is the relation to what is outside—or rather, the impossibility of there being any relation to any outside.

For all these special distinctions, Spinoza shares much the same concepts of the Infinite and finitude as we saw in Descartes, particularly the insistence on the epistemic and ontological priority of the Infinite over finitude. Nonetheless, I think we can find an important shift in their sense of the features of finitude that make for vulnerability. In contrast to Spinoza's emphasis on the relation to what lies outside, Descartes concentrates his attention particularly on the relation of composition between parts and whole. As we saw before, Descartes makes the traditional attribution of divine simplicity: God has no parts; moreover, God has only attributes, not modes. Spinoza, however, grants God both attributes and infinite modes, an infinity of infinite modes flowing from God's substance and attributes. The sharp contrast between Descartes's denial of modes attributable to God's substance, and Spinoza's endorsement of them may be largely explained by both Spinoza's slightly altered notion of mode (which has to do more with conceptual dependence than variability) and his discovery of a notion of infinitude appropriate to modes. But I think it may also reflect Descartes's view that the admission of any sort of mode implies divisibility into some sort of part,[29] on the grounds that the possibility of qualitative change in a substance requires that the substance alter either some of its parts, or at least some of the relations among its parts.

We should recall here Descartes's emphasis on the unending divisibility of matter as a mark of its finitude: because any extended thing is *composed* of smaller and smaller parts, it counts as finite and imperfect. More generally, he takes it that all of the proper parts of a finite thing are smaller than the thing itself, and all the proper parts of the parts smaller still, *ad indefinitum*. The view is an example of the Euclidean axiom that the whole is greater than its parts, which Descartes

---

[27] See Letter 35 in Shirley (2002), esp. pp. 856–7.

[28] Gabbey (2008), p. 47.

[29] Spinoza struggles mightily against this inference when arguing that both the attribute and the modes of extension can belong to God, see *Ethics* I P15s, also the letter to Meyer in Curley (1985), p. 203.

cites several times as an example of a "common notion" (see Letter to Plempius, 20 December 1637, AT I: 476; CSMK III: 77, and to [Mesland], 2 May 1644, AT IV: 111; CSMK III: 231; the axiom also figures in several of Descartes's causal maxims). Like other geometric axioms, the proposition depends on God's creative volition, and so it may well fail to apply in any obvious way to God.[30] Indeed, there is good reason to think that it does not so apply. As we saw before, Descartes denies that God is subject to any sort of change or modification. For this reason alone, God is not subject to division into parts, since Descartes considers the possibility of partition in things to be a kind of modal distinction. Although Descartes refuses to ascribe partitions or modifications to God, he does allow that God has attributes, which we might understand as aspects of God, e.g., God's power, goodness, wisdom, etc. Were these to be considered parts, they would necessarily be parts that are not less than the whole—which is to deny that they are parts in any sense we can comprehend. At the risk of committing an anachronism, we might say that Descartes conceives of the positive Infinite as having *only* the properties of a Dedekind-infinite set, that is, a set the infinity of which is characterized by its possession of proper subsets that have as great cardinality as the set itself.[31] In contrast, the finite—no matter how indefinitely divisible—only has proper subsets that are Dedekind-finite, that is, with fewer members than the set itself.

By putting the point so, I do not mean to ascribe some prescient, yet inaccurate grasp of modern set theory to Descartes; I mean only to emphasize how he builds his conception of finitude on the containment and composition of parts, while denying anything of the kind to the genuinely Infinite. Descartes and Spinoza offer compatible approaches to thinking of finitude.[32] But they divide the conceptual labor rather differently, and the division of labor carries over into their approach to

---

[30] The general claim about dependence on God is meant to be a consequence of Descartes's doctrine of the "eternal truths," a topic of much discussion and no little confusion. That the doctrine is a matter of dependence, however, seems widely recognized among French-language commentators, e.g., Jean-Luc Marion, *Sur la Théologie Blanche de Descartes* (Paris: Presses Universitaires de France, 1981), J-M. Beyssade, *La Philosophie Première de Descartes* (Paris: Flammarion, 1979). Jonathan Bennett also makes this point explicitly, "Descartes's Theory of Modality" in *The Philosophical Review* 103 (1994), pp. 639–67, see especially pp. 641–3. I have examined the significance of the doctrine for the distinction between God's Infinity and the finitude of created things in an unpublished piece "The View from Where We Are: Descartes on Eternal Truths, My Nature, and its Sources," and to a lesser extent in "On the Eternal Truths: A Commentary on Papers by G. Walski, I. Agostini, and L. Devillairs" *Descartes e i Suoi Avverari: incontri Cartesiani II*, ed. G. Belgioiso (Le Monnier Università, Lecce 2004), pp. 61–70.

[31] Roughly, we can say that this means that the members of the set and the subset can be put in one-to-one correspondence with each other; for example, the set of all the counting numbers can be put in one-to-one correspondence with the set of all the even counting numbers.

[32] Indeed, it seems fairly easy to understand the composition out of smaller parts in terms of the relation to a following member of a series, and vice-versa.

the vulnerability our finitude confers. Descartes models finitude on the composition out of smaller parts, and so it makes sense to concentrate on how any finite, extended thing is made vulnerable by interference in the relation between part and whole, or even by the parts' interfering with the operation of the whole. That is just the view that drives the mechanico-medical strategies Descartes advocates: the conditions that create vulnerability are, so to speak, internal to the finite thing, a matter of its composition.

Again, such a view is not incompatible with allowing threats from what lies outside, from what is larger and more powerful than the thing itself. But the emphasis lies elsewhere.. Consider Descartes's word of advice to Pollot (possibly) in 1648:

> [H]owever energetic or healthy we may be, we ought also to be prepared to meet death without regret when it comes, because it may come at any time, and any action we perform may cause it. If we eat a piece of bread, it may be poisoned; as we walk down the street we may be hit by a falling roof-tile; and so on (AT V: 558; CSMK III: 359).

Although flying roof-tiles clearly represent threats to batter us from outside, the example of the poisoned bread is just as clearly a case of disruption from the inside, since it would be harmless unless ingested. In contrast, Spinoza is adamant that "no thing can be destroyed except through an external cause" (E IIIP4). To be sure, on Spinoza's reckoning, a poisoned piece of bread would still count as an "external" cause of death, for it cannot count as a proper part of the singular thing that it harms. Healthful bread, in contrast, can become one of our proper parts when we incorporate it into our bodies to further our conatus. Such distinctions follow directly from Spinoza's individuation of singular things through their conatus, a move that entails that all threats are *ipso facto* "external." Spinoza refuses to countenance the possibility of harm from small, "internal" disruptions—the sorts of disruptions that are the particular province of the medical arts. Of course, Spinoza does not deny the possibility of medicine, since he accords it some instrumental value. But he cannot adopt Descartes's view that the need for medical interventions is intrinsic to our very nature as singular things. Instead, he insists on the rather different point that insofar as we are singular things *in* nature, we will always be vulnerable to damage and destruction. The difference may seem so subtle as to be sophistical, but if I am right, it prompts contrasting conceptions of and responses to our vulnerability.

## Mind-Body Vulnerability and Finitude

To close, I would like to address a somewhat different issue: if it is finitude as such that produces vulnerability, then finite minds should be vulnerable just as finite bodies are. Do Descartes and Spinoza recognize a distinctive psychic frailty? Neither the strategy of political incorporation according to the metaphor of the artificial body, nor that of medical intervention seems directly to address the vulnerabilities of minds. But they might do so indirectly, through the medium of the body. Despite their rather different accounts of the metaphysics of mind and body, I think that both Spinoza and Descartes put great stock in such indirect approaches to psychic vulnerability. Each also directly confronts the vulnerability of finite minds. Because what is at stake is our susceptibility to disturbance and disruption, these direct strategies have a whiff of Stoicism, but because both acknowledge our intrinsic vulnerability, it remains only a whiff.

Once again, Spinoza can provide a touchstone for the discussion, since he not only distinguishes his strategies by divisions in the *Ethics* (political in Part IV, as well as in the *Theological-Political Treatise*, and individual and psychic in Part V), but the parallelism of the attributes requires that much the same issues of vulnerability, passivity and activity arise for minds as for bodies. By the same token, any strategy directed at one will also be effective for the other. Because the order and connection of ideas is the same as the order and connection of things (IIP7), and because the mind is identified as the idea of the body (IIP11–13), strengthening and perfecting the body also strengthens and perfects the mind. Since there is no causal action across different attributes (IIP6), a strong body does not cause a strong mind or vice-versa; rather, they are simply two aspects of the same thing, which increase or diminish their power in tandem. Appealing to the consequences of parallelism may help us make sense of the full import of Spinoza's political strategy for resisting vulnerability. Forming a commonwealth truly does mean that we incorporate our bodies into a larger, "artificial" body. That body counts as an individual striving to maintain itself and increase its powers, insofar as it coordinates our movements towards self-maintenance. The incorporation of the body politic, however, is simply the converse of our psychic identification with a larger self. Rather than being torn by contrary, individual passions, we act on what we have in common with others. When we are not the plaything of passions, we act for our own advantage, or rationally. Reason, however, is what we have in common with others. Insofar as we act rationally, and for our own advantage, that advantage is also common to others, and so we act for the common good. The upshot is that we ally ourselves with what is common, and forge a common identity. To become part of a unified polity is genuine psychosomatic identification with the whole.

Spinoza also recommends techniques that are much more obviously psychic than somatic in character.[33] This is the case with many of the most widely recognized "remedies" for the bondage of the passions that Spinoza advocates. Without going into the often problematic nuts and bolts of those remedies (see VP20 for examples), the trick that they are all supposed to perform is to replace merely passive affects (passions) with active ones—either by countering reactive

33 This aspect of Spinoza's thought seems at odds with his parallelism, and raises difficult questions about how Part V conceives the identity of the mind that achieves salvation; see Rutherford (1999) for a detailed discussion.

passions with stronger affects, or by transforming passions into active affects through a kind of emotional jujitsu. Passions are to be transformed, not because they are inevitably harmful, but simply because they are *passive,* that is, reactive states in us. As such, they are (partly) caused by external objects. The more we are prey to passions, the more we are subject to being battered by outside forces. But converting our passions into genuinely active affects means that we become their adequate causes, and thereby incorporate them into our conatus. As such, these affects both constitute an expression of our power, and work to increase our power. The strategy, then, involves assimilating whatever can be taken in to an increasingly powerful self, and eliminating that which cannot be so incorporated.

That such assimilation constitutes an increase in our power helps explain Spinoza's identification of the growth of the affects with the increase in genuine knowledge (of the "third kind"). That growth in knowledge is identified with the (intellectual) love of God, and ultimately with the state Spinoza calls blessedness [*beatitudo*]. But we achieve such a state, it seems, by identifying ourselves as much as possible with God, or Nature, that is, with the infinite whole. Spinoza argues that the "Mind's intellectual Love of God is part of the infinite Love by which God loves himself" (VP36), and that the wise man is "by a certain eternal necessity, conscious of himself, and of God, …" (VP42sch). This seemingly psychic and individual strategy, then, is analogous to the "political" strategy of identification with a larger whole; indeed, it goes one step further, insofar as it pushes us to identify with the infinite whole. It is no wonder, then, that Spinoza takes such a person to have a mind "whose greatest part is eternal" (VP39).

Of course, we never perfectly achieve our end, for we cannot become solely active, adequate causes of all of our states, any more than we can become fully knowledgeable. Only God can (and is) perfect in these senses; even though we strive to become like unto God, we will necessarily fall short (see VP36). That we will always be imperfect and incomplete is one way in which Spinoza departs from a rigidly Stoic conception of human virtue. Many ancient Stoics proposed an ideal of freedom that involved a full *apatheia*, in which we would not be subject to passions of any sort, but in complete control over our own "internal" states. But Spinoza counts this an impossible ideal; our status as singular things in nature forbids such thorough independence. Our fate as metaphysically dependent entities is not necessarily an unhappy one, however. Passions always have external causes, and those causes can enfeeble us—but they can also increase our power. This is the flip side of our vulnerability: we can be acted upon by forces that strengthen us, and thereby make us *less* vulnerable to damage.[34] We natural things cannot become, or be made, invulnerable. External natural forces eventually will conspire in our downfall, but they can also conspire that—for a time—we have a drive, a force, a conatus that increases through its own operations. Indeed, if we exist at all, then they must have done so.

---

[34] I thank Ursula Goldenbaum for clarifying the importance of the asymmetry in Spinoza's thinking.

Spinoza's treatment of the passions bears many similarities to Descartes's, but here we may find the differences between their projects equally instructive. Descartes is not just concerned with fortifying our defenses against outside intrusion, but in harnessing external forces to our benefit—even while they remain external. For this reason, he is particularly interested in methods for dealing with our vulnerabilities that work through and across the mind and body, without adopting anything like Spinoza's parallelism. Descartes's interest is illustrated in a 1645 exchange of letters with Princess Elisabeth of Bohemia, prompted by concern over a "low grade fever" suffered by Elisabeth. Descartes suggests that she is suffering from melancholy, for which he proposes reading Seneca in the service of reflecting on her mind and its ability to master bodily-based passions. Elisabeth takes some umbrage at what she first sees as Descartes's overly sanguine approach, pleading the "weaknesses" of her body as an example of how bodily conditions, such as illness or damage, may interfere with our reasoning and willing, make us more prone to the passions, and thereby compromise our ability to apply the cure Descartes has recommended. (Elisabeth to Descartes, 24 May 1645, AT IV 208).[35] Elisabeth's point is a direct challenge to any claim of the mind's inviolability: whereas reasoning and willing are activities proper to our nature, we are passive recipients of the effects of bodily malfunction. Such effects, whether passions in the narrow sense, or other kinds of perceptions, are states inflicted upon us by "external" causes—passions in the broadest sense of the term.[36] Indeed, all effects arising in the body (and originating even farther afield) count as passions in this sense. So, the bodily conditions under discussion in the correspondence represent genuine interference with and constraints on our own proper psychic activities. Our finite minds can be disrupted by what lies outside their limits, even to the extent of impairing their proper functioning, although their substance is not be subject to natural destruction. Descartes fully admits our limitations when pressed by Elisabeth, despite maintaining that happiness involves a "mastery" of the passions that allows our rationality and proper willing to flourish.

For this reason, there is real urgency to the question Elisabeth ultimately poses: even if we do manage to overcome the passions and achieve happiness, is it possible to do so "without the assistance of that which does not depend absolutely on the will?" (Elisabeth to Descartes, 16 August 1645, AT IV 269).[37] Descartes's answer is complicated; on the one hand, we do indeed require the cooperation of that which does not depend absolutely on the will, for the same reason that Spinoza admits: finding oneself in the position of strength, health, or power such that one can act to resist intrusions from outside is at least initially a matter of luck—of external forces conspiring in our favour. Unfortunately, we sometimes

---

35 For a translation, see Shapiro (2007), pp. 88–90.

36 This is a use of "passion" endorsed in the *Passions of the Soul* §1–2 (AT XI: 327–8; CSM I: 328). Note that in this late work Descartes has come to restrict our activities solely to willing; see §17 (AT XI: 342; CSM I: 335).

37 For a translation, see Shapiro (2007), pp. 99–101.

find that "a bodily indisposition prevents [our] will from being free" (AT IV: 282; CSMK III: 262–3). But if we manage to have our mind "at liberty," we should find ourselves better able to resist "indisposition" and its attendant difficulties later. Here and elsewhere, Descartes cleaves to a notion of happiness and virtue very similar to that of the Stoics before him, and Spinoza after; these goods involve a kind of autonomy, of acting according to one's own proper nature, so that one escapes fortune's vicissitudes.

This quasi-Stoic aspect of Descartes's thought is most obvious in his identification of a resolute "disposition of the will" as the good for the individual.[38] Descartes fastens on the resolution of the will precisely because he takes it that it is the only thing fully in our control. This is made explicit in his letter of November 1647 to Queen Christina of Sweden, where he contrasts several kinds of goods on the basis of what does and does not depend on us. In general, the goods of the soul are to be preferred to those "of the body and of fortune," because the latter "do not depend at all absolutely on us" (AT V: 83). Even among those proper to the soul, the good of willing that which is good—or at least what we decide to be good—is to be preferred to that of knowing what is good, since "knowledge is often outside our powers [*la connaissance est souvent au delà de nos forces*]" (AT V: 83). Because our will is something "which we can dispose of absolutely" [*notre volonté, dont nous puissions absolument disposer*], it counts as the "sovereign good of the individual" (AT V: 83). For as he declares early in the letter, "we should not consider anything as good, in relation to ourselves, unless we either possess it or have the power to acquire it" (AT V: 82, CSMK III: 324).

This supreme good, however, brings happiness, which Descartes identifies with "contentment" (see letter to Elisabeth, 18 August 1645, AT IV: 275; CSMK III: 261). Such contentment is a pleasure that is both within the soul and related in complicated ways to things outside of it (see AT V: 84–5; CSMK III: 325–6). The ideal of freeing oneself from the slings and arrows of fortune remains; such freedom is just what produces the state of "tranquility," or "contentment," without the pangs of remorse, repentance or regret.[39] But it is important to recognize that this contentment is not a completely dispassionate state. Descartes chides those "cruel" philosophers who "require their sage to be insensible," holding instead that the passions are the sources of "the sweetest pleasures in this life" and "are all good in their nature" (AT XI: 485; modified from CSM I: 403). What Descartes means by "passions" here are a species of perceptions generated by bodily movements; they have external causes and so cannot depend absolutely on the will. Descartes goes on to sketch a complicated relationship between passions,

[38] This may seem problematically circular since the resolute disposition that is good is precisely that to pursue what we judge to be the good. Presumably, Descartes's treatment of the voluntary resolution as the good for the individual represents a meta-stance that plays little role in our concrete practical reasoning.

[39] On these terms, as well as on the notion of "fortune," see Deborah Brown (2005), especially Chapter 7.

virtue and contentment, which illustrates how part of the "strength" and "power" of finite things such as we are lies in harnessing the cooperation of things that do not depend absolutely on our will.

By the time of the *Passions of the Soul*, Descartes has come to treat only our will*ing* as an activity proper to us. Even the perceptions *of* our volitions are passions in a broad sense (see §19, AT XI: 343; CSM I: 335–6). But just because he admits a very broad scope to the passions, Descartes seems to think it a hopeless task to eliminate them. Furthermore, he does not seem to think we can expel from ourselves everything that is *not* one of our proper parts or activities; we cannot push out whatever does not belong to our essential, but finite nature, so that it lies safely beyond our boundaries. In particular, certain kinds of passivity, such as perceptual receptivity, are endemic to our condition as limited beings. This is the analogue to the intrinsic divisibility of all extended things. It belongs to the limitations of finite minds to be not just porous, but riddled with passivity, externality, and a certain kind of otherness. Since we cannot simply fortify ourselves against those intrinsic intrusions (to speak oxymoronically), we need to learn to work with them.

It is on such an understanding of what our finitude involves that Descartes formulates his intricate, ambivalent and dynamic notion of the "remedies" for the passions. He explicitly recognizes that we are always subject to passions that can overwhelm us, and disrupt the firmest resolutions made unilaterally by the will; no voluntary stiffening of the upper lip will suffice to rid us of our susceptibility. Instead, we must equip ourselves with "proper weapons," particularly "firm and determinate judgments bearing upon the knowledge of good and evil, which the soul has resolved to follow in guiding its conduct" (AT XI: 367; CSM I: 347).[40] But this is just the first step, for we should also alter our very *dispositions* to feel the passions, learning new and improved "habits" (AT XI: 369; CSM I: 348). Those habits involve stopping, or transforming "the bodily movements which accompany" certain passions. Moreover, we develop such habits by working on the body, particularly through that part of the brain that Descartes identifies as the corporeal imagination. Imagining different states of affairs, or different responses to the state of affairs causes brain events, which over time can alter the structures and dynamics of the brain by which various passions are generated. Such imaginative practice then becomes an indirect, but voluntary way to reshape our internal bodily "dispositions" so that they produce specific passions under the appropriate, rationally endorsed circumstances.

These practices constitute "remedies" for the passions. But the chief remedy for the passions is itself a *passion*. This is "generosity," which is treated at length in Part III of the *Passions*. It is, in fact, both a passion and a virtue. It is a passion

[40] Descartes goes on in these passages to take back some of what he said in the letter to Christina, noting in particular that "the strength of the soul is inadequate without knowledge of the truth." Here he seems to allow that the very strength of a soul may depend on that which he had previously declared to lay outside of its bailiwick, namely knowledge of the truth. See §49, AT XI: 367–8; CSM I: 347.

because it is a perception "caused, strengthened, and maintained by" bodily mechanisms that are not directly under our control. More particularly, it is a form of esteem, which is itself a species of "wonder," the first of the passions. Generosity is esteem that takes ourselves, particularly our free will, as its object; as a species of wonder, it keeps our attention focused on the experience of our own free will. Feeling the passion of generosity is just what we need to ensure that we resolve to use the will we wonder at properly. Thus, generosity is also a virtue. Because it is both passion and virtue, generosity shows interplay between what is internal to us and what is external, between what is active in us and what is passive. On the one hand, developing the passion of generosity requires focusing on what is in our control; on the other, it is receptive to and dependent on what lies outside. Generosity provides autonomy, so that generous people "have complete command over their passions ...in particular ... over their desires, and over jealousy and envy, because everything they think sufficiently valuable to be worth pursuing is such that its acquisition depends solely on themselves" (AT XI: 448; CSM I: 385). But we develop this autonomy by learning to work with and through our bodies, by exploiting the movement of the spirits to strengthen the habits of generosity, which "are both actions of virtue and at the same time passions of the soul" (AT XI: 453; CSM I: 387–8). Generous, experienced autonomy is not unlimited: it is the autonomy available to a *finite* creature, one who will always be vulnerable to what is alien, yet tries to shape that susceptibility to its own ends.

The nature of the autonomy available to us may provide yet another reason for Descartes's turn to medicine. The "remedies" for the passions, the disciplines of virtue, and the development of generosity are all presented as therapeutic regimens for the soul, designed to correct its weaknesses and increase its power. But this therapy is not so much a technique for fortifying body and soul against external invasion, as it is an art for harnessing the imagination and the rest of the body to work for the good of the soul. By the same token, medicine directed at the good of the body may make use of psychic resources: Descartes insists in several places (including the letters to Elisabeth) that controlling the passions has important consequences for bodily health. Indeed, the rational education of the passions should cultivate bodily health, including proper heat, digestion, and so forth, just as bodily hygiene should seek to "remedy" the passions. Both, however, are open-ended and dynamic processes, for the possibility of disruption—that is, of something for which we will need a remedial treatment—is endemic to our finitude as both mind and body.

The view of Descartes's "medical" response might strike some readers as surprising, especially the contrast it draws to Spinoza's "political" approach. If I am right, the tenor of their strategies for managing the vulnerabilities that come with our finitude inverts their metaphysical postures neatly. On the one hand, Spinoza presents us with a view in which a singular thing in nature acts to reduce its vulnerability by turning its passive affects into active ones, and thereby increases the boundaries within which the singular thing is safe from external threats. It can use materials from outside, that is, its passions, to accomplish its end, but the goal is to throw up a circle of fortifications, and then to enlarge it as much as possible. The strategy is to deter incursions, in spite of Spinoza's position that all finite, singular things are only modally differentiated from other finite singular things, or from the infinite modes, attributes, and substance of which they are an expression. On the other hand, Descartes suggests that we manage the vulnerabilities of our finitude by arranging matters so that what lies outside of our immediate control will be disposed to further our goals, rather than interfere with them. The picture of our autonomy he presents is one woven out of both active and passive elements of our nature. We develop such autonomy by using bodily means to address mental vulnerabilities, and to a lesser extent, applying psychic therapies to bodily infirmities. Descartes's strategy stands even though he differentiates mind and body metaphysically more sharply than does Spinoza, and even though he counts minds as distinct, if finite substances. Still, we should not exaggerate the differences. For both recognize the importance of our vulnerability, and both recognize that it is our status as finite things that makes us vulnerable. These insights are worth remembering.[41]

[41] I'd like to thank a number of people for helpful discussions on topics related to this paper: they include Alan Gabbey, Rebecca Kukla, Don Garrett, and Alison Simmons. I am grateful to the members of the NY-NJ Early Modern Research Group, especially Martin Lin (who presented a paper on the topic), Raffaella de Rosa, Alan Gabbey (again), Dan Garber, Don Garrett and Ursula Goldenbaum, for an extremely informative consideration of Spinoza's "remedies" for our passions—particularly for clarifying just how difficult the issues are. I also extend thanks to Wade Robison, Hale Ethics Chair at Rochester Institute of Technology, and to the Philosophy Department at Vanderbilt University for inviting me to present this material during their colloquia series, and for the lively and fruitful discussion afterwards. I am likewise grateful for the chance to participate in the Symposium on Spinoza, held at the University of Washington, Seattle, in March 2012, which allowed me to clarify some thoughts (and realize some errors) shortly before going to press: particular thanks are due to Michael Rosenthal and Lisa Shapiro, Don Garrett (again), Erica Tucker, Ursula Renz, and Dai Heide. Stephen Pender rendered a great deal of valuable editorial advice. Al McLuckie and Yual Chiek cheerfully helped with research, and Juan Santos Castro with copy-editing. I would also like to remind Aladdin Yaqûb that he prompted much of my thinking about the role of the positive Infinite in Descartes; I appreciate his insights, but he should not be held responsible for what I made of them. Finally, I gratefully acknowledge financial support received from the Social Sciences and Humanities Research Council of Canada and from the University of Alberta.

# Chapter 7
# The Many Rhetorical Personae of an Early Modern Physician: Girolamo Cardano on Truth and Persuasion

Guido Giglioni

One of Cardano's favorite rhetorical moves is to present himself as immune from the temptations of rhetorical display. He claims with pride that he never indulges in affectation or flourish. Indeed, his is the self-portrait of an anti-rhetorical personality: awkward, disagreeable, shabby, rough-mannered, outspoken, sharp-voiced in arguing, inconsiderate, heedless of social or literary convention. Cardano's very peculiar *excusatio* is in fact a wilful disregard for any *excusatio*. When he sets out to tell the story of his life, his professed aim is to recount in a straightforward manner how the events occurred without resorting to literary embellishment or sugar coating. One of Cardano's fundamental beliefs is that a honest examination of one's own nature is always to be preferred to any form of self-delusion. He warns his readers from that particular kind of complacency that is nothing but "an ignoring of conditions, a pretence of not being aware of what we know exists, or a will to set aside a fact by force," particularly common, Cardano claims, when we treat with "our sins and everything else foul, vain, confused and untrue in our lives."[1] In contrast to professional humanists, Cardano shows no interest in stylistic polish; he has no inclination for irony and sophisticated techniques of literary subversion. He admits to have always relied on the written word more than on memory and oratorical skills.[2]

On the other hand, though, Cardano's views of rhetoric, elusive as they are, shedmore than a little light on a number of issues that were particularly dear to him. The place of rhetorical expertise in human learning becomes a question of dramatic urgency every time he discusses the increasingly widening gap that seems to separate knowledge from actuality. Cardano examines the nature of rhetorical persuasion when he explores feasible ways of managing men's violence without impairing their freedom. Finally—and perhaps most importantly for Cardano's frame of mind—rhetorical critique makes sure that actuality, with all

---

1 Girolamo Cardano, *De vita propria*, in *Opera omnia* (hereafter abbreviated as OO), ed. Charles Spon, 10 vols (Lyon: Jean-Antoine Huguetan and Marc-Antoine Ravaud, 1663), I:11a; Id., *The Book of My Life*, transl. by Jean Stoner (New York: *New York Review of Books*, 2002), 51.

2 Cardano, *De vita propria*, Ch. 23.

its tensions and contradictions, is examined bravely and dispassionately without appealing to escapist solutions (including empty intellectualism). Hence Cardano's various characterizations of rhetoric: rhetoric is sometimes seen as a protective device (through the use of simulation and dissimulation), as a demystifying and debunking inquiry (relying on what he calls *scientia animi*), as a therapeutic tool (by providing awareness of the inescapable reality of the passions and their role in human life).

## Cardano on Rhetoric

A number of scholars have explored the ways in which the recovery of the classical tradition during the fifteenth and sixteenth centuries, in particular of Cicero's work, resulted in a wide variety of rhetorical models and how they found suitable application in new social and institutional settings. The early Renaissance ideals of *vita civile*, in particular the Florentine example of civic humanism—what has been called "a civilization of communication and exchange"—re-proposed a form of wisdom programmatically centered on a skilful use of language and accommodated to the concrete circumstances of life and to the interests and passions of real people.[3] Cardano knew the scope and impact of this movement. By and large, he embraced the humanistic agenda of combining *sapientia* with *eloquentia*, and acknowledged the political and social implications of such a project. In keeping with Cicero's famous pronouncement (*De inventione*…, I, i), he agreed that, while eloquence without wisdom could be dangerously effective, wisdom without eloquence was ineffective. This is particularly evident in such works as *De sapientia* and *Proxeneta.*

In a discussion of Cardano's account of rhetoric, it is important to remember that he was not only a very successful medical practitioner and a professor of medicine at the universities of Padua (154—551 and 1559–1560) and Bologna (1562–70), but that he also contributed significantly to such diverse fields as natural philosophy, astrology, mathematics, music, and ethics. Born in Pavia in 1501, he studied both in Pavia and Padua, where he absorbed the fundamentals of a comprehensive view of both nature and history based on the principles of Aristotelian philosophy.[4] Open to influences coming from the Platonic tradition

---

3 Marc Fumaroli, *L'âge de l'éloquence* (Geneva: Droz, 1980). See also Hans Baron, *The Crisis of the Early Italian Renaissance. Civic Humanism and Republican Liberty in an Age of Classicism and Tyranny* (Princeton: Princeton University Press, 1966); Eugenio Garin, *L'Umanesimo italiano* (Rome and Bari: Laterza, 1964); Nancy S. Struever, *The Language of History in the Renaissance. Rhetoric and Historical Consciousness in Florentine Humanism* (Princeton: Princeton University Press, 1970).

4 On Cardano's natural philosophy, see the fundamental studies by Alfonso Ingegno *(Saggio sulla filosofia di Cardano,* Florence: La Nuova Italia 1980), Ian Maclean ("The Interpretation of Natural Signs: Cardano's *De subtilitate* Versus Scaliger's *Exercitationes,*" in *Occult and Scientific Mentalities in the Renaissance* ed. by Brian

and exposed to a series of existential hardships, Cardano elaborated a notion of rationality that was flexible enough to take notice of the important role played by precariousness and contingency in human life. The Averroistic interpretation of Aristotle, which he assimilated in his studies at Pavia and Padua, gave him a clear awareness that figural language, religious devotion and rhetorical arguments were ineliminable components in every political organization. Although he never accepted the Averroistic view of the intellect as one common source of rational knowledge for all human beings, he endorsed Averroes's preoccupations with the cultural and political dimensions of human knowledge.[5]

Cardano's had a complex and nuanced view of human nature. He was convinced that man's tendency to errors and moral lapses, and the resulting need to look for a proper use of the passions in the public sphere, called for rhetorical aids. In *Proxeneta*, he maintained that especially in society one found it difficult to keep a good reputation and to avoid the consequences of other people's envy.[6] In *De sapientia*, he recommended flexibility and circumspection in dealing with the wide diversity of human character. "Since there is a great variety among human natures [*ingenia*]", he pointed out, "some are ruled by prudence, others are subject to ambition, avarice, fear, and shyness, others are weak and feeble." Differences in character demanded different approaches. "Those natures which are governed by prudence are convinced by reasons. You can seduce the ambitious through flatteries, corrupt the greedy with money, fill the lustful with hope, instigate the timid with terrors, incite the shy by using examples." Cardano reminded his readers of the example of Julius Caesar, who, in Lucan's version, had embraced all the above-mentioned techniques in order to take possession of the state.[7]

By and large, Cardano maintains quite a skeptical attitude toward the ability of reason and language to dispel the power of passions and prejudices. In *Proxeneta*, he bluntly defines persuasion, together with simulation and dissimulation, as one of the ways in which other people can be deceived (*genera fallendi*).[8] In *De sapientia*, the picture is even bleaker. Of the several ways to convince other people, he lists force and violence (*vis*) as the most effective. Then he places, in

---

Vickers (Cambridge: Cambridge University Press, 1984), 231–52; "Cardano's Eclectic Psychology and its Critique by Julius Caesar Scaliger," Vivarium, 46 (2008), 392–417), Nancy Siraisi *(The Clock and the Mirror. Girolamo Cardano and Renaissance Medicine,* Princeton: Princeton University Press, 1997) and Anthony Grafton *(Cardano's Cosmos: The Worlds and Works of a Renaissance Astrologer,* Cambridge and London: Harvard University Press, 1999).

5 On Cardano's attitude towards Averroes, see Guido Giglioni, "Nature and Demons. Girolamo Cardano Interpreter of Pietro d'Abano," in *Continuities and Disruptions between the Middle Ages and the Renaissance*, ed. by Charles Burnett, José Meirinhos and Jacqueline Hamesse (Louvain-la Neuve: Brepols, 2009).

6 Cardano, *Proxeneta*, OO I:453b.

7 Cardano, *De sapientia*, OO I:548b. See Lucan, *De bello civili*, V, 319–64.

8 Cardano, *Proxeneta*, OO I:395b.

descending order, terror, money, and words (*oratio*).[9] By violence, Cardano means extorting someone else's consent "through deception or power, or by flashing hope through someone's mind, or by provoking immoderate affects in him, or by abusing his modesty."[10] In one of his characteristically disconsolate and bleak portraits of human affairs, he describes rhetoric as vicious, medicine poisonous, and poetry fatuous (*rhetorica malefica, venefici medici, poësis stulta*).[11] The list of perils that Cardano associates with a canny and unscrupulous use of words is long: vanity, self-delusion, social and political disruption, emotional disorder, economic greed, even self-inflicted physical injuries. Left to itself, rhetoric occupies the domain of violence.

On the other hand, when used properly, rhetoric provides precisely those means necessary to hold the roots of human violence in check. To keep civil society together, one should choose lesser evil and prefer persuasion to violence and fraud. In the short treatise *De inventione*, Cardano displays a positive attitude toward the function of persuasion, understood as a basic requirement for good scientific practice. Reversing the conclusion reached by Socrates in Plato's *Gorgias*, Cardano claims that rhetoric is not only a science, but a universal science that deals with the making of arguments and demonstrations.[12] In *Dialectica*, the Aristotelian model prevails on the Platonic one (Aristotle, *Rhetorica*, I, 1, 1354a–1355b), and truth is defined as not persuasive on its own. In keeping with other contemporary attempts to reform logic by subordinating the level of syllogistic demonstration to that of rhetorical induction (as in Lorenzo Valla's, Mario Nizolio's, and Peter Ramus's projects), Cardano seeks to incorporate dialectic into the universal scheme of rhetoric.[13] In *De utilitate*, in a section devoted to a survey of the main

---

9 Cardano, *De sapientia*, OO I:548b. See also ibid., 535b: "hominibus praesumus, vel vi, vel consensu, vel mixta quadam via. Vi quidem armorum metu, consensu orationis persuasionis et eloquentia, mixta via legibus ac magistratibus, qui quidem hominum consensu constant vi tamen exerceantur." See also *Proxeneta*, OO I:358b.

10 Cardano, *Proxeneta*, OO I:362a.

11 Cardano, *Mnemosynon*, OO I:234b.

12 Cardano, *De inventione*, OO X:93a: "At medij inventio ad persuasionem pertinet. Appello autem persuasionem scientiam veram etiam demonstrativam, non solum quod demonstratio non excludat persuasionem, sed fortuita, sed etiam quia nostra haec scientia persuasio sit et non omnino certa."

13 Cardano, *Dialectica*, OO I:293ab. See also *Contradicentium medicorum libri duodecim*, OO VI:336ab. On Cardano's views on dialectic, see Antonio Corsano, "La 'dialectica' di Girolamo Cardano," *Giornale Critico della Filosofia Italiana*, 40 (1961), 175–80; Ingo Schütze, "La *Dialectica* di Cardano e la rivalutazione enciclopedica della logica," in *Girolamo Cardano. Le opere, le fonti, la vita*, ed. by Marialuisa Baldi and Guido Canziani (Milan: Angeli, 1999), 147–57; Francesco La Nave, *Logica formale e dialettica nella filosofia di Girolamo Cardano* (Rome: Pontificia Universitas Gregoriana), 2004; Id., *Logica e metodo scientifico nelle* Contradictiones logicae *di Girolamo Cardano* (Pisa: Istituti Editoriali e Poligrafici Internazionali, 2006). On the role of rhetoric as an introduction to the use of logic in medicine, see Jean Fernel, *Medicina* (Venice: Baldassarre Costantino,

disciplines specifically written to highlight the benefits that can be drawn from even the most ignoble arts, rhetoric —garrulity apart—is presented as one of the arts of discourse, capable of making people eloquent, improving their memory, and giving them the ability "to search for and find arguments."[14] Depending on the contexts in which one delivers his speech, Cardano recommends a skilful use of figurative language, for "the figurative mode of speaking (*figuratio*)"—*velut pictura quaedam*—is "closer to the image of the mind than any discourse".[15] What is more, there are genuine epistemological reasons that explain the importance of rhetoric for the attainment of truth. Contrary to the Platonic view that truth *qua* truth is self-evident and as such irrefutable, Cardano believes that the purely intellectual love for truth is not sufficient—"thieves, too, desire to know"—and must be supplemented with the ethical, psychological, and physiognomical ability to distinguish between dishonesty and honesty through discerning perception and finesse of judgment.[16]

As already mentioned, anxiety about the widening gap separating knowledge from reality, opinion from truth, words from things is a recurrent theme in Cardano's writings. He describes the rift between being and appearance as a divide between two types of worlds, the world of natural wisdom and that of human learning, the former being the unmediated and uncorrupted expression of the life of nature and its cognitive functions, the latter the result of a series of increasingly more complex and artificial constructions of human astuteness. Cardano explains that, while one may acquire natural wisdom through the exercise of virtue, discipline, faith, and study, the acquisition of human wisdom depends largely on the work of rhetoricians, political thinkers, and poets.[17] The awareness that such a division pervades human culture and the view that human knowledge is a result of both natural and human wisdom represent the principal assumptions behind Cardano's preoccupations with the role of rhetoric in human life and history.

1555), II, sig. [*iiiv]. On the characteristically Renaissance attempts to extend the scope of rhetoric, see: Garin, *L'Umanesimo italiano*, 171–92; Cesare Vasoli, *La dialettica e la retorica dell'Umanesimo. "Invenzione" e "Metodo" nella cultura del XV e XVI secolo* (Milan: Feltrinelli, 1968); P.O. Kristeller, "Rhetoric in Medieval and Renaissance Culture," in *Renaissance Thought and the Arts* (Princeton: Princeton University Press, 1990), 228–46; Brian Vickers, "Rhetoric and Poetics", in *The Cambridge History of Renaissance Philosophy*, ed. by Charles B. Schmitt, Quentin Skinner, Eckhard Kessler and Jill Kraye (Cambridge: Cambridge University Press, 1988), 715–745; George A. Kennedy, *Classical Rhetoric and Its Christian and Secular Tradition from Ancient to Modern Times* (Chapel Hill and London: The University of North Carolina Press, 1999) 241.

14 Cardano, *De utilitate*, OO II:131a.

15 Cardano, *Proxeneta*, OO I:373a.

16 Ibid., 356b.

17 Cardano, *De sapientia*, OO I:553b.

## Uses of Rhetoric

Cardano's ambivalent attitudes are apparent when we examine the various contexts in which he explores rhetoric. Cardano the moral philosopher regards rhetoric as the calculated use of language to persuade other people using oblique strategies. In *De consolatione*, he claims that his aim is to convince the reader of the goodness of his moral arguments not in a rhetorical fashion (*non rhetorum more*), but following a philosophical purpose (*philosophorum instituto*).[18] In *Neronis encomium*, he claims that he could use all the artifices of oratory, but his real intention is not "to prove with the pen" what he could not prove inwardly (*animo*).[19] In *De Socratis studio*, rhetoric is presented as an untruthful practice based on the deliberate use of lies and falsehood. As evidence of the unreliable nature of rhetoric and its dangers, Cardano adduces the example of those states which "favored rhetoricians" and were all ruined by them: "Demosthenes destroyed Athens, Aratus the Achaeans, Cicero the Romans."[20]

Throughout his works, Cardano reveals the many shortcomings and pitfalls deriving from an unscrupulous use of rhetoric. One of the most insidious dangers lies in the rhetorician's ability to instill belief in the lack of difference between "knowing how to speak about things and knowing and taking control about the things themselves", between "talking nonsense and arguing."[21] Among the illegitimate kinds of proof (*probatio*) misused by "vicious orators," he lists those based on profit, prudence, examples, and fables.[22] From a psychological and moral point of view, vanity is one of the defining features of rhetoric and rhetoricians. "Ostentation is part of deception," writes Cardano, "because one pretends to have what one does not have", and people usually show off through words, as they do with dialectic and rhetoric.[23] The treacherous territory of human vanity and its rhetorical implications is finely analysed by Cardano in his preface to *De consolatione*. To whom should he dedicate the book he wrote on consolation, he wonders, without risking offending the dedicatee?

> Initially, I had thought of dedicating this book to one of my friends, but then it dawned on me that, because of the topic, the person to whom I would dedicate the volume was likely to be offended. For all men seem to share this trait, namely, that they consider themselves to be less happy than they are, but nonetheless they desire to appear happy. And so rich people parade their riches, kings show off their power, soldiers their strength, learned men blab about their trifles, even to people who have no intention to listen to them. Such is human effort to appear to other people the most different from what they really are.[24]

18 Cardano, *De consolatione*, OO I:625a. See also *Neronis encomium*, OO I:213a.

19 Cardano, *Neronis encomium*, OO I:194b.

20 Cardano, *De Socratis studio*, OO I:152b.

21 Cardano, *De utilitate*, OO II:131a.

22 Cardano, *Proxeneta*, OO I:396ab.

23 Cardano, *De utilitate*, OO II:175a.

24 Cardano, *De consolatione*, OO I:588.

Vanity is for Cardano the symptom of one's deep dissatisfaction with oneself. It is also a sign of the inability to gauge the level of one's own confidence correctly. People think they are in an unfortunate situation (which is not true, but their vanity makes them believe it is so). On the other hand, they also want to give everyone the impression that they are happy (which, again, is not true, but their vanity tells them that, socially speaking—that is, in terms of *civilis existimatio*—it is more advantageous to look happy than unhappy).

In the dialogue *Theonoston*, the character who plays the role of the Citizen objects to the Hermit's ideal of tranquility by saying that, in fact, human happiness derives from change and alternation of passions, as the example of tragedy also demonstrates from an aesthetical point of view. The Hermit replies by saying that such "dubious sciences" as rhetoric disquiet the mind and provoke conflicts and controversies, instead of providing calmness.[25] In *De sanitate tuenda*, Cardano lists the injuries caused by giving public speeches (*profiteri*) and delivering orations before an assembly (*concionari*). For Cardano the physician, the rhetorician's job may have its physiological drawbacks: as a consequence of straining one's voice, the brain and the stomach are hurt, the intercostal muscles get tired, the chest overheats, and the spirits are disturbed. From a strictly medical point of view, the exercise of singing is healthier than rhetorical projection because it widens the lungs and disperses the black bile.[26]

Judging from all these various critical remarks, one would think that Cardano's attitude towards rhetoric is consistently unfavorable. In fact, as I have said, his position is more complex. His disillusioned and painfully critical perception of reality constantly alerts him to the constitutively political dimension of human affairs. A sworn enemy of any form of intellectualistic optimism, Cardano considers dissimulation and lies (and not just noble lies) to be an ineradicable component of public life, an integral part of the worlds of *civilis negociatio* and *humana sapientia*. More specifically, he theorizes the social expediency and advisability of controlling the outward expression of one's inner life, to the point of recommending the achievement of a condition of emotional indifference.

> I have accustomed my features always to assume an expression quite contrary to my feelings: thus I am able to feign outwardly, yet within know nothing of dissimulation. This habit is easy if compared to the practice of hoping for nothing, which I have bent my efforts toward acquiring for fifteen successive years, and have at least succeeded. And now, trained to pretenses of a sort, I sometimes go forth clad in rags, but just as often elegantly dressed; sometimes

---

25 Cardano, *Theonoston*, OO II:341b–342a. See also *Proxeneta*, OO I: 400b.

26 Cardano, *De sanitate tuenda*, OO VI:66a–67a. On the structure of public speech (*publica professio*), see *De sapientia*, OO I:526a. On Cardano's views on singing, see Guido Giglioni, "'Bolognan Boys are Beautiful, Tasteful, and Mostly Fine Musicians': Cardano on Male-Sex Love and Music", in *The Sciences of Homosexuality in Early Modern Europe*, ed. by Kenneth Borris and George Rousseau (London and New York: Routledge, 2008), 201–20.

> I am taciturn, and sometimes talkative; sometimes gay, sometimes sad. From these moods all things acquire double aspects.[27]

Hoping for nothing represents for Cardano the ground zero of man's expressiveness. Emotional indifference does not mean a form of Stoic rational impassiveness, nor an attitude of jaded callousness acquired from being repeatedly disappointed in life. Rather, emotional indifference is for Cardano the psychological and physiological condition *sine qua non* for reticent and guarded behavior in society. Intriguingly, emotional suppleness finds a counterpart in physiognomy. Cardano tells how his "truly commonplace" physical appearance proved to be a nightmare for more than one painter, who took great pains in making his portrait.[28]

Cardano's view of rhetoric is closely linked to his conception of language. Language is first of all a social medium. Since man is a "talking", "gregarious", and "civic" animal, he needs other people's "homage", "help", and "opinion". Indeed, Cardano believes that man's knowledge and power are increased by glory, honor, fame, friends, and means, that is, by the whole spectrum of social relationships that goes under the name of *civilis conversatio*. To Cardano, the praise of cognitive solipsism and moral self-sufficiency sung by the Stoics sounds false ("because they live in a way which is different from what they teach"), vain ("because their deeds do not correspond to their words"), and impious ("because they impute to the mortals what pertains to the gods").[29] Although deliberately offered as a rhetorical paradox, Cardano's presentation of Nero as a victim of Seneca's initiation to the paradoxical views of Stoic philosophy is nonetheless significant.[30] Cardano often repeats the Aristotelian saying (*Pol.*, I, 2, 1254a) that a solitary man is either a god or a beast. He counters Diogenes' inane gestures of ascetic exhibitionism with the concrete heroism of Marco Antonio Bragadin, the Venetian governor of Cyprus killed in 1571 in the attempt to defend Famagusta from the Turks, and the contrast has a clear political and civic meaning. In the end, philosophical rigor is for Cardano synonymous with folly.[31]

The whole system of social and political interactions (*civilis negotiatio*) is thus based on the way in which one's own reputation and conformity to shared values (*civilis existimatio*) is improved by a skilful handling of the many opportunities offered by public life (*civilis conversatio*). The natural world of plants and animals has no part in artifice and deceit; the intelligible world of the blessed souls is an unadulterated reflection of sheer truth: only man's middle world is "the seat of fickleness and falsehood."[32] But this is precisely the reason why knowledge

---

27 Cardano, *De vita propria,* OO I:10b; *The Book of My Life,* 47–8.

28 Cardano, *De vita propria,* OO I:5a; *The Book of My Life,* 19.

29 Ibid., 355–56, 400b.

30 Cardano, *Neronis encomium,* OO I:198b. Cardano's praise of Nero stands in the same tradition of Gorgias' praise of Helen.

31 Cardano, *De vita propria*, OO I:11b.

32 Cardano, *De Socratis studio*, OO I:152a. See also *De vita propria*, OO I:9a; *De inventione*, OO X:95a.

of rhetoric is essential. In a world in which deception and violence hold sway, the art of detecting deceit and protecting oneself from abuse has necessarily a positive value: "we must hide not only things and words, but also our mind," is a characteristically Cardanian maxim.[33] There is latitude, in his opinion, in the extent to which simulation and dissimulation may be allowed, and it depends on particular circumstances, the people with whom we are dealing, and the ends we wish to achieve.[34]

Because of the discrepancy between thoughts, words, and deeds, nothing seems to be more appropriate and convenient than to live "cautiously, moderately, and discreetly," to become experienced and dexterous in the many situations of life, and to establish a rich network of social relationships (*conversatio familiaritasque cum multis*), "especially if someone lives at the court of a prince or in big cities."[35] When it cannot be manifested overtly, dissent needs to follow the circuitous paths of simulation and dissimulation. In *De sanitate tuenda*, Cardano suggests that our thoughts be "joyful and cheerful" so that "they can be less subject to the distrustful scrutiny of princes and magistrates" and "we can live better with our fellow citizens."[36] The art of conversation, meant as a harmonious blend of ethics and etiquette, is another key aspect in Cardano's view of civic life. At court, the language of conversation must be smooth and adapted to the various kinds of people with whom one deals. One should be able to speak of "beauty and style" with women, of politics with magistrates, of heroic virtues with military officers, of estate and business with wealthy people.[37] Even one's gait can be a telling indicator of one's character.[38] In social intercourse, he recommends not to appear "sad, thoughtful, or more joyful than is appropriate." During conversation, it is important not to touch on public events, civil laws, or God, and to focus instead on "common talk" such as the weather, the site of the city, weddings, matters of economy, common friends, and one's own studies. When talking, it is not appropriate to lower one's eyes—"which many people do —to speak in a loud or in a low voice, or to laugh like a madman or a scoffer. Recalling Solomon's rules (*Prov*. 12:13–14; 13:15; 16:23), Cardano suggests that one can improve one's own social status (*civilis existimatio*) by learning to control one's own gait, attire, and words. In *Proxeneta*, he sings the praises of the virtue of *comitas*, understood as a combination of courteousness, affability, and kindness.[39] Attention to every little detail is crucial. In the spirit of the tradition of handbooks on good manners, a tradition that counted Erasmus among its most illustrious exponents, he warns

33 Cardano, *Proxeneta*, OO I:374b.

34 Ibid., 394a–395b.

35 Cardano, *De utilitate*, OO II:219a.

36 Cardano, *De sanitate tuenda*, OO VI:37b.

37 Cardano, *De sapientia*, OO I:555b.

38 Cardano, *De vita propria*, OO I:14b–15a.

39 Ibid., 369b–370a. See also *De sapientia*, OO I:523b: "In vestitu, risu, et ambulatione decorem servabit."

people involved in conversations against being too close to the mouth of their interlocutor and, above all, he recommends checking that one's own mouth "does not smell bad." [40]

Cardano appreciates the aspects of critical inquiry characteristic of rhetorical knowledge. He embraces the demystifying power of rhetoric: together with physiognomy, chiromancy, and astrology, rhetoric is an integral part of what Cardano calls *scientia animi*. Rhetoric furnishes the linguistic skills "to detect the friendly, hostile, or sychophantic disposition of he who is talking with you." The first impression we receive from the conversation with someone, his or her appearance and expressions, especially his or her "eyes, face, and gestures," is often crucial.[41] For Cardano, conversations have a precise cognitive function, namely, "to put other people's intentions (*animus*) to the test" and "to discern their habits." In *Proxeneta*, the traditional distinction between demonstrative, deliberative, and forensic rhetoric is presented as a tool of social inquiry to examine divisions in society: equals, superiors, and subordinates.[42] We could say that, for Cardano, rhetoric and medicine share a fundamental critical attitude. Like rhetoric, medicine is a demystifying art. "Not only does this divine art free the bodies from illnesses", writes Cardano in his *Encomium medicinae*, "it also frees the mind from superstitions."[43]

## Cardano's Praise of Medicine

Cardano's stress on the civic and political implications of rhetoric derives from his understanding of the important role that action and execution play in human affairs. *Civilis negociatio* rests on what he calls the "transmutations" between words, things, and actions. The interplay of language, thought, and action can be seen in all those circumstances of life where decisions need to be made, a delicate job that requires timely and careful planning and the ability not to lose sight of the right moment, the *occasio*.[44] In *Ludo aleae*, Cardano asks whether "a learned (*sciens*) physician is also a skilled (*expertus*) one." His answer reaffirms the urgency of timely action and delicate judgment: "[i]n those matters which give time for reflection, the same man is both learned and successful, as in mathematics, jurisprudence, and also medicine, for very rarely does the sick man

---

[40] Cardano, *Proxeneta*, OO I:412b, 442b, 446a. On the Erasmian notion of civility, see Dilwyn Knox, 'Erasmus' *De civilitate* and the Religious Origins of Civility in Protestant Europe', *Archiv für Reformationsgeschichte*, 86 (1995), 107–135.

[41] Cardano, *Proxeneta*, OO I:390a, 391b–392a. For the astrologer's ability to detect human characters and physiognomy, see *Commentaria in Ptolemaeum de astrorum iudiciis*, OO V:102ab.

[42] Cardano, *Proxeneta*, OO I:372b, 399b.

[43] Cardano, *Encomium medicinae*, OO VI:4.

[44] Cardano, *Proxeneta*, OO I:375a, 388b–389a: "occasionem in omnibus actionibus ac sermone observare decet."

admit no delay." There are activities, such as gambling, war, dueling, commerce, the appraisal of gems and paintings, and the recognition of counterfeit or genuine money, in which knowledge, practice, and a certain physical ability are expected to converge in one's mind in a well-timed and expedient manner, for if "no time is given", "guile prevails."[45] As words have the power to move people to action, Cardano admits that rhetoric has something divine in its persuasive power (*in publica autem concione divinum quiddam inest*). Indeed, when a speech is successful, it functions as collective enchantment where "everyone understands the speech as if it were specifically prepared to persuade him, so that even the words do not seem the same for the one and the others and that everyone draws to the better part of what he is listening to, which sometimes depends on good luck."[46] In the same way, physicians, like rhetoricians, make things with words (they exchange things for words, *verba rebus commutare*).[47]

As a whole, Cardano's praise of medicine reflects his ambivalent attitude toward rhetoric. Sometimes he addresses the question of the value of the medical art in the form of a rhetorical encomium, in which medicine is overtly contrasted with rhetoric. Cardano's position is part of a time-honored tradition of *paragoni* between different arts and disciplines, but in his case it is also a rhetorically crafted representation of medicine as a non-rhetorical activity. He often characterizes the decision to devote his life to medicine as a choice in favor of service and social commitment against a vacuous search forpublic recognition. While the life of the physician may be more trying and ethically more challenging than that of the rhetorician, in the end it is also more rewarding:

> Amongst the great majority of nations, the rhetorician is unwelcome; his work is never unanimously appreciated even in the course of the same lawsuit; more often than not he provides unjust rather than just advice; very frequently he finds himself in awkward situations. He may achieve glory or reach his target, but this happens not without using a large number of words, studying hard, great intelligence and tenacious memory—in short, not without the greatest amount of mental and physical energy.

The picture of the physician looks very different. For him:

---

45 Girolamo Cardano, *De ludo aleae*, ed. by Massimo Tamborini (Milan: Angeli, 2006), 82; Engl. transl. by Sydney Henry Gould, in Øystein Ore, *The Gambling Scholar* (Princeton: Princeton University Press, 1953), 225–6. On this aspect, see Guido Giglioni, "Una nuova edizione del *De ludo aleae* di Girolamo Cardano", *Rivista di Storia della Filosofia*, 25 (2008), 75–8.

46 *Proxeneta*, OO I:432a.

47 Ibid., 358b. On the relationships between medicine, law, moral philosophy, and rhetoric in the humanistic context, see Lynn Thorndike, "Medicine versus Law at Florence", in Id., *Science and Thought in the Fifteenth Century. Studies in the History of Medicine and Surgery, Natural and Mathematical Sciences, Philosophy and Politics* (New York: Columbia University Press, 1929), 24–58.

> all places turn into sources of help and protection, whether these come from a garden while he is strolling around, or from uncultivated lands while he is travelling, or from his country while he consults apothecaries. His intelligence is ordinary, so is his memory and the effort he puts in his work, but he does not lack determination, nor does he set goals higher than he can achieve. As an objection to this choice, one might mention the untimely toils, the sleepless nights, the invidious judgements coming from people who criticize with malignant intention what has been done properly, as if it were done in a reckless manner; not to mention unexpected events, plots orchestrated by other physicians and slanderers, and—what is the greatest drawback of all— the hard and regular servile work, so much so that medicine is more wretched than any other discipline. Indeed, medicine always deals with loathsome and painful matters. No wonder it once was a task performed only by slaves. This is all true and I acknowledge it. But is it not also true that we carry with us and have within us everything we see and that you call filthy and loathsome?[48]

As he recounts in his autobiography, Cardano was led to opt for a medical career—thus contravening to his father who would have preferred him to study law—by the expectation that the study of medicine would have provided him with a more universal and philosophical demeanor, being "of a more concern to all the world in every age," "a profession of sincerer character than law; and a pursuit relying rather upon reason and nature's everlasting law, than upon the opinions of men."[49]

On the other hand, every time Cardano feels the need to vindicate the worth of medicine against the liberal disciplines, he is quite willing to acknowledge the rhetorical dimensions of medicine. After all, since Hippocrates' times, the ability to persuade had been recognized as an integral part of the physician's art. In addition, Cardano often recognizes the epistemological features that medicine shares with rhetoric, such as the emphasis on inductive reasoning and the attention to particulars. For him, though, the most positive contribution offered by rhetoric to medicine lies in the treatment of human passions. Rhetoric can be seen as the medicine of the affects. By and large, at the level of the *civilis negociatio*, Cardano's ethical strategies draw on a whole range of therapeutic techniques from the past masters of moral philosophy, such as countering the effects of one emotion with those of its opposite, pre-empting possible future relapses, restraining the power of desire by gauging one's opinions with his or her perception of the external objects, and diverting one's attention from the focus of disorderly passions. However, more than a philosophical therapy based on the exercise of the intellect, Cardano recommends a rhetorical awareness of the affective conditioning of human judgment. Expanding on Aristotle's renowned definition of tragedy, he points out that a well-constructed oration has the same power to arouse and "heal"

48 Cardano, *Encomium medicinae*, OO VI:5–6.

49 Cardano, *De vita propria*, OO I:8b; *The Book of My Life*, 38.

fear and compassion as tragedy.[50] Reliance on the cathartic power of words is what unites rhetoric with poetics and medicine. In Cardano's general account of human disciplines, rhetoric has the same ambivalent status as music. Like music and musicians, rhetoric and rhetoricians capture other people's attention by enticing their senses and the most corporeal faculties of the soul. A rhythmical oration moves the mind more than a loose one because its parts are held together by the law of proportion, and the harmony of the speech softens the passions in the same way as poems and music do.[51] As he argues in *De subtilitate*, the passions of the mind alter the body in the same way as the sounds alter the passions.[52] If we want "to move men's affects," says Cardano, the first rule in oratory is conciseness (*brevitas*). (The only exception is when the audience we are addressing is a large crowd. In this case, "Asianiast" bombast and turgid style are allowed, which is another instance of Cardano's eclecticism in matter of rhetoric).[53]

What is more, Cardano assumes that the very exercise of the process of *inventio* may have a therapeutic influence on the afflicted soul. As he argues in *De sapientia*, the best remedy to free the mind from oppressive thoughts consists in devoting oneself to light-hearted concerns (*curae iucundae*), and "nothing is more delightful than the faculty of invention," with the important disclaimer, though, that excessive absorption into creative activities can turn itself from remedy into poison. Cardano looks at *inventio* as an exercise in controlled alienation, which can set the mind free from impending anxieties, but which can also alter one's mental balance irreparably when pushed too hard. In addition, "as a result coming from the habit to demonstrate," *inventio* makes men "ingenuous". For this reason "those who have applied themselves to mathematics … alienate themselves from the conventions of practical wisdom and from the habits of the rest of human beings, and, because they know how to demonstrate what other people do not know, they come to believe that they are wiser than the rest." The same happens to poets, who, in Cardano's opinion, sometimes are ruined by the very effort they invest in their inventive process.[54]

Sticking to the mutually stipulated rules of practical wisdom (*humana prudentia*) represents for Cardano the key to a successful social life. *Inventio*, as a treatment for the passions, works only when it is controlled and moderated by

---

50 Cardano, *Proxeneta*, OO I:433b. See Arist., *Rhet*, III, 1, 1403b. On Cardano's therapy of the passions, see Guido Giglioni, "Girolamo Cardano on the Passions and Their Treatment", *Bruniana & Campanelliana*, 12 (2006), 25–40.

51 Cardano, *Theonoston*, OO II:348b; *Proxeneta*, OO I:473.

52 Cardano, *De subtilitate*, OO III:585b. On the relationship between passions and music see Ingo Schütze, "Cardano und die Affektenlehre der Musik", *Bruniana & Campanelliana*, 7 (2001), 453–67; Giglioni, "'Bolognan Boys are Beautiful, Tasteful, and Mostly Fine Musicians'. Cardano on Male Same-Sex Love and Music," in *The Sciences of Homosexuality in Early Modern Europe*, ed. by Kenneth Borris and George Rousseau (London and New York: Routledge, 2008), 201–220.

53 Gardano, *Proxeneta*, OO I:372b.

54 Cardano, *De sapientia*, OO I:575ab.

the requirements of *civilis conversatio*. The rigor of demonstrative science and the outbursts of poetical inspiration are not always compatible with the demands of everyday life. In addition to making mathematicians and artists unhappy, lost in a world of intellectual hubris, mathematical abstraction and creative tension produce social outcasts.

## Rewriting Plato's *Gorgias*

Cardano's ambivalence toward rhetoric is at its highest in the *Antigorgias*, a philosophical dialogue that he wrote after the pattern of Plato's *Gorgias* and published in 1566 (in Basel, through Heinrich Petri). The very title is significantly ambiguous. One wonders whether the *anti* of the title means that Cardano's dialogue is a reference against the Platonic dialogue or against Gorgias himself. In other words, did Cardano write an anti-Platonic or an anti-Gorgian dialogue? The most disconcerting but engaging aspect of the dialogue is the fact that both interpretations are tenable and that, throughout the work, condemnations of rhetorical practice alternate with appreciations of its good political uses. Sometimes concern about truth (*cura veritatis*) is shown to pertain exclusively to the philosopher, while rhetoric is dismissed as a useless art; indeed, it is dismissed as not being even an art but a natural skill (*peritia*). At other times, it is the civic function of rhetoric that is brought to the fore, so that rhetoric is presented as the most suitable discipline to master the complex interplay of human decisions and external circumstances in a world of unpredictable contingencies. However, it seems safe to say that Cardano's principal aim in writing *Antigorgias* was to emphasize once again his characteristic anti-Socratism.[55]

Cardano transports the Platonic dialogue to a Renaissance setting and re-enacts the duel between Socrates and Gorgias. He describes his dialogue as taking place the day after Plato's dialogue. The narrative differences between the two works are striking. In Cardano's dialogue, Gorgias appears to be less on the defensive than he was in Plato, while Socrates is presented as an unreliable character, as if, in a way, he were the real sophist. Cardano's *Antigorgias* is seen from the point of view of Gorgias and his friends rather than Socrates', so much so that one could say that the roles are reversed. Socrates looks like Gorgias and Gorgias like Socrates. This time, Socrates and Gorgias appear to be evenly matched and the reader has a hard time deciding the victor. Gorgias asks the questions and Socrates is told to limit himself to giving the answers. The dialogical setting is framed in such a way that Gorgias shows the limits of Socrates' intellectualism, whereas Socrates points to the shortcomings of Gorgias' voluntarism. As a whole, Cardano's attitude is genuinely dialectical, sometimes even more so than Plato's.

---

[55] On Cardano's Socratism, see Ingegno, *Saggio sulla filosofia di Cardano* (Florence: La Nuova Italia, 1980); Micaela Valente, "Per una storia dei rapporti tra retorica e politica nel Cinquecento: Socrate e Cardano", in *Socrate in Occidente*, ed. by Ettore Lojacono (Florence: Le Monnier, 2004), 189–99.

One might argue that Cardano has failed to understand the many nuances of Socrates' irony in the Platonic dialogues and that he has deliberately stiffened the subversive character of the Socratic inquiry to the point of abstract intellectualism. More than anti-Socratic, it would be more correct to say that Cardano's attitude is anti-Senecan, which is a recurrent trait of his ethical investigation. However, this is not the point I want to make here. As a writer, Cardano seems to be quite refractory to the use of irony and in general he has no time for stylistic and rhetorical techniques of argumentative subversion. More than Plato, he acknowledges the practical value and the theoretical legitimacy of rhetoric, because persuasion is useful in itself (*persuadere utile est per se*). In *Gorgias*, Plato questioned the practice of persuasion for the reason that, roughly speaking, truth is convincing in its own right, and therefore any technique that pretends to mediate between the truth and its reception is redundant or deceitful (based as it is on a purely instrumental and formal use of the language).[56] By contrast, Cardano is convinced that the search after truth is never a simple and straightforward enterprise and therefore it is of the utmost importance that one tries to improve one's own persuasive skills. Significantly, at the end of Cardano's dialogue, Gorgias has the final word, and his concluding remarks favor rhetoric. Relying on his ethical program of drawing profit from adversity and dismissing Plato's rejection of the educational, cognitive, and political implications of rhetoric, Cardano holds a more relativistic and flexible view of truth: "It is expedient to compare the goods with the ills and to choose what contains more good and less evil, since among men nothing is anywhere exempt from evil."[57]

Cardano's Gorgias explains that the main problem with Socrates is not the supposedly vicious nature of his character (*pravitas*), but his intellectual arrogance (*iactantia*) and "a vain desire to become famous, combined with a lack of knowledge of all the useful disciplines."[58] Socrates' irony has lost its charm and has become abrasive and sarcastic. Cardano's Socrates looks smug and sounds pompous: "Didn't I say that opinion is of the many and truth of the few?".[59] The thesis is an old one, but here, in the mouth of this Socrates, it sounds irritatingly elitist. Socrates advocates a sort of "philosophical license" that limits the pursuit of truth only to those who have the intellectual capacity to afford it. Talking about the use of images and similes in philosophical arguments, he claims that only philosophers are entitled to tell fables to inculcate the truth:

---

[56] See, for instance, Plato, *Gorgias*, 473B. On Plato and his critical attitude toward rhetoric, see Struever, *The Language of History in the Renaissance*; Fumaroli, *L'âge de l'éloquence*; Kennedy, *Classical Rhetoric*, 58–66.

[57] *Antigorgias*, OO I:665b. In *Proxeneta*, Cardano acknowledges Plato's rhetorical ability in debunking rhetoric's claims: "Adeo vero Gorgiam in Dialogo omni autoritate ac dignitate artis dicendi (in qua princeps habebatur) spoliat; ut ille quum Dialogum legisset, dixerit: Pulchre novit Plato male dicere" (OO I:398a).

[58] *Antigorgias*, OO I:641b.

[59] Ibid., 642b.

> SOCRATES: In their search after truth, many actions are permitted to philosophers that are not allowed to ordinary people.
>
> GORGIAS: Do you think that you are the only philosopher, and, if that is the case, that only philosophers should care about the truth?
>
> SOCRATES: Sure, unless you can name other professional categories.
>
> GORGIAS: What about judges, mathematicians and craftsmen?
>
> SOCRATES: But they don't recognize that as the aim of their profession![60]

Socrates' intellectual elitism culminates in his vindication of the cultural superiority of the Greeks over the 'barbarians'. Gorgias' reply is worth quoting in full:

> GORGIAS: Mind that you and your learned friends are not mistaken thinking that human beings are not human because either they do not talk your language or they do not live in the same way as you, but they are slaves, and therefore for you an injustice perpetrated against this kind of men is not an injustice. To me all human beings seem to be worthy of the obligations of humanity (*Mihi homines omnes humanitatis officio digni esse videantur*). And if a difference needs to be introduced, I believe that this must not derive from one's country, language, money or social status, but from conduct, a favorable disposition towards mankind, and wisdom.[61]

So it is up to Gorgias, who echoes the characteristically humanist ideals of reason and virtue, to defend the legitimacy of a more universal form of wisdom, not contingent upon differences of class or nationality.

Generally speaking, Gorgia's appeal to common sense prevails over Socrates' use of paradox. In Cardano's dialogue, Gorgias reiterates two fundamental questions already examined in Plato's dialogue: whether the ability to persuade rests on a specific discipline (*ars*) or only on practical knowledge (*peritia*), and whether the art of persuasion is useful for the state.[62] As in Plato's dialogue, Gorgias criticizes Socrates for maintaining two paradoxical theses. The first is that "those who have all the means at their disposal" are said by Socrates to be unhappy, while "those who find themselves in the direst and most unfortunate conditions" are characterized by him as happy men. The second thesis—"which is even more surprising"—is that "those who got possession of the supreme power through violence and despotic rule" are unhappy. And yet, Gorgias presses his interlocutor, "you urge your friends to unjust power, like Alcibiades who has ruined his and your country with the power of eloquence." In response to this objection, Socrates repeats Plato's classical ethical argument that happiness is virtue, and

60 Ibid., 643b.

61 Ibid., 645b.

62 Ibid., 644a.

virtue is knowledge. However, rather than making his point with inductive flair and increasing stringency, he shapes his arguments in the form of fatuous syllogisms: "Everything that is evil is reason for unhappiness; every shameful act is evil; therefore every shameful act has ruinous consequences." While Socrates syllogizes mechanically, Gorgias shows his mastery in the art of dialectic. Under the pressure of his antagonist's arguments, Socrates reveals the extent to which his ideas rely on abstract generalizations. By contrast, Gorgias has an easy time in showing the real power of beliefs and opinions in shaping men's identities and their sense of happiness. It is precisely at this point that Gorgias asks Socrates to be more specific about the nature of human happiness by recalling the case of the tyrant Archelaus, a case already familiar from Plato's dialogue:

> GORGIAS: Tell me, to whom does Archelaus look unhappy?
>
> SOCRATES: What do you mean?
>
> GORGIAS: I mean, granted that he is unhappy, who is the one to whom he looks unhappy? That is to say, does he look unhappy to himself, or to the people, or to the courtiers or to the gods?
>
> SOCRATES: By the dog, you don't sound like the same person as yesterday, so shrewd is the way you are prattling now. In any case, to your question I will answer that he does not look unhappy to you, to the courtiers, to the people, or to the gods. Maybe he looks so to wise people, but I am not sure about this.
>
> GORGIAS: Ha, ha, ha! This is indeed a clever answer, if our happiness is not to be valued by us, by other people, not even by the gods. Is it not a great part of one's happiness to value oneself happy, or a great part of one's misfortune to value oneself unhappy? What is your answer to this, Socrates?
>
> SOCRATES: That these thoughts are not true, but foolish.

Cardano's Gorgias argues that a realistic account of human happiness cannot leave elements of subjective evaluation—such as opinions, beliefs, and judgments—out of consideration. With his sharp contrast between knowledge and ignorance, Socrates flattens the whole argument: either one knows or does not know; if he knows, he cannot be unhappy. Subjective opinions find no place in Socrates' magic circle of knowledge, virtue, and happiness.

> GORGIAS: So in the end what will be this life of ours?
>
> SOCRATES: No doubt, it is miserable to consider yourself miserable, for if it is true, you are miserable; if it is not true, you are foolish. A fool is miserable.
>
> GORGIAS: Now I have what I want.
>
> SOCRATES: Not really, because once the very opinion is taken away, he who thinks he is miserable as a result of being deceived and mistaken is not miserable.

Gorgias is not impressed by Socrates' argument. He insists that someone who is convinced he is unhappy—regardless of whether his happiness rests or not on objective grounds—is unhappy. Once again, Socrates' distinction between objective reality and subjective opinion sounds too abstract, a distinction that contradicts common sense. In Socrates' opinion, it is not the presence of real adversity that makes one unhappy, but simply one's misperception of the events affecting his or her life. Gorgia then can easily object:

> GORGIAS: The fact remains that he is miserable.
>
> SOCRATES: I admit that.
>
> GORGIAS: Therefore one's own opinion has a great power.
>
> SOCRATES: But not with respect to real misery.
>
> GORGIAS: Is not a foolish person really miserable?
>
> SOCRATES: Yes.
>
> GORGIAS: Therefore, he who thinks he is miserable he also is really miserable.
>
> SOCRATES: But not for the reason that he thinks he is miserable, for instance, poverty or prison, but because he is mistaken.
>
> GORGIAS: O what an extraordinary piece of subtlety! He is and he is not. But for me it is sufficient to say that he is really miserable because he thinks he is miserable. Would you deny even this?
>
> SOCRATES: No.[63]

In his analysis of the famous Platonic argument that happiness is simply the result of one's knowledge of virtue, Cardano insists on *aestimatio*. Later in the dialogue, Gorgias explains that one's feeling of being happy is also inextricably intertwined with social attitudes (including ones that are not very noble) and with the perception of other people's happiness or unhappiness. Vanity, envy, and feelings of inadequacy inevitably obfuscate the way people assess their own happiness: "The greatest part of unhappiness depends on judging oneself unhappy. But this belief presupposes that other people are happy. However, when someone finds out that the powerful are not happy, and he learns this fact not through cavils and disputations on the nature of the beautiful and the honest, his soul finds peace and becomes tranquil, and this is the greatest part of happiness."[64] As already acknowledged in the preface to *De consolatione*, one's feeling of happiness is

63 Ibid., 644b.

64 Ibid., 648a.

constantly measured with the perception of other people's happiness. Happiness is a social good and is inevitably tinged with envy and schadenfreude.

Combining Stoic and Machiavellian arguments, Cardano's Gorgias proclaims the superiority of public good over the pursuit of private happiness. God and nature, he argues, have endowed human beings and some other animals with an instinct for the general good (*utilitas totius generis*) and the means to attain it, so much so that, if a ruler, in order to maintain the security and unity of the state, kills other people or commits wicked crimes, he must not be seen as "evil" or "unjust".[65] Through Gorgias, Cardano establishes a notion of human happiness which takes into account both the reality of private appetites and the social implications of public good. According to Gorgias, human beings are driven by appetites and not by the knowledge of the good. The only way of maintaining the social and political organization of a state is the ruler's control of the citizens' appetites with any means, even resorting to the use of force. *Tranquillitas animi* remains one of the highest targets for a human being, but a secure condition of happiness can only depend on the mastery of appetites. In such a picture, virtue rests not on knowledge, but on *aestimatio* understood as a delicate balance of self-judgement and evaluation of social appearances. In *Antigorgias*, Gorgias' arguments take into account concrete situations, legal implications, and the consequences of human actions. In contrast, Socrates focuses on matters of knowledge, conscience, and abstract morality. In Gorgias's opinion, wrongdoers and criminals are tormented by their evil actions not because of their mental and virtuous disposition (*ingenium*, *prudentia*, and *fortitudo*), but because their ambition and lust for power are insatiable (*immensa cupiditas*) and the consequences of their actions are frustratingly unintended. Their behavior does not depend on virtue and is not an expression of good intentions. Consequently, the regret and chagrin related to their bad behavior simply derives from the realization that they cannot proceed with their evil intent, that the expansion of their will is bound to encounter inescapable limits. To Socrates' optimistic view that knowledge is sufficient to direct the course of one's life, Gorgias opposes real situations in which decisions are to be made taking the power of the will into account and accepting the possibility that compromises are to be made. It is when someone loosens the reins of social control based on virtues, ideals of truth, and notions of good, and succumbs to his own inordinate desires, that he falls into a boundless sea of misfortunes and greediness (*vastum calamitatum pelagus .. illud vastum pelagum incontinentiae*).[66]

## Conclusion

Cardano's work as a whole provides ample and varied evidence that he took rhetoric very seriously, and not only with respect to the circumscribed field of medicine. He seems to have been perfectly aware of the many links connecting

[65] Ibid., 646b, 647b.

[66] Ibid., 647a.

medicine and rhetoric. He did not discount the rhetorical components of medicine, nor did he downplay the medical (diagnostic and therapeutic) aspects of rhetoric. In his opinion, both disciplines shared the fundamental concern that truth, however powerful in itself, may become effective only when the physician or the rhetorician adopt plausible means of persuasion. Such a close entanglement of medical and rhetorical motives in Cardano's work is the result of a number of basic assumptions: that the human soul is in a condition of natural embodiment within a world of material necessities, that human knowledge does not have the effortless and impeccable timing of either God's or nature's wisdom, and, finally, that human appetites are insatiable and violent and need to be curbed with determination.

In *Proxeneta*, Cardano characterized persuasion as a "friendly deceit" that, unlike violence and genuine deceit, does not leave behind physical injury and desire for revenge.[67] All in all, he acknowledged the ambivalent power of words and the "hidden tyranny" of eloquence.[68] He did not rule out the possibility that truth may be reached by practicing a severe exercise in philosophical asceticism (resonating with the typical accoutrement of Neoplatonic philosophy), but he thought that such a possibility belonged to a different epistemological avenue. Here and now, in this world, where fraud and deceit, lust and greed hold sway, those who are in charge of dispensing the *pharmakon* of truth must convince their audiences to buy their goods. In *Antigorgias*, Cardano resorted to a "medicinal" image to describe the predicament of truth and persuasion:

> SOCRATES: Human affairs, lifestyles and opinions concerning God are like the prices that apothecaries put on their drugs: usually, only a third of their price goes into the expenses, for if the apothecary asked only what is due, his business would soon die. If someone declares only the truth of his thoughts about God, human affairs, virtue and the order of this world, once that third is taken away, there will be no profit. Therefore, we are compelled to add something more to the truth.
>
> GORGIAS: No doubt, if you did as you say, but you seem to take away precisely the knowledge about God, the immortality of the soul and the care for human affairs.
>
> SOCRATES: Gorgias, Gorgias ... Then we need someone who can persuade people to follow their customs (*consuetudo*) rather than truth. For, if I talk about God and the immortality of the soul, since the way men are persuaded is a very different one, they will say that a cause which can be defended only through fables is preserved badly indeed. For this reason, it is necessary to resort to virtue, honor and subtle cavils, and to add to them from the fictitious arguments only that much that we lost from the truth because of the inflexible attitude of some people.[69]

---

67 Cardano, *Proxeneta*, OO I:359b-361a.

68 Ibid., 416a. See also *De sapientia*, OO I:535b.

69 *Antigorgias*, OO I, p. 646a.

If Plato used fables and myths to make truth more accessible to the philosophical layman, Aristotle (and Averroes following Aristotle) emphasized the social relevance of various traditions of fables and myths pertaining to the cultural heritage of every nation.[70] In the quotation above, by adding a new twist to a well-known argument, Cardano's Socrates makes clear that, at a time when skeptical attitudes seem to prevail, the 'fables' of virtues and values are more believable than the 'fables' of the gods. In so doing, this new incarnation of Socratic wisdom goes beyond Averroes' culturally-sensitive rationalism and seems to anticipate the form of disillusioned rationalism characteristic of the Enlightenment. To prolong the 'medicinal' metaphor, philosophers know the 'active ingredient' in the *pharmakon* of truth, but they can sell it and make a profit out of it only by adding the 'excipient' of subjective and cultural values.

For Cardano, the philosopher is an apothecary of the will more than a physician of the soul. It is undoubtedly a sign of the times—one may think of the growing importance of apothecaries, barber-surgeons, and midwives in the medical marketplace—that in Cardano's view both the physicians of the soul (philosophers and rhetoricians) and the philosophers of the body (physicians, but also a whole host of "artisans" of the body) acknowledged the need for more sophisticated forms of mediation between knowledge and action.[71]

---

[70] On Cardano's subtle use of characteristic Averroistic themes in his political and moral philosophy, I refer again to my essay "Nature and Demons".

[71] On the notion of "artisans of the body", i.e., early-modern professions dealing with the care, comfort, and appearance of the body, see Sandra Cavallo, *Artisans of the Body in Early Modern Italy. Identities, Families and Masculinities*, Manchester: Manchester University Press, 2007. I would like to thank David Marshall and Stephen Pender their comments and stylistic suggestions. Many thanks also to Clément Godbarge and Nicholas Holland for discussing with me the ideas contained in this essay.

# Chapter 8
# You've Got to Have Soul: Understanding the Passions in Early Modern Culture

Julie R. Solomon

Separating the Humors from the PassionsWe are indebted to recent scholarship on the passions in the early modern period to re-opening our eyes to the material and environmental components of early modern psychology.[1] Such work has focused on the physiology of the four humors, on the nature of the four temperaments, the character of the three spirits (natural, vital, animal), and on the manner in which climate, nature, and nurture shape the humors, that in turn shape human emotional states.[2] These contemporary critics, hand in hand with contemporary neuroscientists and cognitive theorists, have hammered away at those post-Cartesian views concerning the separation of mind and body that have distorted our understanding of the contributions of bodies and the passions to the workings of the early modern mind.[3] From Gail Paster we learn that within the human body, a given flow of bodily spirits and humors produced a particular temperature and degree of humidity, that, taken together, constituted a person's emotional temperament. She advises the importance of "keeping the materiality of the passions in our minds," for "bodily fluids" could "carry the full weight of a character's destiny. " Indeed, "to alter the character and quantity of a body's fluids was to alter the body's passions and thus that body's state of mind and soul," for the early moderns

1 See Michael Schoenfeldt, *Bodies and Selves in Early Modern England: Physiology and Inwardness in Spenser, Shakespeare, Herbert, and Milton* (Cambridge: Cambridge University. Press, 1991) and Gail Paster, "Unspeakable Deeds: The Comic Actor and the History of Shame," *Elizabethan Theatre* XIII (1994): 63–77; "Nervous Tension" in *The Body in Parts: Fantasies of Corporeality in Early Modern Europe*, ed. David Hillman and Cara Mazzio (New York: Routledge, 1997), 107–25; "The Body and Its Passions," *Shakespeare Studies* 29 (2001): 44–50; and *Humoring the Body: Emotions and the Shakespearean Stage* (Chicago: University of Chicago Press, 2004).

2 For an overview of these topics, see Nancy G. Sirasi, *Medieval & Early Renaissance Medicine: An Introduction to Knowledge and Practice* (Chicago: University of Chicago Press, 1990).

3 See for example, Antonio R. Damsio, *Descartes' Error: Emotion, reason and the Human Brain* (New York: Putnam, 1994) and Mark Johnson, *The Body in the Mind* (Chicago: University of Chicago Press, 1987).

held to a "materialist psychology." As Paster contends, only a "conventional and theologically accommodating" physician like Helkiah Crooke would feel "obliged" to mention the "soul" before discussing the emotional meteorology and hydraulics of the body.[4] Michael Schoenfeldt has argued that the "humors and affections are the same phenomenon in different psychological media," and that early moderns pursued a study of the "physiology of inner emotion." To support his contentions, Schoenfeldt quotes *The Optick Glasse of Humours* by Thomas Walkington, who promotes Galen's view that the soul "'follows'" the "'crafts and temperature of the body. " ' He bolsters his claims with Nancy Sirasi's comment that the balance of humours "'was held to be responsible for psychological as well as physical disposition.'"[5]

Schoenfeldt complicates the biological genesis of what he sees as a Adeeply materialist and incorrigibly determinist" account of the passions and the behaviour it sets in motion. So too does Paster. They do so by acknowledging the environmental and cultural conditions that shape the humoral body. Both writers discuss the importance of the regulation of the six non-naturals—air, exercise and rest, sleep and waking, food and drink, repletion and excretion, and the passions—within hygienic practice.[6] Paster points out that the humoral subject maintains a "full immersion in and continuous interaction with a constantly changing natural and cultural environment." And Schoenfeldt admits that "in actual practice it was possible to manipulate the humoral fluids and their concomitant behaviors through diet and evacuation."[7] Schoenfeldt's primary interest is in understanding the regimes of "self-discipline" that the humoral understanding of the bodily passions precipitated. Schoenfeldt acknowledges that early moderns made important distinctions between the material mechanisms—the humors, spirits, the bodily vessels—that the passions enlist to their service, and the immaterial soul itself. Hence, he endorses Walkington's view that "'we must not imagine the mind to be passible, being altogether immaterial, that it self is affected with any of these corporall things, but onely in respect of the instruments which are the hand-maids of the soule." '[8]

If we dig a little deeper in the critical record, we find that the claims of Paster and Schoenfeldt have been anticipated, although with much less finesse and

---

4 Paster, "The Body and Its Passions," 46 and "Nervous Tension," 113.

5 Schoenfeldt, *Bodies and Selves*, 2, 7, 9, 49.

6 On the non-naturals see Sirasi, *Medieval & Early Renaissance Medicine,* 101 and Andrew Wear, "Health and the Environment in Early Modern England" in Andrew Wear, *Health and Healing in Early Modern England: Studies in Social and Intellectual History* (Aldershot, Hampshire: Ashgate, 1998). Robert Burton appeals to the non-naturals in *Anatomy of Melancholy* (1621), stating that "A clear air cheers up the spirits, exhilarates the mind; a thick, black misty, tempestuous, contracts, overthrows. Great heed is therefore to be taken at what times we walk, how we place our windows, lights and houses, how we let in or exclude this ambient air" (Cited in Wear, "Health and the Environment," 135).

7 Schoenfeldt, 2; Paster, "The Body and Its Passions," 456.

8 Schoenfeldt, 9.

sophistication, by Patrick Cruttwell. In 1951, Cruttwell argued in "Physiology and Psychology in Shakespeare's Age" that the psychology of Shakespeare's age "may almost be called behaviorist," for it evinced a Arigorous physical determinism." Cruttwell based his argument largely on a reading of the physiological references in Shakespeare's plays, leading him to claim that from "this physiological basis, the step is a very short one to thinking of humours as composing the character men."[9] Though rarely cited, Cruttwell's view has come to typify the preponderance of early modern scholarship on the passions in early modern English drama. Like Paster, who wants us to read Hamlet's call for the drinking of "hot blood" literally—to mean that Shakespeare and his character believe that drinking blood will increase Hamlet's choler and his quest for vengeance—Cruttwell wants us to read allusions to the humors in Shakespeare's plays as indicators of Shakespeare's firm adherence to a simplified humoral materialism.[10]

One aspect of Cruttwell's reading of *Henry IV, Part II* and *Othello* makes me highly suspicious of these kinds of claims, at least insofar as Shakespeare is concerned. As evidence of Shakespeare's materialist psychology, Cruttwell points to the excuses that Falstaff makes for his disorderly behavior in his conversation with the Chief Justice in act one, scene two of *Henry IV, Part II.* Falstaff blames his behavior on the humoral and qualitative complexion of young men's bodies in comparison with those of older men. Falstaff thus reminds the Chief Justice that "you that are old, consider not the capacity of us that are young: you measure the heat of our livers with the bitterness of your galls."[11] According to Cruttwell, by this "Falstaff means: Your gall has adequately performed its physiological function of 'receiving the choleric superfluities,' but mine (I being young and hot) has not. I therefore am passionately choleric; you are a tame and respectable old man."[12] As to *Othello*, Cruttwell refers us to the passage where Othello comments upon the "moist" complexion of Desdemona's hand as indicative of her lechery:

> Give me your hand. This hand is moist, my lady . . .
> This argues fruitfulness and liberal heart.
> Hot, hot and moist–this hand of yours requires
> A sequester from liberty; fasting and prayer,
> Much castigation, exercise devout,
> For here's a young and sweating devil here
> That Commonly rebels. (3. 4. 34–41)

---

[9] Patrick Cruttwell, "Physiology and Psychology in Shakespeare's Age," *Journal of the History of Ideas* 12 (Jan 1951): 85, 78.

[10] Paster, "The Body and Its Passions," 48–50. For another example of reductive humoralism see Joseph R. Roach, *The Player's Passions: Studies in the Science of Acting* (Newark: University of Delaware Press, 1985).

[11] All references to the plays of William Shakespeare are taken from the *Riverside* Shakespeare, ed. G. Blakemore Evans (Boston: Houghton Mifflin, 1974).

[12] Cruttwell, 78.

Cruttwell's readings are obviously flat-footed from a dramatic perspective if they are to be taken as evidence of Shakespeare's so-called belief in Amaterialist psychology." For in either case, whether it be Falstaff's humoral excuse for his unseemly behavior, or Othello's belated humoral diagnosis of the origins of Desdemona's (non-existent) immoral behavior, Shakespeare means his theatre audience to see beyond the frame of humoral materialism. In the case of the aged Falstaff, the humoral claims to youth are deceitful, ludicrous, ironic, even inane; for the misguided Othello, the supposed humoral evidence is non-indicative of Desdemona's character, and the wrong belief it supports will culminate in tragedy and Othello's ruin. Rather than supporting the idea that Shakespeare simply endorses the materialist psychology of his age, Shakespeare's ironic representations of humoral explanation, at least in these two instances, suggest that early modern psychology was not simply reducible to a material base. Cruttwell himself acknowledges that "there was, of course, an essential difference between this [humoral psychology] and modern behaviorism—the fact that Shakespeare's age believed in the soul, in a part of man that was wholly spiritual in nature and divine in origin. . . . it is a little difficult to see how the soul was fitted in. And, in fact, the precise relationship between body and soul was one of the most debated questions of the age."[13]

What is crucially missing from recent analyses of the material bases of early modern psychology is a meaningful sense of this vigorous debate over the nature of, and relation among, body, soul, reason, and passions in philosophical, moral, religious, literary, as well as medical discourse. Unfortunately, such an omission risks eviscerating the role of the art of moral persuasion or rhetoric in the disciplining and cultivating of the passions in the realms of medicine, politics, religion, courtesy, and drama. But the art of rhetoric is in large measure the cultural form or tool that both reflects and informs the workings of faculty psychology in this era: for, it is in the language of rhetorical acts and machinations that the thinkers of this period discuss the interactions among reason, imagination, sensation, passions, will, and body that lead to both rational and irrational human behavior. And it is the passions in particular, with their ability to respond to both sensation, will, imagination, and reason that make possible much of the rhetorical functioning of the mind and become the focus of those thinkers, sermonizers, and dramatists who which to describe and represent its frequent troublesome character.

One problem with the current a-rhetorical analyses of the passions has been their over-reliance on the literature of Galenic hygiene, their selective use of the medical literature, as well as over-valuation given to Galenic works such as Juan Huarte's *The Examination of Men's Wits* (London, 1594). The latter work, dedicated to the Portuguese monarch, promotes a simplified Galenic perspective that makes conceivable an elaborate program of monarchical social control of minds, trades,

[13] Cruttwell, 85.

and professions.[14] True, Galen advocated a hygienic regime—including diet and exercise—for maintaining a healthy temperament in body and mind. True also that Galen in "That the Faculties of the Soul Follow the Temperaments of the Body" advances the idea that human "behavior depends on his somatic constitution and disposition" and that "even moral philosophers might well profit by a regimen, he Galen, would be willing to prescribe." But, nonetheless, as Owsei Temkin informs us, even Galen never became a total moral determinist, and he remained uncertain, "an agnostic," as to whether the soul was immortal or incorporeal.[15] We find one example of this uncertainty about the moral temperament in Galen's *On the Passions and On the Errors of the Soul.* In this work, Galen does not condone purges or bloodletting to control the concupiscible passions. Rather, he suggests a self-regulating, rhetorical, ethical solution—that we use our irascible passions to offset our overly desirous ones.[16] Of importance from a historical perspective, Temkin explains that the Bishop Nemesius of Emesa was the first to "establish" Galen as a medical "authority" for Christian theologians in his book entitled *De Natura Hominis*. However, in doing so, Nemesius explicitly rejected Galen's notion that the soul could be regarded a temperament of the body. Hence, while Galenism and its materialism was an important influence in the early modern period, it was markedly tempered by a Christian culture that valued the incorporeal character of the soul.

---

[14] Juan Huarte, *Examen de ingenios. The Examination of Men's* Wits (1594), intro. by Carmen Rogers (Gainesville, FL: Scholars' Facsimiles & Reprints, 1959). For Galenic hygienic regimes see Thomas Elyot, *Castel of Helthe* (1541), ed. Samuel A. Tannenbaum (New York: Scholars' Facsimiles and Reprints, 1937); Levinus Lemnius, *The Touchstone of Complexions,* trans., T. Newton (London, 1565); William Vaughn, *Directions for Health, Naturall and Artificiall* (London, 1626); and Leonard Lessius, *Hygiasticon, or The Right Course of Preserving Health* (Cambridge, 1634). For major secondary works on the relation between reason and the passions in ancient, medieval, early modern, and contemporary thought see Damasio, *Descartes' Error: Emotion, Reason and the Human Brain*; Jon Elster, *Alchemies of the Mind*: *Rationality and the Emotions* (Cambridge: Cambridge University. Press, 1999) and *Strong Feelings: Emotion, Addiction, and Human Behavior* (Cambridge: MIT Press, 1999); Peter Goldie, *The Emotions: A Philosophical Exploration* (Oxford. Oxford University Press, 2000); William V. Harris, *Restraining Rage: The Ideology of Anger Control in Classical Antiquity* (Cambridge, MA: Harvard University Press, 2001; Bennett W. Helm, *Emotional Reason: Deliberation, Motivation and the Nature of Value* (Cambridge: Cambridge University Press, 2001; Martha Nussbaum, *The Therapy of Desire: Theory and Practice in Helenistic Ethics*(Princeton: Princeton University Press, 1994) and *Upheavals of Thought* (Cambridge: Cambridge University Press, 2001); Timothy Reiss, *Mirages of the Self: Patterns of Personhood in Ancient and Early Modern Europe* (Stanford: Stanford University Press, 2003); and Robert C. Solomon, *A Passion for Justice* (Lanham, MD: Rowman and Littlefield, 1995).

[15] Oswei Temkin, *Galenism: Rise and Decline of a Medical Philosophy* (Ithaca: Cornell University Press, 1973), 83, 86–7. Temkin also discusses Galen's view that by taking hygienic measures, we promote moral virtue in ourselves (84).

[16] Galen, *On the Passions and On the Errors of the Soul*, trans. Paul Harkins (Columbus: Ohio State University Press, 1963), 46.

To sum up, we should be wary of swallowing uncritically this newly biologized, medicalized, a-rhetorical version of the early modern passions. True, early modern Europeans did believe that the bodily humors helped to create emotional, complexions, dispositions, tendencies, even ruling temperaments by affecting the bodily organs and spirits through which the soul operated. Moreover, when suffering from disease, the bodily humors—through the spirits and "'sympathetic connection'"—could induce emotional disease or indisposition.[17] However, diseased passion was the exception, not the norm. Moreover, emotional predispositions, ethical tendencies, or mood states were distinguished from occurrent passions by most early modern philosophers, divines, physicians, moralists, and dramatists, as I will discuss below. In general, ancients and early moderns reserved the label "passion" for those occasions when the sensitive soul responded—with awareness—to temporary external or internal stimuli.[18] For this reason, the emotions that inspired numerous writers were referred to as the passions of the sensitive soul. Early moderns viewed the sensitive soul, that functioned as an intermediary between the rational soul and the bodily spirits, as the body's caretaker. The sensitive soul's "cogitative faculty" received sensory information concerning external or internal events. After evaluating the information as good or ill, the "cogitative faculty" would generate those movements or perturbations—the passions—that would spur the body to take appropriate action. These soulful passions stirred the humors and spirits that in turn created the bodily changes and gestures that we associate with the emotions.

To be sure, in accord with Aristotle and Aquinas, early moderns believed that the mind and the body together, what Susan James has called a "body-soul composite," experienced the affections.[19] But until Descartes and even after, most thinkers believed that the emotions were first stirred in the sensitive soul and only then registered in the body. We should not discount the fact that most writings on the passions published in English between 1500 and 1700 refer to these disturbances as passions of the soul or mind. Aristotelian-Thomist views of the soul's primacy in originating and generating the passions in the healthy human being were alive and well in the sixteenth and seventeenth centuries. Views of the soul's role in originating the passions appear in the works of the natural philosopher, Walter

---

17 On the material, spiritual, and sympathetic causes of mental disorder see Michael McDonald, *Mystical Bedlam: Madness, Anxiety, and Healing in Seventeenth Century England* (Cambridge: Cambridge University Press, 1981), 177–87. For an example of the way in which physical and mental causes often became entangled in medical cases see "Observation LXIX" in *John Hall and his Patients: The Medical Practice of Shakespeare's Son-in-Law*, ed. Joan Lane (Stratford-Upon-Avon: Shakespeare Birthday Trust, 1996), 315–9.

18 Jon Elster, *Alchemies of the Mind*,, 65–6.

19 Susan James, *Passion and Action: The Emotions in Seventeenth-Century Philosophy* (Oxford: Oxford University Press, 1997), 42. Descartes argues that passions are initiated in the body [*Passions of the Soul* (1649), in *The Philosophical Writings of Descartes*, 2 vols, trans. John Cottingham (Cambridge: Cambridge University Press, 1985), I, 337–443]. See also Susan James, 259.

Charleton, and medical men such as Timothy Bright and Marin Cureau de La Chambre. The protestant theologian Philip Melanchthon offers a particularly thorough account of the soul's generation of the passions, alongside a robust Galenic discussion of the role of the humors and spirits in his commentary on Aristotle's *De Anima*.[20] Moralists, prudential writers, and theologians (as will be argued below) all acknowledged that the passions first arise in the soul. Where the passions originate—in soul versus body—is not a trivial matter. Rene Descartes, in his *Treatise on the Passions,* argued decisively that the passions originated in the body and only then registered by the soul. In doing so, he effectively separated out his notion of a rational immaterial soul from a non-rational, material body.[21] Prior to Descartes, however, the passions, though in many respects sub-rational, were thought to partake of reason in important ways because they originated in the sensitive part of the soul—a part thought susceptible to the dictates of reason. Moreover, as this essay will establish, the early modern passions were conceived as particularly human re-presentations of the world that were imbued with cognitive content. A short sketch of Aristotelian-Thomist epistemology will help me begin to clarify these complicated matters.[22]

## The Workings of the Aristotelian-Thomist Soul and Its Passions

Within Aristotelian-Thomist epistemology, the soul was divided into three parts: intellectual, sensitive, and nutritive.[23] All parts of the soul were thought to

---

20 Philip Melanchthon, *On the Soul,* in *A Melanchthon Reader,* trans., Ralph Keen (New York: Peter Lang, 1988).

21 For Descartes's notion that the physical motions of the spirits cause the passions see *Passions of the Soul*, I, 337–43. On the notion that the "passions are ideas" but "ideas rooted in the body" see Deborah Brown, "The Rationality of Cartesian Passions" in *Emotions and Choice from Boethius to Descartes*, ed. Henrik Lagerlund and Mikko Yrjönsuuri (Boston: Kluwer Academic Publishers, 2002), 259–61. Walter Charlton disputes the Cartesian allocation of the passions to the body in *A Natural History of the Passions* (London, 1674) where argues for the existence of two distinct souls—one rational, the other sensitive—in human beings.

22 Of course there were varied understandings of Aristotelianism during these and subsequent years. See for example Brian Copenhaver, "Aristotelianisms," In *The Columbia History of Western Philosophy,* ed. Richard H. Popkin (New York: Columbia University Press, 1999) and Charles B. Schmitt, *John Case and Aristotelianism in Renaissance England* (Montreal: McGill-Queens University Press, 1983).

23 See Aristotle, *On the Soul* (*De Anima)* in *The Complete Works of* Aristotle, 2 vols., ed. Jonathan Barnes (Princeton: Princeton University Press, 1984), 1. In the *Timaeus,* Plato argues, in contrast to Aristotle, that human beings possess both an immortal and a mortal soul. The latter is made up of two parts: one part of the mortal soul contains the spirited passions like anger and ambition, and is receptive to reason. The other, part contains lustful passions and is unreceptive, to reason *Timeaus* in *Plato: The Complete Works*, ed. John M. Cooper (Indianapolis: Hackett Publishing, 1997, 1271–2).

be immaterial, but the nutritive and sensitive parts of the soul were thought to be receptive to material impressions generated by external and internal bodily environments. However, the intellectual part of the soul was thought to be, as Lodowick Bryskett relates, "impassible," i.e., not susceptible to being impressed or affected by any material component of the physical world.[24] Its role instead was to judge the species—images denuded of corporeality—relayed to it by the imagination, and thus to be said to know. This knowing, as far as Aristotle was concerned, functioned in two ways. The intellect could both "become all things" and "make all things." The making of all things suggests the mind's self-directed agency and action and its imperviousness to external impression. Aristotle attempts to circumscribe the passivity of the intellectual soul's "becoming all things" by describing that "becoming" as operating like a type of "lighting" or illumination. Rather than passively receiving the immaterial species brought by the imagination into itself, the intellectual soul illuminates these species—in a sense becomes luminous with them, somewhat as a light source realizes the existence of material objects in a previously darkened room.[25]

Aristotle's efforts to shelter the soul's intellectual capacities from material impressions would seem to have eliminated rational process from the sensitive and nutritive parts of the soul. This may be to a large extent true for the nutritive soul, but it was certainly not the case for the sensitive soul, that Aristotle and later thinkers believed to be both the seat of the passions, the location of the estimative or cogitative faculty (what Bryskett would later call the "passible understanding"), as well as a field for the operations of imagination and some aspects of memory. To a large extent, what philosophers called prudence was an operation of the sensitive soul, informed by the power of soul's higher intellect.[26] The workings of the sensitive soul were multi-faceted. From the external world, material impressions were relayed through the operation of the five outer senses and processed by the inward senses or wits located (wholly or in part) in the brain. Building and elaborating upon Aristotle, Thomas Aquinas lists four interior powers: the common sense, the imagination, the estimative or cogitative faculty, and the memory. According to Aquinas, the faculties of common sense and the imagination would, respectively, receive and retain the sensory images delivered by the external senses. But because of the need to apprehend the "advantages

---

[24] Lodowick Bryskett, *A Discourse of Civill Life* (London, n.d.;rpt. New York: Da Capo Press, 1971), 274.

[25] Aristotle, *On the Soul,* 682–4.

[26] For a discussion of practical thought or prudence informed by the appetite of the sensual soul see Aristotle, *On the Soul,* 688–90. St. Thomas Aquinas argues for a judging or "cogitative faculty" within the sensitive soul (*The Summa Theologica of Saint Thomas of Aquinas,* 2 vols, trans., Fathers of the English Dominican Province (Chicago: Encyclopedia of Britannica, 1952), 1, 412–13. Aquinas argues that the "speculative and practical [prudential] intellects are not distinct powers," but they do seem to have distinct fields of operation since the speculative intellect relays what it apprehends to "the consideration of truth, while the practical intellect is that which directs what it apprehends to operation" (425).

and uses, or disadvantages" that the sense impressions of external objects pose—what Aquinas labels "intentions"—the sensitive soul's "estimative faculty" (in animals), or the "cogitative faculty" (in humans), is required. The passions of the soul then arise in the sensitive soul in response to the cogitative faculty's judicial apprehension of the positive or negative "intentions" contained within sensory images.[27] Impressions signaling the interior state of the body could be carried more directly by means of spirits and humors to the sensitive part of the soul itself. At certain unusual times, or when a disease state was present, the humors and the spirits could set off passions in the soul without the intervening step of "judgement" normally carried out by the sensitive soul. Only in this latter case would passions appear to be generated by no reason at all, or with little relation to the local environment or situation at hand.

By passions, Aristotle meant the capacity to receive, to suffer, to respond to, and be moved by impressions external to the sensitive soul. Passions were opposed to actions that were initiated by the soul's own internal agency. However, passion did not mean being totally inert or passive without energy, awareness, or response. In Aristotle's sense, passion meant what Timothy Reiss terms the soul's "passibility"—its capacity to receive, suffer, and respond to its own embodiment, as well as the natural and cultural environment surrounding that body. For Reiss, passibility names the "essentially interactive" character of the relation between body and soul, the fact that "passible mind was somehow *with* impassible mind, the living body affected its physical surrounds as they affected it." In other words, passion involved responsive activity, and action was in large measure dependent on the nature of human responsiveness to its environment.[28] Reiss argues that the rational mind (made up of impassible and passible components) was similar to the imagination in being "simultaneously active and passive."[29] Aristotle, in *On the Soul*, further aligns the capacities of thinking and imagination in arguing that one "may venture to regard imagination as a kind of thinking; for many men follow their imaginations contrary to knowledge, and in all animals other than man there is no thinking or calculation but only imagination." And elsewhere in the same text he claims that judgment is impossible without "imagination."[30]

Clearly, for Aristotle, appetite, passion, and imagination were to one degree or another interwoven with one another as well as with the human capacity to judge and reason. For example, in *On the Soul,* Aristotle claims that the appetitive

[27] Aquinas, *The Summa Theologica*, 1, 412–13. Avicenna influenced Aquinas's views. On the former, see Simon Knutilla, "Medieval Theories of the Passions of the Soul" in *Emotions and Choice from Boethius to Descartes*, ed. Henrik Lagerlund and Mikko Yrjönsuuri (Boston: Kluwer Academic Publishers, 2002), 58–61.

[28] Timothy Reiss, *Mirages of the Self*, 2, 93, 97. "Passibility, " claims Reiss, is the frame through which we must conceive notions of the pre-modern subject- and self-hood. On passion and action see also Susan James, 1997.

[29] Reiss, 93.

[30] Aristotle, *On the Soul,* 688, 680.

part of the soul where the passions arise is incapable of functioning without the "imagination." Furthermore, human beings possess both "sensitive imagination" (that merely reproduces sensory images) and "calculative" or "deliberative imagination"—that is capable of a certain degree of rational assessment and measuring of the goodness or badness of the images perceived.[31] Although the deliberative imagination does not possess the capacity to make a full rational "inference," it does possess a rational calculative capacity that Aquinas, as mentioned above, will label as the estimative or cogitative faculty. This cogitative faculty of the sensitive soul seems to merge at times with Aristotle's notion of the prudential part of the rational soul that contemplates "variable things" that he discusses in the *Nicomachean Ethics*.[32] For the most part, I believe that Aristotle reserves the heavy duty prudential lifting to the intellectual soul proper, although it is very difficult to draw the line between where the cogitative functioning of the sensitive soul leaves off and that of the intellectual soul begins.

Just as the intellectual and imaginative functions of the soul are enmeshed in the healthy mind-body composite, the passions of the sensitive part of the soul, according to Aristotle, partake of the rational principle to some extent. In the *Nicomachean Ethics*, Aristotle explains that there is in the soul "something beside reason" that works in "resisting and opposing" reason. This something else are those habits of action and reaction that have been shaped by our passions in their response to what they perceive as apparent good or bad as delivered to them by the sense organs. But Aristotle goes on to say that passion "seems to have a share in reason, as we said; at any rate in the continent man it obeys reason—and presumably in the temperate and brave man it is still more obedient: for in them it speaks, on all matters, with the same voice as reason." Thus, Aristotle claims that the "appetitive and in general the desiring element in a sense shares in it [reason], in so far as it listens to and obeys it; this is the sense in which we speak of paying heed to one's father … not that in which we speak of 'the rational' in mathematics. That the irrational element is in some sense persuaded by reason is indicated also by the giving of advice and by all reproof and exhortation."[33]

Anger is the passion that Aristotle most explicitly links to reason. In the *Politics*, Aristotle makes clear that the passion of anger is more stirred up in us by "our friends and acquaintances than against those who are unknown to us, when we think that we are despised by them."[34] Elsewhere he states that "Anger seems

[31] Aristotle, *On the Soul,* 689, 690

[32] Aristotle, *Nicomachean Ethics* in *The Complete Works of Aristotle,* ed. Jonathan Barnes, 2 vols. (Princeton: Princeton University Press, 1984), 2, 1798. Later Aristotelian scholastic commentators, such as Toletus, associated the imagination with prudence. See Dennis des Chene, *Life's Form: Late Aristotelian Conceptions of the Soul* (Ithaca: Cornell University Press, 2000), 29.

[33] Aristotle, *Nicomachean Ethics,* 741–2.

[34] Aristotle, *Politics* in *The Complete Works of Aristotle,* ed. Jonathan Barnes, 2 vols. (Princeton: Princeton University Press, 2, 2107.

to listen to reason to some extent, but to mishear it, as do hasty servants who run out before they have heard the whole of what one says, and then muddle the order, as dogs bark if there is but a knock at the door, before looking to see if it is a friend. . . . For reason or imagination informs us that we have been insulted or slighted, and anger, reasoning as it were that anything like this must be fought against, boils up straightway; while appetite, if reason or perception merely says that an object is pleasant, springs to the enjoyment of it. Therefore anger obeys reason in a sense . . . .[35] In other words, we feel anger only when reason or some other faculty of judgment has first given us a "reason" to feel anger. Hence, paradoxically, as Aristotle explains, the "man who is incontinent in respect of anger is in a sense conquered by reason,"[36] since reason initiated his descent into irrational passion.

In his *Summa Theologica*, Aquinas argues that both the irascible and concupiscible passions have the capacity to hear and obey the directives of the Aparticular reason"—i.e. the "cogitative faculty." And this "cogitative faculty" is capable in turn of being directed by the universal principles contained in the speculative or higher intellect.[37] In the views of both Aristotle and Aquinas, much of the confusion and contrariety that we experience between reason and the passion is a result of our temporal and bodily condition and the fact that there are times when our bodies need to act and we need to make prompt decisions and cannot await the full judgment of the intellect. When this happens, we rely on the swift workings of our passions to make immediate decisions for us. Then there are other times when our passions quickly encode the judgments of our cogitative faculty and the body over-responds—for example, generating rage or mad grief instead of judicious anger or stately mourning.

Stoic philosophers, building upon the ideas of Plato and Aristotle, also acknowledged a significant relation between reason and passion.[38] The Stoic Roman philosopher Seneca, for example, largely accepted Aristotle's definition of anger and its relation to reason. According to Seneca, "wild beasts and all animals, except man, are not subject to anger; for while it is the foe of reason, it is, nevertheless, born only where reason dwells."[39] Seneca even makes a distinction between true anger and "mock anger": true anger requires some kind of rational

---

35 Aristotle, *Nicomachean Ethics,* 2, 1815.

36 Aristotle, *Nicomachean Ethics,* 2, 1816. For a sixteenth-century account of Aristotle's ethics see John Wylkinson, *The Ethiques of Aristotle*, London, 1547.

37 Aquinas, *The Summa Theologica*, 1, 430–1, 507, 815, 825. Aquinas also argues that the passions of the sensitive appetite obey the rational will (1, 431).

38 On the Stoics' view of reason in relation to passion see Nussbaum, *The Therapy of Desire,* 316–401. On Plato's view of the passionate part of the soul see *Timaeus,* 1271–2. For Augustine's discussion of the Stoic view of the pre-passions and their conversion into rue passions only with the assent of rational judgment, see *City of God,* trans. Henry Bettenson (New York: Penguin Books, 1984), 345–9. For an examination of Stoicism's influence on the Christian fathers, see Knutilla, 49–83.

39 See Seneca, *On Anger* in *Moral Essays,* trans. John W. Basore, 3 vols (Cambridge: Cambridge University Press, 1928), 1, 113–14.

assessment of a situation, whereas those who suffer from "mock anger" are like "children, who, if they fall down, want the earth to be thrashed, and who often do not even know why they are angry—they are merely angry, without any reason and without being injured.... " Seneca proceeds to argue that animals do not suffer from the kind of passions that human beings do because "in them the ruling principle"—i.e. reason—"is lacking in fineness and precision." While animals may suffer from "violent outbreaks and mental disturbances, they do not have fear and anxiety, sorrow and anger, but certain states similar to them."[40] Human passions, like anger, according to Seneca, only occur with the assent of the rational mind:

> For to form the impression of having received an injury and to long to avenge it, and then to couple together the two propositions that one ought not to have been wronged and that one ought to be avenged – this is not a mere impulse of the mind acting without our volition. The one is a single mental process, the other a complex one composed of several elements; the mind has grasped something, has become indignant, has condemned the act, and now tries to avenge it. These processes are impossible unless the mind has given assent to the impressions that moved it. [41]

Because rational assent is necessary to the constitution of anger, Seneca believes that we can use reason and will to eliminate anger. When we received the "first prompting" or involuntary impulse that would prepare us for the passion, it is incumbent upon the rational man to refrain from assenting to this impulse and thus to suppress the emotion of anger.[42] Hence, as Martha Nussbaum notes, the Stoics want their followers to engage in a "toning up of the soul–developing its [rational] muscles" in order to enable it to refrain from assenting to involuntary impulses or irrational pre-passions.[43]

Descartes' delegation of the passions to the body and its mechanical mode of functioning contributed greatly to the neglect of the rational aspects of the emotions and their involvement with reason so evident in earlier philosophy. The anti-cognitive stance of the pragmatic psychologist William James, and his near contemporary George Lange, helped solidify the tendency to ignore the rational components of emotion. For, as James claimed, "our feeling of the same [bodily]

---

40 Seneca, *On Anger,* 113, 117.

41 Seneca, *On Anger,* 169.

42 Seneca, *On Anger,* 175. Seneca also argues that A delay is the "best corrective of anger" [229]. On Stoic view of passions as "perverse judgments" and on the role of reason in suppressing passions, see Harris, *Restraining Rage,* 107; Nussbaum, *The Therapy of Desire;* and Nussbaum, *Upheavals of Thought.* For Stoic views about anger and an argument for the notion that the passions are on ideas or beliefs, see Cicero, *Tusculan Disputations,* trans. J. E. King. Loeb Classical Library (Cambridge, MA: Harvard University Press, 2001), 255, 309, 343.

43 Nussbaum, *The Therapy of Desire,* 317.

changes as they occur" that "follow directly the perception" of a fact, situation, or object "is the emotion."[44] However, within the last fifteen years, philosophers and theorists such as Robert Solomon and Martha Nussbaum have revisited Aristotelian and Stoic views on how the emotions participate in, and are susceptible to, the operation of reason to promote a cognitive theory of the emotions.[45] Others have formulated theories of emotions in terms of intentionality, evaluative import, cognitive antecedents, and conative-cognitive interpenetration that, while refusing to define emotions as entirely cognitive, fully explore their cognitive dimensions.[46]

Recent cognitive theorists of the passions have stressed that emotions are relational and perspectival. For example, Michael Meyers claims that emotions involve a reflexive "intersubjective relationship" with other people and the world around us. They involve the way that we imagine ourselves imagining each other and of others imagining ourselves in differing social situations.[47] And for Martha Nussbaum, emotions "see the world from my point of view."[48] I would argue that such formulations, while essential, fail to make explicit a vital aspect of the passions—at least so far as early modern culture goes—namely that the passions of the soul are primarily representations in the fullest sense of that term. In a sense, for early modern philosophical and, even aesthetic culture, they are primary representations—the first entities that consciously or intentionally re-constitute or re-present the world from an individual human perspective. Unlike the senses, that merely reflect external sense data, the rational soul, that understands the universal species of things, or even the imagination that, at least initially, simply records the images of things, the passions of the soul are the product of a deeply personal reassessment or re-staging of the way things are or look to us from our viewpoint. Passions indicate that we each contain within ourselves a kind of proscenium arch through which we view our world. Human beings are not simply all actors, as Shakespeare would have it, but also playwrights of a sort—constantly

---

44 William James, "What is an Emotion" (1884), in *The Emotions* (New York: Hafner Publishing, 1967), 13. See also Carl George Lange, "The Emotions" (1885) in *The Emotions* (New York: Hafner Publishing 1967).

45 Solomon, *A Passion for Justice;* Nussbaum, *The Therapy of Desire* and *Upheavals of Thought.*

46 See for example Jon Elster, *Alchemies of the Mind* and *Strong Feelings*; Goldie, *The Emotions*; and Helm, *Emotional Reason.*

47 Michael Meyer, *Philosophy and the Passions,* trans. Robert F. Barsky (University Park, PA: University of Pennsylvania Press, 2000), 50, 49. For the social character of the emotions, see also Thomas Buoni, *Problemes of Beautie and All Humane Affections* (London, 1606), 84

48 Nussbaum, *Upheavals of Thought,*, 52. See Goldie, *The Emotions* and Martin Heidegger, *Being and Time*, trans. John Macquarrie and Edward Robinson (New York: Harper, 1962), 172–82.

re-presenting the external world in terms of our own frame of reference as to the good and the bad.[49]

Passions are in a sense mini-narratives, internal rhetorical ploys or justificatory stories that we construct about our relations with other people and the world around us. As mini-narratives, they are temporal in character, taking place in, being about, and surveying the range of past, present, and future. The Stoics, in fact, organized their understanding of the passions in terms of past, present, and future. The passion of delight is a response to present good, whereas grief is the response to present loss or evil. Lust involves the anticipation of future good, whereas fear anticipates looming evil. Anger, that for the Stoics was a combination of distress and desire for revenge, was forged out of the belief that one had been just injured or insulted.[50] From the philosophical perspective of Aristotle and the Stoics human beings can and should be the authors of the mini-narratives we call the passions. If human beings are authors, then they are also agents, and talk of the passions of the soul will necessarily involve talk about human agency, will, and decision-making. It is to early modern writings that handle these topics that I now turn.

## Early Modern Views of the Passions

Early modern views of the relation among the passions and the humors, the soul and the body, are layered and rich. They are robust in offering variations on Aristotelian-Thomist accounts of the soul's incorporeal operations alongside full Galenic descriptions of the material workings of the spirits, humors, and bodily organs. In these accounts, soul is not reduced to bodily material, nor is the body, its humors, and its subtle spirits given short shrift. Philip Melanchthon's *Commentary on Aristotle's Ethics*, Book I (1546) and *Commentarius de Anima* (1540)—that, according to Ralph Keen, became "one of the major philosophical texts of the reformation"—are exemplary of this robust approach.[51] Like Aristotle

[49] See Meyer's comment that passion is "nothing else than the impression that we have of what is essential." (43) On the question of whether Aristotle thought passions were initiated by impression or belief see *On the Soul,* 681 and Elster, *Alchemies of the Mind,* 57. Cicero, following the Stoics, argues that passions are "a matter of belief" (309). Examining the social character of the passions, Jacqueline T. Miller argues for an externalist view of their construction. Rather than being formed internally, passions result from the external imitation and representation of the behavior of other people. In that sense imitation and representation "precede[s] and produce[s] the passion" ["The Passion Signified: Imitation and the Construction of Emotions in Sidney and Wroth," *Criticism 43*(no. 4, 2001): 407–21.]

[50] On Stoic passions see Cicero, 339. Also Nussbaum, *The Therapy of Desire*.

[51] Philip Melanchthon, *On the Soul* (*Commentarius de Anima, 1540*) in *The Melanchthon Reader,* trans. Ralph Keen (New York: Peter Lang, 1988). For Melanchthon's interest in natural philosophy see Sachiko Kusukawa, *The Transformation of Natural Philosophy: The Case of Philip Melanchthon* (Cambridge University Press, Cambridge 1995).

and Aquinas, Melanchthon claims that the passions are powers of the sensitive appetite of the soul "which impels the mind to pursuing those things which seem right and fleeing those things which offend."[52] While the vegetative faculty of the soul cannot "obey judgment" or reason," the "sense" and the "appetite" are "able to obey." Thus "affects of the heart, like anger and sadness, are subdued by reason and deliberation."[53] The passions, or those appetites "which do not come about through" physical means "follow thought, and have their rightful place in the hart." For the "order of nature must be taken into account, that cognition precedes the movements of the hart, as it is said: What remains unknown is not desired by those ignorant of it."[54] While acknowledging the role of cognition and the sensitive soul in the generation of the passions, Melanchthon, following in the footsteps of the fourth-century Bishop of Emesa, Nemesius, also recognizes the relevance of Galen's thought to Christian understanding of the mind and its passions. The German reformer argues that the sensitive soul works through physical organs like the brain or heart. The brain is the seat of the sensitive soul's common sense (that for Melanchthon includes fantasy), prudential thought (the estimative faculty), and memory.[55] As Melanchthon explains, the passions of the sensitive soul constitute physical movements of the heart that follow upon cognition and initiate other material operations and movements: "thus when we apprehend an object and judge whether it is good or bad the spirits in motion strike the heart upon recognition, which, as it is beat and impelled, is moved and either seeks or flees the object. For such is the coupling of the forces of nature, that the movements of the heart respond to cognition, as a man will either acquiesce in things that he knows, or sense punishment and destruction." Melanchthon, in Galenic fashion, also acknowledges that it is important to know the temperament of the heart because "the warmer and drier it is, the quicker and more vehemently it burns in anger." The affections of the heart in turn set in motion some of the humors. For example, anger, "which comes from an inflamed heart, moves the most firey humour, namely red bile, and when it is poured out it infests the rest of the blood, which is otherwise set on fire by the spirits of an irate heart."[56]

Melanchthon's comprehensive view of the passions as an Aristotelian faculty of the soul that sets in motion the spirits and humors of the Galenic body is replicated in the works of later writers. Juan Luis Vives would adopt Aristotle's view that the passions are faculties of the sensitive soul that "follow the judgement's conclusions, no matter how quick and hasty they might be, since the soul is not

[52] Philip Melanchthon, *Commentary on Aristotle's Ethics* in *The Melanchthon Reader*, trans. Ralph Keen (New York: Peter Lang 1988), 217.

[53] Melanchthon, *Commentary on Aristotle's Ethics,* 200.

[54] Melanchthon, *On the Soul,* 243.

[55] See Melanchthon, *On the Soul,* 240–1 for his description of the brain as the seat of operations of the three inner senses of the soul: common sense, thought or composition, and memory.

[56] Melanchthon, *On the Soul,* 247.

moved unless the object has previously been judged to be good or bad."[57] But Vives also pioneered the notion of *ingenium* or intellectual temperament, that owed much to Galen. Moreover, Vives complained that "the more our judgment is infected by its contact with the body and the deeper it is immersed into it, the more grave and numerous do the 'passions' grow, upsetting and distorting not only the intellect but even the external senses of the soul."[58] The ex-Jesuit, Thomas Wright, in *The Passions of the Minde in general* (1604), sites the passions in the sensitive soul, "bordering upon reason and sense" and underlines their cognitive character by repeating the well-worn dictum that "We may love an ill thing, but wee cannot love an unknowne thing." He mixes Galen with Aristotle in describing the contributions of humors, spirits, and the organ of the heart to the operation of the passions.[59] He also comments on the on the "diversities of complexions [that] wonderfully increase or diminish Passions" and states that the passions can be raised in the soul "by humours arising in our bodies, by externall senses and secret passage of sensuall objects, [and] by the descent or commandement of reason."[60] However, Wright makes clear that, for the most part, the passions of the soul impel the humors rather than the other way around:

> "for there is no Passion very vehement, but that it alters extreamly some of the foure humours of the body. . . for although it busieth their [doctors'] braines, as also the natural philosophers, to explicate the manner how an operation that lodgeth in the soule can alter the body, and move the humours from one place to another (as for example, recall most of the blood in the face, or other parts, to the heart, as we see by daily experience to chance in fear and anger) yet they consent that it may proceed from a certain sympathy of nature, a subordination of one part to another, and that the spirits and humours wait upon the Passions, as their Lords & Masters. "[61]

Similarly, in his *Anatomy of Melancholy* (1621), the Anglican clergyman Robert Burton speaks of the sensitive soul, its passions, and its cognitive functions, including

---

[57] Juan Luis Vives, *The Passions of the Soul: the third book of De Anima et Vita,* trans., Carlos G. Noreña (Lewiston, NY: E. Mellen Press, 1990), 3. Vives acknowledges, however, that ASome of the soul's motions are nevertheless so abrupt and violent that they do not give any time to notice them, and seem therefore to precede judgment. Still, a properly educated and well-trained mind is able to increase, decrease, repress, and change the direction and power of its affections (3). "

[58] Vives, 5. For Vives's notion of *ingenium* see Carlos G. Noreña, *Juan Luis Vives and the Emotions* (Carbondale, IL: Southern Illinois University Press, 1989). See also Lorenzo Casini, "Emotions in Renaissance Humanism" in *Emotions and Choice from Boethius to Descartes*, eds. Henrick Lagerlund and Mikko Yrjönsuuri, 205–228. Reiss examines some of the complex origins of the term *ingenium,* 282–3,304–305.

[59] Thomas Wright, *The Passions of the Minde in generall* (London, 1604; rpt. Urbana: University of Illinois Press, 1971), 8, 35–45.

[60] Wright, 8, 31, 46, 149.

[61] Wright, 4.

that of imagination. Like Melanchthon, he discerns three cognitive faculties of the sensitive soul operant in the brain: the common sense, the phantasy, and memory.[62] Melancholy has many causes, Burton notes. "Bad humours, troubling the spirits, sending gross fumes into the brain" can induce melancholy, but the "passions and perturbations of the Mind" are the "greatest of all." Passion is "a most frequent and ordinary cause of melancholy" for the "mind most effectually works upon the body, producing by his passions and perturbations miraculous alterations, as melancholy, despair, cruel diseases, and sometimes death itself: insomuch that it is most true which Plato saith in his Charmides. . . all the mischiefs of the body proceed from the soul."[63]

Some moral theorists and contemporary clergyman, such as William Perkins, Pierre de La Primaudaye, J.F. Senault, and Thomas Cooper, focus on the passions of the soul and the healing powers of God's grace instead of the workings of the humoral body. The protestant minister, William Fenner, perhaps following in the footsteps of Pierre de la Primaudaye, goes so far as to locate the passions in the will—a faculty of the rational soul. But others—both protestant and Catholic—including Pierre Charron, F.N. Coëffeteau, and Edward Reynolds—follow Melanchthon in drawing upon both Aristotle and Galen.[64] They take an Aristotelian tack in assigning the passions to the sensitive soul and noting their cognitive antecedents; yet each recognizes to a greater or lesser degree the validity of Galenic views on temperament, the spirits, and the humors.[65] Charron, for example, combines Aristotelian and Galenic arguments in describing the workings of the mind. He argues that the human soul is "an invisible substance" and is, as Aristotle would have it, the "forme" of the body. Except for its highest spiritual reaches, the soul is "passible," that is "capable of suffering" bodily impressions."[66] For Charron, the faculties of the "reasonable soule"—understanding, memory,

---

62 Robert Burton, *The Anatomy of Melancholie* (1628), Part II, ed. By Holbrook Jackson (New York: Vintage Books: 157–69.

63 Burton, Part II, 250.

64 William Fenner, *A Treatise of the Affections; or the Soules Pulse* (London, 1641); Pierre de al Primaudaye, *The French Academy*, trans. T. B. (London, 1586), 31, 35. For the meshing of Aristotle and Galen see Edward Reynolds, *A Treatise of the Passions and Faculties of the Soul of Man* (London, 1650); William Perkins, *The Whole Treatise of the Cases of Conscience*, London, 1606, 188–9; Pierre Charron, *Of Wisdom*, trans. Samson Lennard [London, n.d. (before 1612); rpt., New York: De Capo Press, 1971]. Walter Charlton, *A Natural History of the Passions* (London, 1674) ; F.N. Coëffeteau, *A Table of the Humane Passions,* trans., E. Grimestone (London 1621); Thomas Cooper, *The Mysterie of the Holy Government of our Affections* (London, 1620); Marin Cureau de La Chambre, *Les charactères ces passions,* 5 vols. (Paris, 1660–62); J. F. Senault, *The Use of the Passions*, trans. Henry Earle of Monmouth (London, 1649); Juan Vives, *The Passions of the Soul*, trans. Carlos G. Norena (Lewiston, NY: Edwin Mellen, 1990); and Thomas Wright, *The Passions of the Minde in generall* (London, 1604).

65 Charron, Coëffeteau, Reynolds.

66 Charron, 25, 29.

imagination—reside in the three ventricles of the brain, for the soul needs a "corporall instrument to exercise it [sic] functions." Human beings understand "not alike and after one maner, but with great diversitie" because of the "change and alteration of the state of the organ or instrument." The "temperature of the Braine," Charron claims, affects the operations of the part of the reasonable soul—understanding, memory, and imagination—that uses the brain as its instrument. Thus, "drunkenness, the bite of a mad dog, a burning fever, a blow on the head, a fume rising from the stomacke, and other accidents pervert and turn topside turvy the judgement, intellectual spirit, and all the wisdom of Greece .... These accidents being purely corporall cannot touch nor arrive to this high spirituall facultie of the reasonable soule, but only to the organs or instruments, which being corrupted, the *Soule* cannot well and regularly act & exercise it [sic] functions." Clearly appreciative of Galenic views of the workings of the mind, nonetheless, Charron, like Aristotle, locates the passions in the sensitive part of the soul, for the affections "follow that which the *Soule* thinketh to be good for it, or to flie that which it takes to be evill."[67]

The doctor Timothy Bright, to whom recent scholars of the humoral psychology frequently turn, and the French physician Marin Cureau de La Chambre follow the Aristotelian-Thomist synthesis in describing the normal upwelling of the passions. According to Cureau, all "Passions are impermanent actions which are formed in the Soul before she agitates the Body, and principally the humours."[68] For Bright, the "first occasion riseth from outward things, wherein we either take pleasure, or wherewith we are offended: this object is caried to the internal senses [common sense, cogitative faculty] from the outward; which if it be a matter sensuall onely, the minde useth to impart it to the hart, by the organicall internall senses [e.g., the cogitative faculty] which with joy embraceth it, or with indignation, and mislike refuseth it; if of such points as it self [i.e., the rational mind] liketh, without their [internal senses] help it giveth knowledge thereof to the hart by the spirits, which either embraceth the same, impelled by the minds willing, or rejecteth it with mislike and hatred, according to her nilling." Under normal circumstances external stimuli, not the humors, cause the passions; and the passions move the humors, not the other way round. Only ill health allows the humors to affect the soul and its passions, and then only indirectly, by altering the bodily organs and the spirit, thus becoming the "occasion" but not the "cause" of passion.

Bright believes that temperament does not derive simply from an excess, or cyclical surge and ebb, of a particular bodily humor. Rather, nature, nurture, diet, climate, habit, occupation, and humors create varying kinds of dispositions, that, over time, congeal to form the temperamental inclination of a particular individual. Bright argues that "neither purgations of humour alter complexion, a fixed thing ingenerate by nature, & not overthrown but by some venimous qualitie

---

67 Charron, 48, 46, 47, 71.

68 Timothy Bright, *A Treatise of Melancholie* (London, 1586) and La Chambre, 2, 313–14.

direct opposite against it, or long custome of other disorder, whereby nature is supplanted in time."[69] Bright contends that this "ingenerate" complexion disposes individuals to certain moods or feelings—but does not mechanically cause the passions.[70] In an extended, complex passage, Bright argues against the idea that we may "with reason referre" the normal arising of the passions to the "humours" or to the way in which the humors shape the complexion of the heart itself. First, he denies that it is possible for four humors to give rise to only two primitive passions, that is "love or liking, or hate or mislike," for if "we with reason referre them to the humours, which are foure: and if the perturbations should rise of humour, then should they aunswer ech other neither mor nor fewer …." Second, if passions arise from the humors then "should those parts wherein humours most abound, be instruments of passions," such as the "gall of anger" and the "splene of sadnesse," but it is not these sites, but the "hart, which is the seat of all those affections." Third, even if "you will say: these affections rise of the temper of the hart, and the temper of the humour," this is "Not so: for either the affections rise of the frame alone of the hart, or else at the least joyned with the temper." However, "the humours have so small force in making temper, and framing the complexion; that themselves are all thereof framed …." And fourth, "these passions being wrought of the heart by a certain enlarging of it self, if it be pleased, and closing, if it be contrarily affected: which be actions not of complextion, but of frame & shape…." For complexion can transform things that it "toucheth" directly, such as "victuals," that it "can make into humors" and subsequently into the "substance of the body, which it indueth with the same complexion."[71] In sum, insofar as the body's physical contribution to the character of the undiseased passions, Bright gives pride of place to the "frame" or physical shape of the heart, not the humors.

To explain how it is that "melancholicke persons are more sad than other, & cholericke more angrie," Bright again distinguishes the normal rising of the passions upon "an outward occasion" that occurs "if the bodie be well tempered, and fautles in his instruments" and those diseased, "unnaturall, and disordered" states when the passions rise "of no outward occasion, but from inward delusion" or "by the fault of the report of the senses, or evil disposition of the hart" in which the "humours seeme to have greatest rule."[72] But outside of the diseased state, Bright is adamant that the humors follow the passions rather than the other way

[69] Bright, 81, 99, 85–6.

[70] In *Shakespeare's Brain*, Mary Thomas Crane notes that Bright combines a "material theory of humoral psychology and an idealizing theory of an immaterial and transcendent soul" (Princeton: Princeton University Press, 2001), 120.

[71] Bright, 84–6,

[72] Bright, 86. According to Bright, during disease states the humors can affect the instruments of the body, the "corporall organs of the body or spirit" or the ingenerate complexion in such a way to affect the course of the passions or to induce disturbing passions (91–3).

around. He thus answers his own rhetorical question in this fashion through an appeal to an illogical metonymy:

> But why then say you have the Philosophers defined anger as a boyling of the blood about the hart? If it be according to that definition, then the more cholericke a man is, so much the more angry is he: because the choler is first apt to boyle, as it were brimstone to the match, in respect of the other humours. That definition of anger, is to be taken not by proper speech, but by a metonymical phrase, whereby the cause is attributed to the effect. For first the heart moveth, kindled with anger, then the bloud riseth, which being cholericke encreaseth the heate, but addeth nothing to the passion: now because we sensibly feele an extraordinarie heate about our hearts when we be moved to angrie pasions, therefore they have defined anger by that effect: which boyling, riseth not of the quality of the bloud, but by a strife of a contrary motion in the heart at one time.[73]

It is thus not surprising that Bright claims that "all manner affection thereof" is not "to be subject to the phisicians hand." He is outraged that some have "esteemed the vertues themselves, yea religion, no other thing but as the body hath ben tempered, and on the other side, vice, prophanesse, & neglect of religion and honestie, to have bene nought else but a fault of humour." He comments satirically that "if either humour, or excrement should have part in moving affections, no counsel of philosophy, nor precept of wise men were comparable to calm these raging passions" than "the purging potions of Phisitians," unconscionably making the physician stand "above all the schools of Divinitie and Philosophy." Instead, he commits himself to "correcting the judgement of such as so greatly mistake the matter" and explaining the difference "betwixt natural melancholie, and the heavy hande of God upon the afflicted conscience, tormented with remorse of sinne."[74] Bright here clearly rejects an a-rhetorical view of the passions.

Arguably, one of the most intriguing legacies of the early modern synthesis of Aristotelian-Thomist and Galenic theories of the passions appears in the not uncommon notion of what I term false or "pseudo" passions. Generally, pseudo-passions owe their occurrence to disease and chance. Pseudo-passions are by nature a-rhetorical. Listening to music can also lead to the stirring of fabricated passions. In the case of disease, they arise when the humors and/or spirits are aroused by physical means, without the prior instigation of the passions, that themselves are normally raised by the cognitive powers of the sensitive soul. Because the sensitive soul notices that the humors and spirits have been aroused, it presumes that some situation worthy of attention must exist. Consequently, the sensitive soul raises those passions thought appropriate to the mix of humors or spirits detected. The result is the raising of a defective, false, or pseudo-passion.

---

[73] Bright, 87–8. Bright goes on to argue that if passion were caused by humor, then "why is not then the hart always affected without intermission, with such passions as the bloud enclineth unto, seeing it is always present, & keepeth his disposition alike" (89)?

[74] Bright, *iii–*iii$^{v}$, 89.

For example, Marin Cureau de La Chambre begins by explaining that the natural appetite initiates movements akin to the passions of the soul. But unlike the sensitive appetite, it possesses "une connoisance moins exacte [a knowledge less exact] " that "ne discerne pas si justement le objects que l'imagination [does not discern objects so justly as does the imagination]", so that the passions it cause are "si imparfaites, qu'on peut dire que ce no sont que des images grossieres & comme les esbauchmens [so imperfect, that one could say that they are only gross images & like the rough-hewn outlines]" of true passions. La Chambre then remarks that: "Car la peine que souffre la Nature … qui suit les indispositions du corps, ne sont a vrayement parler que de foibles commencemens, ou des crayons imparfaits de la vraye Douleur; Comme ces espanouissemens secrets & ces agreeable ressentimens qui accompagnent les actions naturelles ne sont les ombres de la Joye & du Plaisir. [Because the discomfort that nature experiences which follows from bodily indisposition are only, to speak truly, the weak beginnings, or the imperfect sketches of true Sadness; as are the secret blooms and the pleasant feelings which accompany the natural actions are only the shadows of Joye and Pleasure]." Thus, "ces mouvements ne meritent pas le nom de Passions; n'estant conduits par aucune connoissance, laquelle est absolument necessaire pour former les Passions [these movements do not merit the name of Passions being not conducted by knowledge which is absolutely necessary to produce the Passions]."[75]

To illustrate his points, La Chambre describes how during a diseased state the bodily passions can induce false passions in the soul. We learn that the soul has an interior, care-taking sense provided by nature through which it knows all that occurs within the bodily organs. This interior sense communicates its knowledge of the body's interior state to the imagination. If disease or environmental distress has led to the raising of the humors and spirits, this fact is communicated to the imagination for consideration, even though the soul does not know distinctly the physical nature or type of disturbance that has caused this raising. However, the soul does know that it is a hot and ardent humor and thus the imagination represents to itself those qualities that correspond to the bilious humor. Moreover, the imagination retrospectively constructs fictions—passionate objects and reasons—that would justify the raising of this bilious humor:

> Et parce qu'elle scait encore que cette humeur sert a là Colere & a là Hardiesse pour destruire l'ennemy qu'elles attaquent; la voyant en l'estat où elle a accoustume d'estre en ces Passions, elle s'en propose incontinant les objects & les desseins, & forme ainsi des enemis, des assauts & des combats [And because that it knows that this humour serves the passions of Choler and Boldness in order to destroy the enemy that they attack; seeing that it is in the condition where she is accustomed to be when in these Passions, she freely proposes to herself the objects and the designs, & hence forms the enemies, assaults, and combats].[76]

---

75 La Chambre, 2, 388–9.

76 La Chambre, 2, 459.

In addition to physical disease, chance can contribute to the formulation of pseudo-passions. La Chambre notes that if by chance the contrary emotions of sadness and boldness are raised in the soul, even though no external injury to the self has occurred, the mixing of the two can produce the complex passion of anger when the imagination fabricates a cause or reason for their simultaneous rise.[77] Music too can adventitiously and artificially induce passions, or in Thomas Wright's words, "semblable passions." The cause of these seeming passions is either some "sympathie, correspondence, or proportion betwixt our soules & musicke," "Gods generall providence," or that "the very sound itselfe, which according to the best Philosophie, is nothing else but a certaine artificiall shaking, crispling or tickling of the ayre ... which paseth thorow the eares, and by them unto the heart, and there ... tickleth it in such sort, as it is moved with semblable passions."[78]

## Passion as Representation

My brief survey of sixteenth and seventeenth century writings on the passions reveals that the preponderance of moral and theological writers, as well as a number of medical writers, take a robust perspective on the passions that embraces both the Aristotelian-Thomist view that the passions arise first in the soul and a Galenic appreciation of the role of the humors and spirits in their generation. Now, I would like to turn to a matter that I believe was central to early modern views of the passions and that depended on this complex view for its conceptualization: namely, the idea that the passions were representations imbued with rhetorical significance. Juan Luis Vives emphasizes the representational character of the passions in arguing that in most cases passions are generated by the "visions" that the imagination constructs in the process of judging external sense data. Thus, "a formal judgment stating a conclusion based on the pondering of some reasons is not always required to excite an emotion; in most cases it is enough that our imagination be moved by its visions. A mere commotion of our fantasy bearing some resemblance to an opinion or judgment that a given object is good or bad, is enough to disturb our soul with all emotions."[79]

The claim that the passions are representations means not simply that they are imitations in another medium of something outside themselves, although notions of sympathetic relation among humors, elements, and fundamental qualities were rampant in the period. Nor that individuals learned and constructed their passions through the imitation of other people, although this too was popularly believed to be the case. What I want to advance here is the idea that passions "re-presented" or "re-framed" the information that they received from the external senses so as to view it from the perspective of the bodily and psychic well-being—as well as

---

[77] La Chambre, 2, 58 and 486

[78] Wright, 168ff.

[79] Vives, *The Passions of the Soul,* 3.

the values—of the person doing the viewing. Passions are necessarily perspectival and hence rhetorical; they are views of the world through the lens formed by the values held by the individual and with which he or she reads the external and internal world. Moreover True passions (as opposed to pseudo- or false passions) are intrinsically tied to re-presentation, to the way things in the material dimension appear to us in the ethically, culturally, and experientially saturated dimension of a mind that knows, feels, and imagines. Hence, passion in this period involves the notion of a crossing between different ontological dimensions—in this case the "re-presentation" of physical/material conditions as "intentions," either positive or negative, depending upon an individual's psychic awareness, agency, and values. Without a comprehensive notion of the separate, though intertwined, existence and operations of body and soul, this kind of re-presentation would not exist. For, as Francis Bacon states, the "mother" of "affection, passion, or perturbation" is "nothing els but the object of apparent good [intention] in the eies of Appetite" (sensitive soul).[80]

Writers in this period characterize the passions in axiological and representational terms. They often treat the "apparent" nature of these representations as indicative of their perspectival nature: the fact that they are good or bad according to us. Hence, F.N. Coëffeteau sees passion as "but a motion of the sensitive appetite, caused by the apprehension or imagination of good or evill, the which is followed with a change or alteration in the body, contrary to the Lawes of nature." For, first the "Exterior sences" transmits the "forme of things" to the "common sence" that "judgeth them, and distinguishe them." Second the common sense, presentes them "to the Imagination" to "preserve them in the absence of their objects." Third, the imagination "propounds them unto the Appetite, under the apparance of things that are pleasing or troublesom, that is to say, under the forme of Good and Evill." Fourth, "at the same instant the same formes enlighted with the Light of the understanding, and purged from the sensible and singular conditions, which they retaine in the Imagination" become "capable to be imbraced by the understanding, the which under the apparance of things which are profitable or hurtfull, that is to say, under the forme of Good and Evill, represents them unto the Will." Fifth, the "Will" being "blind referres it selfe to that which the understanding proposeth unto it. And then as Queene of the powers of the soule she ordaines what they shall imbrace, & what they shal fly as it pleseth her." And finally, "the Sensitive Appetite yeelding a prompt obedience to excute her [the will's] command, from the which it never straies, so long as it containes it selfe within the bounds and order prescrib'd by Nature, quickeneth all the powers and passions over which shee commands, and sets to worke those which are necessary to that action, and by their meanes commands the moving power, dispersed over all the members, to follow or fly, to approch or to recoyle, or to do any other motion which it requireth."

---

[80] Francis Bacon, *The Wisdome of the Ancients,* trans. Sir Arthur Gorges (London, 1619; rpt., New York: Garland Publishers, 1976), 109.

But of course, as Coëffeteau points out, things do not often work the way they are supposed to, for "oftentimes hee [man] overthrows and perverts this order, either by bad education, or by custome, or the organs being unsound, or for that his will hath bad inclination; so as reason cannot enjoy her power, & subject the Sensuall Appetite unto her; but contrariwise hee abandons himselfe in prey unto this disordered Appetite, and suffers himselfe to bee transported by his furious motions so as suddenly when as fantasie offers to the Appetite, the formes which shee receives from the Sences, under the shew of Good or Evill; he without stay to have them judged by the discourse of understanding, and chosen by the will, commands himselfe the moving power, & makes it to act according to his pleasure. And herein consistes the disorder which the passions cause in the life of man, which divert him many times from the lawes of Reason."[81]

Similarly, Pierre de la Primaudaye recognizes the good and bad aspects of passionate representation. He claims that our "weake" or mild passions inspired by faith tend towards accurate representation, for they are "good and holie, aspiring and rejoicing in that which is truly good, " whereas our Astrong" ones are Aevil and pernitious, coveting . . . a good falsly so imagined." We should thus "labor by good and sound reasons to overthrow and confound these false and erronious opinions, perswading our selves that whatsoever we imagine to be good or evill in the world ... is indeede neither good nor evil, and so consequently, that it ought not in any sort to breed passions within us." Hence passions arise in the soul only for what "fooles do falsely call good, and what the philosophers call the goods of the bodie and of fortune."[82]

While Coëffeteau and Primaudaye present highly balanced accounts, other writers focus heavily on the negative consequences that arise from the fact that the judging powers of the sensitive soul (whether the faculty of the common sense or that of the imagination), being so attentive to the concerns of the body and enveloped in corporeal organs, would lead us astray from, and even compete with, reason.[83] By collapsing the Aquinian distinction between cogitative and imaginative faculties, Robert Burton constructs the very disorder that he fears. He starts with the claim that the cognitive judgment of the imagination sets the passions in motion:

> Thus, in brief, to our imagination cometh, by the outward sense or memory, some object to be known ...which he [imagination], misconceiving or amplifying, presently communicates to the heart, the seat of all affections. The pure spirits forthwith flock from the brain to the heart ...and signify what good or bad object was presented; which immediately bends itself to prosecute or avoid it, and ... draweth with it other humours ... so in pleasure, concur great store of purer spirits; in sadness, much melancholy blood; in ire, choler. If the imagination

[81] Coëffeteau, 2, A5$^{v}$-A7$^{r}$, A7$^{r}$-A7$^{v}$. On Senault's view on the role of the imagination in constructing representations that direct the passions see 17–19.

[82] Primaudaye, 30, 35–7.

[83] Burton, Part II, 257.

> be very apprehensive, intent, and violent, it sends great store of spirits to or from the heart, and makes a …greater tumult …so that the first step …of all our grievances in this kind is *loesa imaginatio* [a disordered imagination], which, misinforming the heart, causeth all these distemperatures, alteration and confusion of spirits and humours ….. [hence] the cause of melancholy to be ascribed to this [imagination] alone, than to the distemperature of the body.[84]

Pierre Charron too underscores the dangerous character of passionate re-presentation. He starts off simply by stating that: "Every passion is moved by the appearance and opnion [sic], either of what is good, or what is ill." But in the same passage he suggests that the "apparent" character of passionate representation makes them suspect and to be avoided, for, "Thus you see the principall windes from whence arise the tempests of our *Soule*, and the pit whereout they rise is nothing else but the opinion (which commonly is false, wandring, uncertaine, contrary to nature, veritie, reason, certaintie) that a man hath, that the things that present themselves unto us, are either good or ill: for having conceived them to be such, we either follow them, or with violence flie from them. And these are our passions."[85] To exemplify the normal workings and pitfalls of passionate representation, Charron makes use of a political analogy between a royal commonweal. While the rational soule is "Soveraigne," it requires "under-magistrates" that the soul constrains and directs by "lawes and ordinances, reserving unto himselfe the censuring of the greatest and most important occurrents." But if these "magistrates," which are akin to a "power estimative, and imaginative," should "suffer themselves either to be deceived by facilitie, or corrupted by favour; and …shall use their owne authoritie in the execution of their affaires, they fall all with disorder and confusion." For "That which molesteth and corrupteth this power [estimative and imaginative], are first the senses, which comprehend not the true and inward nature of things, but only the face and outward forme," and thus carry with them a "prejudicate opinion of their qualities," and secondly, "the false and indifferent judgement of the vulgar sort." These two false guides impel the imagination to forgo "the commiting of anything to discourse and understanding," and they come to control "our imagination, and as within a Citidell, holdeth the fort against right and reason…. "[86]

Perhaps it is Senault who best describes the representational and rhetorical tumult that freewheeling passions can induce. As he points out, the business of rationally reframing or re-representing the passions oftentimes becomes corrupted, particularly when the passions, egged on by the senses, and supported by imagination, manage to out-maneuver—"out-represent"—or hoodwink the understanding, that then perverts the will. Senault uses the analogy of a courtroom trial to describe a virtual theatre of cognitive corruption:

---

84 Burton, Part II, 159, 252–3.

85 Charron, 71.

86 Charron, 71–3.

> These Passions arising from the senses side alwaies with them; when ever Imagination presents them to the understanding, he pleads in their behalf, by means of so good an Advocate they corrupt their Master, and win all their causes. The understanding listens unto them, weigheth their reasons, considereth their inclinations, and lest he may grieve them, oft times gives sentence to their advantage; he betraies the will, whereof he is the chief officer; he Cozens his blind Queen, and …makes unfaithful reports unto her, that he may draw unjust commandements from her." Therefore, as long as passions "are awakened by objects, solicited by the senses, and protected by Imaginations self, they have no other craft then what they draw from corrupted nature; But when the understanding overshadowed by their obscurity . . . perverts the will, and obliges this soveraign to take upon her the interest of her slaves, she makes them guilty of her sin, [and] she changes their motions into rebellion . . . . [87]

Elsewhere, in speaking of efforts to mortify and govern the passions, Senault again imagines the soul as internally divided constituting a veritable rhetorical theatre of competing players. For in trying to control our passions we "do at once [ourselves] the office of a common soldier, and of a commander." thus, in regards to anger "we fight against a part of our selves that our forces are divided, and that nothing encourageth us in this war, but duty and integrity." Moreover, "when we assail our Passions, our troops are wakened by division; we operate but by one part of ourselves: let vertue …animate our courage with the best reasons she can; our love to our enemies, makes us faint-hearted, and we are afraid of a victory which must cost us …our delights."[88]

Clearly, as Burton, Charron, and Senault suggest, there are many slips between the mouth and the cup when it comes to the proper functioning of passionate representation. Nonetheless, as I argue below, the rational soul, as agent, was thought to be capable of seizing the reins, rectifying the passions, and reestablishing representational hegemony.

## Representation and Agency

Early modern passion registered a relation between entities of different dimensions—immaterial and material—and simultaneously activated two powers of the soul, passive and active. In passion, the soul activated its passive power as a recipient of material impressions and cognitive information, but it was also the agent that re-presented that information in terms of its own concerns and values. In passion, the soul passively suffered, but it also actively responded and moved itself to further action. In other words, in passion, the soul displayed an agency that came into existence only because it was also capable of passivity. If the soul's passions were rightly ordered, its responsive, representing agency could take the form of creative transformation or transcendence of material conditions, for example in the

---

87 Senault, 15–17.

88 Senault, 88–9.

form of righteous anger or charitable compassion. But if the soul's passions were poorly disposed, its agency could take the form of self-enslaving obsession with those very material conditions. As William Fenner avers, citing an old proverb the "Affections" could be the "wings of the Soule" that can transport human beings to higher reaches, but "if the birds wings bee limetwigd and glued to the ground, shee cannot flye up."[89] Using a striking metaphor, Fenner, like Primaudaye before him, describes the agency of ill-disposed affections as if they were nails with which the soul hammers itself to the material world, for the passions are "the nayles of the soule, whereby it's nayled to the things of the body."[90]

The idea that the passions of the soul could and should be rightly ordered underscores the fact that many contemporary writers embraced the idea that the soul could and should maintain its status as a responsible, rational agent even when faced with the "passive" suffering of bodily disease or the perturbations induced by the passions. For William Perkins, in all human actions the soul is the agent and the body the instrument. "Vertue" is "a gift of the Spirit of God" that reforms the "will," and that in turn enables the soul to rightly order the passions.[91] Pierre de la Primaudaye maintains that "reason worketh in the soule of a prudent man" in "curing passions." Indeed, as far as Primaudaye is concerned, the passions of the soul are more dangerous to the body than those of the body are to the soul, because the soul can resist the "corporal passions" because it is "ruled by reason," whereas "the bodie is constrained to alter and change with every infirmitie of the soule. ...The diseases of the bodie hinder not the soule from effecting all good & vertuous actions: yea many have brought forth the fruits of wise philosophers and great captaines, when they were vexed with diseases, which they could never do, at least verie few of them, that were corrupted and defiled in soule."[92] Edward Reynolds argues that "*Education, Custome,* and *Occasion*" empower the soul to exert its "predominancy of the *Body*."[93]

One of the main ways that the rational soul can cure or properly dispose the disturbing passions of the mind is through a strategy of re-representing the cognitive content of the passions themselves. In other words, through the agency of reason, passionate representation of the external world must be re-framed or re-staged once more in order to achieve a rational calm. Hence, Robert Burton contends that the first step in the cure of melancholy is not medicinal, but a matter of taking charge of one's own thoughts and behaviour in order to "rectify these passions and perturbations of the mind." Burton acknowledges that "our passions are violent, and tyrannize of us, yet there be means to curb them; though they be headstrong, they may be tamed .... " According to Burton, it is from "the patient

---

89 Fenner, 10.

90 Fenner, 15; Primaudaye speaks of the passions as those "infinite perturbations fastened in the midst of it [the soul] with the naile of pleasure and griefe" (28).

91 Perkins, 188–9, 470–508.

92 Primaudaye, 34.

93 Reynolds, 10–11.

himself [that] the first and chiefest remedy must be had." To be the agent of his own cure, the patient "must do his utmost endeavour to resist and withstand the beginnings" by engaging in strategic cognitive re-representation: "Whatsoever it is that runneth in his mind, vain conceit, be it pleasing or displeasing, which so much affects or troubleth him, 'by all possible means he must withstand it, expel those vain, false, frivolous imaginations, absurd conceits, feigned fears and sorrows … by doing something or other that shall be opposite unto them, thinking of something else, persuading by reason, or howsoever, to make a sudden alteration of them.'" The patient must "strive against with all his power, to the utmost of his endeavour, and not cherish those fond imaginations which so covertly creep into his mind." Even if the sufferer "be far gone, and habituated unto such phantastical imaginations, yet, as Tully and Plutarch advise, let him oppose, fortify, or prepare himself against them, by premeditation, reason, or, as we do by a crooked staff, bend himself another way." To control one's passions one need only control one's structure of belief:

> Thou thinkest thou hearest and seest devils, black men, etc., 'tis not so, 'tis thy corrupt phantasy; settle thine imagination, thou art well. Thou thinkest thou has a great nose, thou art sick, every man observes thee, laughs thee to scorn; persuade thyself 'tis no such matter: this is fear only, and vain suspicion. Thou art discontent, thou art sad and heavy; but why? upon what ground? Consider of it: thou art jealous, timorous, suspicious; for what cause? Examine it thorougly, thou shalt find none at all, or such as is to be contemned, such as thou wilt surely deride, and contemn in thyself, when it is past. Rule thyself then with reason, satisfy thyself, acustom thyself, wean thyself from such fond conceits, vain fears, strong imaginations, restless thoughts.[94]

While Burton places the burden of self-cure on the patient, Thomas Wright recommends the use of the arts of music and rhetoric to reframe, re-present, and thus rectify the passions.[95] As a representational art or discipline rhetoric, in particular, was well suited to re-frame and reconstitute passionate representation. Wright notes that the effective orator had to engage in theatrical representation, for according to Cicero, "it is impossible" for an orator "to stirre up a Passion in his auditors, except he bee first affected with the same passion himselfe" and Horace contends that "he which will make me weepe must first weepe himselfe."[96] The "action" of oratory involves the imitation or projection of passions through the sound of the voice, the posture of the body, the gesture of the limbs, and the expression of the face:

> for action is either a certaine visible eloquence, or an eloquence of the bodie, or a comely grace in delivering conceits, or an external image of an internall minde, or a shadow of affections, or three springs which flowe from one fountaine,

---

94 Burton, Part 2, 102, 104,106.

95 Wright, 172.

96 Wright, 172.

> called *vox, vultus, vita,* voice, countenance, life, that is, the affection pureth forth it selfe by all means possible, to discover unto the present beholders and auditors, how the actor is affected, and what affection such a case and cause requireth in them: by mouth hee telleth his minde: in countenance he speaking with a silent voice to the eies; with al the universall life and body he seemeth to say, Thus as we move, because by the passion thus wee are moved, and as it hath wrought in us so it ought to worke in you … for it seemeth, that the soule plaieth upon these three parts, as a musitian upon three strings, & according to his striking so they sound.[97]

According to J.F. Senault, the "better part of sciences seem only to have been invented to regulate" the passions.[98] Senault also holds the view that the right use of rhetoric could rectify the passions through the use of artful re-representations. For "as their [rhetoricians] chiefe end is to preserve the truth, they are inforced to imploy all their cunning to beat down such Passions as are contrary thereunto; and in discharging themselves of their duty, they play the part of the Physitian, curing their auditors of all their maladies; If their choler be too much irritated, they appease it; If their courage be too much supprest, they raise it up; they make love exceed hatred, Piety revenge; and repressing one motion by another they draw a calm from out a storm…. Orators who will work upon the soul by the sences, cloth their good reasons in handsome language, tickling the ear that they may touch the heart, and using Tropes and figurative speeches, to move affection. They set upon the two parts whereof man is composed, they make use of the weakest to subdue the stronger; and as the divel undid man by the means of the woman they gain Reason by the means of Passions." Senault notes that efforts have been made by "true religion" to create a "reformed Poetry" that will aid in the rectification of the passions: so that the "very rules imposed upon" playwrights and poets "will not suffer them to be obscene; and by a happy necessity it behoves that those who infuse a soul into the scene, take part alwaies with virtue."[99] Nonetheless Senault, as well as Wright, laments the efforts of Alight and wanton Poets, "[100] and remains pessimistic about poetry's ability to move the passions to virtue through their specific forms of representation for Ait unfortunately fals out (the which I rathor attribute to the disorder of nature, then to the like of Poetry)

[97] Wright, 175–6. Of course the best way for the orator to represent the passions is to imitate the natural passions seen in the course of everyday life. According to Wright, "Thie first is, that we looke upon other men appassionate, how they demeane themselves in passions, and observe what and how they speake in mirth, sadnesse, ire, feare, hope, Etc., what motions are stirring in the eyes, hands, bodie, etc. And then leave the excesse and exorbitant levitie or other defects, and keepe the manner corrected with prudent mediocritie: and this the best may be marked in stage plaiers, who act excellently; for as the perfection of their exercise consisteth in imitation of others, so they that imitate best, act best" (170)."

[98] Senault, 165. For his view of the regulatory role of music and poetry see 166–70.

[99] Senault, 170–172.

[100] Wright, 333.

that chastity appears not so beautiful in verse, as does uncleanness; and that the obedience of the Passions seems not so pleasing as their rebellion. Men betake themselves more usually to violent affections, then to such as are answerable to Reason. "[101] In other words, in the poetic context, vice possesses more allure, more representational *enargeia* than virtue. Consequently, Senault contends that only the educated can gain control over their passions through the benefits bestowed by the representational efforts of poets. The common people will only be mislead by such free-wheeling representations: AIn fine, let what care soever will be had, comoedies are only Schools of vertue for such gallant men, as can discern between appearances and truth, and who abhor vice even then when it comes presented in vertues ornaments. But if you will examine the Common people, they will confess that stage Poetry doth strangely move them, and that it imprints in their souls the feelings of those personages that they represent.[102]

Wright and Senault's rejection of theatre as a tool for assisting self-regulation of the passions tells us more about the stratified nature of the disbursement of early modern culture capital than it does about the theatre's ability to instill moral education and mortify the passions. What critics like Wright, Senault, and the likes of Stephen Gosson underscore is that theatre can pose an ethical danger to the uneducated because their lack of cultural exposure leaves them Arepresentationally challenged, " so to speak.[103] In other words, they have not been allowed to flex their intellectual and ethical judgments through the interpretation and manipulation of texts, arguments, symbols, images, and language in educational settings. And hence, they have not developed those ethical muscles of discernment that would enable them to assess the ethical benefits and deficits of the perspectival representations offered up by the public theatre. Proponents of the theatre, of course, held different views on the matter, arguing that the theatre in fact could provide that very education and opportunity for intellectual flexing that the less educated required.[104] I would like to end this paper with a brief consideration of Shakespeare's *Macbeth*, a play that I believe embraces the view that theatre—because of its metadramatic capacity to re-present the representational and perspectival workings of the passions themselves—was the most potent instrument for rectifying these troubling forces of the sensitive soul.

One of the prime purposes of oratory is of course to persuade an audience to embrace a particular argument, perspective, or course of action. To effect this

---

[101] Senault, 170.

[102] Senault, 171.

[103] On Stephen Gosson's view that theater is dangerous for the uneducated masses rather than the educated elite, see *A School of Abuse* (1579) in *Markets of Bawdrie: The Dramatic Criticism of Stephen Gosson,* ed. Arthur Kinney (Salzburg: Instut für Englische und Literatur, Universität Salzburg, 1974), 77–108 and *Playes Confuted in Five Actions* (1582) in *Markets of Bawdrie,* 164.

[104] See for example Thomas Heywood's *Apology for Actors* (London, 1612; rpt. New York: Garland Publishers, 1973).

purpose, the orator uses rational justification, demonstration of his/her own ethical character, as well as techniques for arousing passions in the audience that would favor the orator's viewpoint. The orator, in a word, must understand the workings of the passions in order to enlist them in service to his/her aim of advancing a particular perspective. Theatre's purposes are generally less narrowly instrumental and focused. Rather than simply constructing a given perspective or view, theatre offers us the opportunity to examine the way that given representations and perspectives are constructed, enter into conflict with one another, and are or are not resolved. Consequently, theatre is an ideal medium for exploring four cognitive aspects of the passions that recent scholarship that has focused more narrowly on the humors has occluded. First, it is suited to the consideration of the generation of the passions, particularly of those internal and external re-framings of perspective conducted by those competing faculties of the soul and body: reason, passion, imagination, spirits, and humors. Second, theatre is also eminently capable of exploring the way that an already established ethical disposition interacts with occurrent passions and vice-versa. Third, it is equally adept at exploring workings of what I have termed pseudo-passions, as well as false or simulated ones. And fourth, given its ethical and representational character, theatre, at least as typified by Shakespeare, is well-suited to explore the cognitive and ethical dimensions of the passions. I now turn to Shakespeare's *Macbeth*, since at several junctures both the play and the character do much to explicate early modern ideas about the emotions.

Macbeth's response to the news that he is now Thane of Cawdor dramatizes the point that a complex interaction among reason, imagination, spirits, and bodily humor is involved in the generation of the passions. Macbeth's sensitive appetite responds to his apparent good fortune with pleasure and perplexity—the "truths" told are "happy prologues"—but try as he might, he cannot come to a clear determination as to whether the witches' predictions are Agood" or Aill. " The Acogitative faculty" of his sensitive soul has been stumped. Unable to make a clear decision, his imagination responds to the external stimulus by raising that Ahorrid image"—the Asuggestion" of Duncan's possible murder. That image serves in lieu of cognitive judgment to induce a passion in his sensitive soul, seated in the heart, that then Aknocks" at his Aribs" and in turn agitates the spirits and humors that "unfix" his hair." Plagued by inner turmoil, Macbeth appears stupefied, or as Banquo remarks, Arapt"—rapt in the representational competition among his thoughts, imaginings, and incipient passions, as well as the physical throes of his bodily humors (1.3.128–43).

The great banqueting scene in which Macbeth displays a traumatic reaction to Banquo's ghost exemplifies the second point concerning the distinction between a settled temperament and an occurrent passion based on new cognitive content. The reason for Macbeth's fear, frustration, and anger are evident to an audience who knows of Banquo's murder and sees a ghostly actor on stage. But Macbeth, thinking the ghost is visible to all on stage, is puzzled by the fact that his other guests remain unperturbed. Hence, Macbeth wonders whether he possesses what he thought he did possess—a courageous "disposition" or settled temperament, distinct from the occasional experience of passionate fear:

> Can such things be,
> And overcome us like a summer's cloud
> Without our special wonder? You make me strange
> Even to the disposition that I owe,
> When now I think you can behold such sights
> And keep the natural ruby of your cheeks
> When mine is blanched with fear. (3.4.111–17)

Macbeth's fearful reaction to Banquo's ghost is an emergent passion of the soul, a Aspecial wonder, " that runs against his usual courageous disposition that his nature, nurture, humors, habits, and intentions have shaped over time. To Macbeth, a passionate response to an unusual sight would be normal even for one with a courageous temperament. But because his other guests have not reacted passionately to what he assumes they see too, Macbeth begins to doubt his emotional sense of himself—"the disposition that I owe. " What recent humoral scholarship occludes, and Shakespeare makes visible (besides the ghost), is the early modern distinction between an occurrent passion of the soul and a settled temperament—a distinction essential to our accurate understanding of this scene.

Shakespeare's *Macbeth* exemplifies the distinction between true and false passions by representing several instances in which characters either discuss or engage in the dissembling of passions. King Duncan, to his sorrow, knows: AThere's no art / To find the mind's construction in the face" (1.4.11–12). Similarly, his son Malcolm knows how easy it is ATo show an unfelt sorrow" (2.3.134). And Macbeth effectively premeditates a Afury" that AOutrun the pauser, reason" (2.3.106- 109) to justify his massacre of Duncan's grooms. Lady Macbeth clearly has this duplicitous gift at the beginning of her murderous exploits. In addition, the play also registers the contemporary view that when passions rise without cognitive antecedents they are perhaps labeled untrue or pseudo-passions rather than true emotions. Indeed, this is Lady Macbeth's view of what has happened to Macbeth in the banquet scene. She chastises Macbeth for his hallucinatory fit of passion by declaring AThis is the very painting of your fear, " these are Aflaws and starts, / Imposters to true fear" (3.4.62, 65–66). For like La Chambre, Lady Macbeth appears to believe that the mind can suffer from false passions when the soul's knowledge of the body is Aobscure and confused, " so that the imagination Aforms no perfect images which respect things as they are. "[105]

And finally, Shakespeare's play underscores the way that management of passions of the soul in the early modern period presumed a capacity for ethical responsibility that current theorists of the Ahumoral passions" tend to ignore. Following the footsteps of Aristotle, early moderns believed that achieving virtue involves not just acting morally, but also feeling properly about one's moral actions. It is not enough to act generously and feel miserly, to act honorably

---

[105] La Chambre, 2, 370–371.

and feel cravenly. In 1620, Thomas Cooper, author of *The Mysterie of the Holy Government of our Affections*, associated Epicurean immorality with the belief that the A*Affections*" are Aonely the effects of the *Complexion* and *Humours* of the body. " In contrast, Christian theologians claim that the affections AProceede immediately from the *disposition of the Divine Soule*, either qualified with *grace*, and so expressing. . . *Affections,* as tend to *good*, or else oppressed with corruption, and so discovering it selfe in those *affections* of *Malice, Envie,* &tc. "[106] For Cooper, the apathetic Stoick philosophy blocks the development of ethical virtue because virtue only exists where the soul both feels the pull of earthly passions and desires and learns to rein in the direction and force of that pull. To fully embody virtue, one must cultivate the passions proper to moral acts. Practice and the instilling of habit lends stolidity to ethical affections. Imagination also influences the emotions. The rational soul induces appropriate passions by instructing the imagination to use compelling images to move the passions in a proper direction.

Shakespeare as a dramatist had good reason to endorse the view that our passions are largely a consequence of the ethical choices we have made rather than the humoral dispositions we have acquired through nature or nurture. Theatre remedies the ethical soul rhetorically, not through purging the passions, as Aristotle would have it, but by imagining the consequences of the ethical choices that characters make as they wrestle with their own occurrent passions, inbred character, and particular circumstances. Unsurprisingly, Shakespeare takes jabs at the art of medicine in *All's Well*, where the king's disease baffles the physicians but is healed by the virtuous young Helena. To cure his melancholic frenzy in the *Winter's Tale*, Leontes accedes to Paulina, an ethical Aphysician, " who uses the healing arts of enforced patience, rather than the humoral remedies of bloodletting or purging. But Shakespeare gets to the core of the matter in *Macbeth*, where the doctor forthrightly declares that Lady Macbeth's mental Adisease is beyond my practice" (5.2.58) for she AMore needs" the Adivine than the physician" (5.2.73). Macbeth later half commands and half pleads with the doctor to ACure her" of her Athick-coming fancies":

> Canst thou not minister to a mind diseased,
> Pluck from the memory a rooted sorrow,
> Raze out the written troubles of the brain,
> And with some sweet oblivious antidote
> Cleanse the stuffed bosom of that perilous stuff
> Which weighs upon the heart? (5.3.40–47)

The doctor's reply—"Therein the patient / Must minister to himself" (5.3.47–8)—reinforces the ethical rather than medical significance of her anxious sorrow.[107]

---

[106] Thomas Cooper, *The Mysterie of the Holy Government of our Affections* (London, 1620), 11ᵛ, 7v

[107] Paul Kocher, "Lady Macbeth and the Doctor," *Shakespeare Quarterly* 5 (Autumn, 1954): 341–9.

In act one, scene three, the witches' prediction that Macbeth would become Thane of Cawdor has been realized, and Banquo remarks: AThat, trusted home, / Might enkindle you unto the crown" (1.3.121–22). Of course, Macbeth's ambitious passions, now inflamed, do just that. Yet by play's end, his brutality has so hardened him that he becomes virtually passionless. He has Aalmost forgot the taste of fears" (5.5.9), and is unable to grieve for his dead wife. AOut, out, brief candle, " can refer to the death of Macbeth's passions as well as to human mortality. Time, all those Atomorrows, " weigh heavy upon those who have lost the capacity to feel for the world and the people around them. Without ethical passion, meaningful passion, life becomes a Ashadow" of itself. One may continue to be a mechanical Aplayer, " an apparent actor Awho struts and frets his hour upon the stage" in an idiot's Atale" that contains Asound" and the doubly false passion of Afury. " False, because in this play, Macbeth's fury has been dissembled and because fury is generally viewed as an inadvertent humoral consequence of the true passion of anger. To the mind of the fictional Macbeth, as well as his real contemporaries, the passions of the soul that power our impulses towards good and evil, those passions that lead us to think and feel in deep ways about the people and events in the world around us, are what makes our lives meaningful. Without those soulful passions, our humoral body Asignifies, " if not Anothing, " then very little indeed.

# Chapter 9
# "The Babel Event": Language, Rhetoric, and Burton's Infinite Symptom

Grant Williams

Impatient to grasp the meaning of melancholy in Burton's treatise, readers give short-shrift to his conceptualization of the symptom. Yet at every turn symptoms mediate our engagement with the disease, the author, and his world and go so far as to exceed the medical discourse that strives to secure their signification. Even as he pursues his Galenic methodology, Burton is at pains to point out and reflect upon this semiotic excess through several tropes of linguistic disorientation. He exclaims frustration at not being able to manage an ever-expanding collection of symptoms that do not so much thwart one's ability to identify melancholy as impair the medical method from building up knowledge about the disease and making treatment feasible. In other words, melancholy appears less as a definable disease than as something endlessly symptomatic. The tropes of linguistic disorientation Burton repeatedly invokes to describe his vexed experiences with reading the text of the body and the body of the text suggest that *The Anatomy of Melancholy*'s peculiar phenomenology of language emerges from an epistemological crisis that plagues Burton's world.

On the face of it, *The Anatomy*'s organizational scheme conforms to basic Renaissance Galenism. After defining the disease, Burton lays out the pathway of the text's first two partitions: "the three precedent species are the subject of my present discourse, which I will anatomize, and treat of, through all their causes, symptoms, cures, together and apart" (1:169).[1] Underscored by the text's title and by the headings of its major sections, the categories through which he organizes his approach to the disease speak to the orderliness of demonstration so integral to traditional Galenism,[2] whose therapeutic method seeks to establish four genera: the disease, the damage done to the body's activity or "special symptom," the peculiar symptoms or what one might call side-effects, and the causes of the

1 *The Anatomy of Melancholy* is cited by volume and page number.

2 For extended discussions of Burton's Galenism, see Christopher Tilmouth, "Burton's 'Turning Picture': Argument and Anxiety in *The Anatomy of Melancholy*," *Review of English Studies* 56.226 (2005): 531–35, and Angus Gowland, *The Worlds of Renaissance Melancholy: Robert Burton in Context* (Cambridge and New York: Cambridge University Press, 2006), 50ff. Gowland locates Burton's medical categories within Galenism too (72).

disease.[3] In order to make fine discriminations between similar and different bodily signs, the medical practitioner leverages Aristotelian logic, which inserts a thing into its genus and then adds the differentiae, the attributes by which a species is distinguished from other species of the same genus.[4] According to Galen, the goal of this inquiry into the nature of a disease—its definition, causes, and symptoms—is to empower the practitioner to discover its cures.[5] At the end of the preface, Burton expressly commits himself to breaking melancholy down into its constitutive components for therapeutic purposes (1:110). His acceptance of the ordering potential of Galenic categories places him in the company of many Renaissance medical writings dedicated to alleviating diseases through the practice of a systematic method.[6] For Burton, symptomology accordingly fits into an overall logical process of working toward the restoration of health.

At the beginning of the section on symptoms, Burton renews his commitment to the Galenic scheme by distancing himself from empiricism. Burton recounts a grisly exemplum out of Seneca about Parrhasius, an Athenian painter who tortured a captive "to expresse the paines and passions of his Prometheus, whom he was then about to paint" (1:381). Burton tells readers that he need not torment any melancholy man, because sufferers' "symptomes are plaine, obvious and familiar" and "there needs no such accurate observation or farre fetched object" (1:381). In minimizing the relative importance of observation afforded by experimentation, he appears to side less with empiricism than with its major rival in classical times, the medical sect of "Dogmatics" or "Logical Physicians."[7] The dogmatists built up knowledge of the human body through a logical procedure departing from the a priori premise of humoralism, which assumed the invisible disease to be an imbalance of the four humours; empiricists relied on evidence only from the senses, disputing the notion that the implementation of logic could supply any knowledge of what went on inside the body.[8] The Senecan exemplum of the

---

3 Galen, *Galen on the Therapeutic Method; Books I and II*, ed. R. J. Hankinson (Oxford: Clarendon, 1991), 33.

4 Aristotle, *Topica*, in *Posterior Analytics/Topica*, trans. Hugh Tredennick and E.S. Forster (Cambridge, MA.: Harvard University Press, 1960), 6.139–30. Galen's implementation of logical procedures derives chiefly from Aristotle. See Luis Garcia Baellester, "Galen as a Medical Practitioner: Problems in Diagnosis," in *Galen: Problems and Prospects*, ed. Vivian Nutton (London: Wellcome Institute for the History of Medicine, 1981), 15, 19–20.

5 Galen, *Galen on the Therapeutic Method*, 64. Burton quotes Galen approvingly, "*It is in vaine to speake of Cures, or thinke of remedies, untill such time as we have considered of the Causes*, so *Galen* prescribes *Glauco*" (1:171).

6 See, for instance, Philip Barrough's *The Methode of Phisicke* (1583) and Walter Bruel's *Praxis Medicinae or the Physician's Practice* (1632).

7 Vivian Nutton, *Ancient Medicine* (London and New York: Routledge, 2004), 124.

8 For an account of the empiricists, see Nutton, *Ancient Medicine*, 148–49; and Alan Bailey, *Sextus Empiricus and Pyrrhonean Scepticism* (Oxford: Clarendon Press, 2002), 88–91.

tortured body exaggerates empiricism's fixation on capturing the sensible and the peculiar, and may allude to the semiotic distinction that the Stoics made between epilogism and analogism: empiricism accepted the former "being an inference from a commemorative or hypomnestic (associative) sign, which is observed in conjunction with what it signifies" and rejected the latter being "an inference from an indicative sign which is unverifiable by experience."[9] Burton does not need to conduct any special experiment to wring melancholic symptoms from an individual. The signs of melancholy "are plaine, obvious and familiar" because logic has no problems with laying hold of the hidden. For Galen as well as dogmatists, who were influenced by the Stoical conception of the sign, symptoms pointed to an unobservable disease and thus made diagnosis possible.[10]

But as soon as Burton directs his attention to gathering and managing symptoms, his discourse repeatedly registers an inability to control its subject matter. Alerting readers to trouble ahead, Burton deflates the confidence of the opening exemplum about Parrhasius while replicating his findings in the previous section: "as the causes are diverse, so must the signes be, almost infinite" (1:381). "Infinite," a veritable symptom of Burton's symptom, recurs most pressingly throughout this section, signifying "innumerable," that which is indefinitely great in number but also for early modernity meaning "indefinite in nature, meaning, etc.; indeterminate" (*OED*).[11] On its own, the "infinite" is a sign of an excess

---

9 Ian Maclean, *Logic, Signs, and Nature in the Renaissance: The Case of Learned Medicine*. (Cambridge and New York: Cambridge University Press, 2002), 159–160. See also Umberto Eco, *Semiotics and the Philosophy of Language* (Bloomington: Indiana University Press, 1984), 31.

10 According to R.J. Hankinson, ed., *Galen on the Therapeutic Method; Books I and II* (Oxford: Clarendon Press, 1991), xxix–xxx, Galen is not "indiscriminately hostile to medical Empiricism." At the same time, according to Baellester, "Galen as a Medical Practitioner," 37, "between what was manifest to the eye and what was obvious to reason, Galen, when it came down to it, chose the latter. In this sense, he only found experience convincing when he was able to interpret it in the light of the premises of his own theory."

11 Symptoms appear both quantitatively and qualitatively indefinite, as the section on bodily and on mental ones unfold. Quantitatively speaking, Arculanus will have the mental symptoms "to be infinite, as they indeed are ... *for scarce is there one of a thousand that dotes alike*" (1:384). The melancholic man "fears an infinite number of dangers, disasters, etc." (1:385). Qualitatively speaking, Burton renders suspect two sources of bodily symptoms quite significant for humoralism. Galen was a key proponent of extensively using the pulse in diagnosing diseases. See Nancy G. Siraisi, *Medieval & Early Renaissance Medicine* (Chicago: University of Chicago Press, 1990), 125–27, and Owsei Temkin, *Galenism: Rise and Decline of a Medical Philosophy* (Ithaca: Cornell University Press, 1973), 49. Burton discounts this practice: "in such Chronick diseases the pulse is not so much to bee respected, there being so much superstition in it, as Crato notes, and so many differences in Galen, that he dares say they may not bee observed, or understood of any man" (1:383). Later in partition three, Burton, however, finds no problems with depending upon it for diagnosing love melancholy (3:142). He also dismisses the diagnostic capability of urine "as uncertaine as the other [pulse], varying so often according to severall person, habits,

incapable of being reduced to a comprehensible order and, for a text concerned with humoral logic, it is a fitting abstraction of all that jeopardizes the salutary balance in the world. As such, this modifier concentrates anxieties about understanding melancholy even as it seems to characterize the condition. At the conclusion to his subsections dealing with the general symptoms, he states,

> They will act, conceave all extreames, contrarieties, and contradictions, and that in infinite varieties. Melancholici plane incredibilia sibi persuadent, ut vix omnibus saeculis duo reperti sint, qui idem imaginati sint (Erastus de Lamiis) scarce two of two thousand, that concurre in the same symptoms; The Tower of Babel never yeelded such confusion of tongues, as this Chaos of melancholy doth variety of Symptomes. (1:395)

The task of assembling melancholy's symptoms in one place exceeds the chaotic proportions associated with the Tower of Babel.[12] The "infinite varieties" of symptoms to which Burton attests resemble God's confusion of tongues that thwarted the proud builders from continuing their enterprise of erecting an edifice that could reach heaven and establish the name, fame, and linguistic integrity of their city. The Babel trope underscores the epistemological impossibility of Burton's medical purpose, reiterating similar admissions in the preface: "[T]o anatomize this humour aright" is comparable with the conundrums of squaring the circle, of finding the Northwest Passage, and rectifying the Gregorian calendar (Preface:23). Like the Babel endeavour of competing with the divine, defining melancholy, Burton seems to suggest, is a futile task, because, religiously speaking, the disease, akin to the mortal limitation of original sin, cannot be eradicated by human means. Burton identifies God as the primary cause of melancholy (1:171–74), implying that the disease is woven into the fabric of creation. Semiotically speaking, the infinite marks a Babel-like eruption within language. In its proliferation of chaotic symptoms, melancholy recreates for the ambitious medical compiler the moment in biblical history when a desire for symbolic order yields unexpectedly linguistic chaos. Language serves neither as a channel of truth nor as a technology for constructing civilization but, flood-like, disperses any unity and all identities, interposing itself as an impediment to communication.[13] Its heterogeneous opacity leaves the auditor bemused and

---

& other occasions" (1:383), even though, for early modern humoralism, "the surest aid to diagnosis was inspecting the patient's urine," claims W.S.C. Copeman, *Doctors and Disease in Tudor Times* (London: Dawson's of Pall Mall, 1960), 118. If the four humors and their corruption could be analyzed at all, urine would supply the best fluid sample. In the subsection on mental symptoms, Burton even renders "indeterminate" fear and sorrow, the two primary symptoms of the disease and the only differentiae included in the disease's definition—the "most assured signs, inseparable companions, and characters of melancholy" (1:384), these last two epithets also occurring earlier in the subsection on the definition (1:163).

12 See Genesis 11.

13 In the Bible, the Babel story follows the flood as though linguistic chaos were a variation on this natural disaster.

alienated from divine revelation and human interchange. Burton's invocation of Babel raises the possibility that the infinite variety of melancholic symptoms rivals—if not exceeds—the infinite and unmanageable potential of linguistic semiosis. What was once "plaine, obvious, and familiar" (1:381) has become, over the course of the two subsections, "diverse, intricate, and hard to be confined" so much so that Burton resolves "to bring them [symptoms] into some order, & so descend to particulars" (1:396). He will not abandon the therapeutic method.

But, as much as to be expected, his two subsections on particular symptoms settle on a conclusion similar to that of general ones. Through a string of rhetorical questions, he doubts the possibility of depicting melancholy's symptoms at all, utterly refiguring the exemplum of the painter Parrhasius, which opened the main section:

> Who can sufficiently speake of these symptomes, or prescribe rules to comprehend them? as *Eccho* to the painter in *Ausonius*, *vane quid affectas &c.* foolish fellow what wilt? if you must needs paint me paint a voice, *& similem si vis pingere, pinge sonum*; if you will describe melancholy, describe a phantasticall conceipt, a corrupt imagination, vaine thoughts and different, which who can doe? (1:407)

Rules can no longer comprehend those boundless symptoms, which earlier had been self-evident. To drive home Burton's point, the Senecan exemplum's assumed faith in painterly representation gives way to Ausonius's Epigram XXXII, "In Echo Pictam," a poem about the aporia of visualizing "Air and Speech, mother of empty utterance."[14] In Epigram XXXII, Echo, the nymph who, for the love of Narcissus, pined away until only her voice remained, decries a painter's attempt to limn her face. The second rhetorical question vertiginously carries within it at least a triple ventriloquization. Burton ventriloquizes Ausonius's witty ventriloquization of Echo in order to ventriloquize melancholy. He echoes Ausonius who echoes Echo to echo Melancholy's challenge to those who would presume to comprehend her symptoms: "if you must needs paint me, paint a voice," but one—here's the catch—not mediated by other voices. Echo denies her representability through representing herself through other voices. Burton's task of compiling symptoms has again terminated with Babel: the lone voice of melancholy scatters into the many. However, Burton adapts the aporia embedded in Echo's challenge to suit his own specific purposes. For Ausonius, the impossibility of painting her lies in visualizing the auditory, since the nymph possesses no bodily form, amounting to nothing more than intangible, disincarnated sound; for Burton it lies in speaking comprehensively about the infinite variety of symptoms produced by the disease. If one wants to circumscribe melancholy's signs, one may as well describe the faculty of the imagination or that of the intellect, since these apparatuses of tireless sign production, like that of the voice, cannot be frozen in an image, either one or many.

Melancholy's symptoms, then, are less a static collection of letters, signs, or utterances than the vast territory of languages playing out their possible variations—

---

[14] Decimus Magnus Ausonius, *Ausonius*, vol. 2, trans. Hugh G. Evelyn-White (London: Heinemann, 1949), 175.

endless semiosis. Melancholy is an organ, a faculty, a semiotic generator, whose utterances cannot be anticipated. It should be no surprise that Burton again alludes to the Babel event directly after elaborating the aporia of Ausonius's Echo:

> The foure and twenty letters make no more variety of words in divers languages, then melancholy conceipts produce diversity of symptomes in severall persons. They are irregular, obscure, various, so infinite, *Proteus* himself is not so divers, you may as well make the *Moone* a new coat, as a true character of a melancholy man; as soone finde the motion of a bird in the aire, as the heart of man, a melancholy man. (1:407)

Neither the output of the 24 letters of the alphabet, in many languages no less, nor the divine shape-shifting of Proteus can compete with the diversity of symptoms conceived by melancholy thinking. The "true character," a pun on "letter" no doubt, has as much chance of being interpreted as impossible tasks have of being accomplished, perhaps because the disease, unable to be enunciated for once and for all, resides in an inexhaustible process of combination and permutation akin to rearranging the letters of the alphabet.

Burton's conclusions on the infinite semiosis of melancholic symptoms significantly deviate from Galenic assumptions about the alphabet's role in forestalling linguistic chaos. When taking issue with the empiricists who refuse to admit logical categories, Galen's *On the Therapeutic Method* cites the example of letters to show how we rely everyday on types to make sense of tokens:

> And for this reason when we say that there are seven vowels in our language, and twenty-four elements of the alphabet in all, clearly we are considering the common form underlying them all, and not individual tokens of them written on papyrus, wood, parchment, and stone, and which are indefinitely numerous, incapable of enumeration, indeed which stretch virtually to infinity.[15]

Faced with different tokens in radically different media, we still recognize the forms of the 24 letters so that we can intelligently read the words, since "no one teaches children a multiplicity of alphas, betas, and gammas, but only one of each."[16] Whereas for Galen the basic elements of writing enable us to comprehend innumerable inscriptions, those same elements for Burton release the confusion of language's semiotic variability. So persuaded by the alphabet's foundational rationality, Galen refers to it in another treatise when imagining the dogmatist quarreling with the empiricist disparagement of the logos:

> Do you think that they [empiricists] do not know that in the almost endless variety of their diseases and the symptoms of them the sick themselves differ from one another as well as in the above-mentioned respects—seasons of the year, lands, and similar things? Or is it that their hearts are blind and their minds too dull to understand this? Or is this something which they know full well, but

---

[15] Galen, *Galen on the Therapeutic Method,* 66.

[16] Galen, *Galen on the Therapeutic Method,* 66.

> desire to comprehend that which is infinite by bringing it into the category of temporal experience without making use of the logos? Should they really wish this, then let them know that the sounds of speech, though endless in number, could not be retained and comprehended by mere memory, but that a wise man grasped them and limited them, because, having reflected upon them and examined them, he discovered that the principles and elements of which these sounds are composed—I mean the letters—are twenty-four in number according to Greek reckoning.[17]

Again the letters stave off infinity, but this time the infinity in question concerns the sounds of speech. Without the wise man's reliance on the logos, there would never have been a way of mastering writing, because the innumerable sounds could never have been delimited and consequently remembered. Likewise, the physician can use the logos to limit the infinite manifestations of diseases and symptoms by finding the representative types. Just as the logos, that is, the alphabet, enables the language user to master inscriptions and sounds, rational categories provide medicine with the means of carrying out a therapeutic method, of which diagnosis comprises an important stage. Galenism does not release the babel inherent in language, but endeavours to contain it.[18]

In effect, what Burton has done by appealing to the infinite variety of melancholy's symptoms is reach an empiricist-sounding conclusion inconsistent with the deployment of the method characterizing medical dogmatism or rationalism. Nevertheless, Burton should not be called an empiricist. However much he may support, according to Angus Gowland, a "therapeutic particularism grounded in experience"[19] through invoking the authority of Hippocrates against Galenic generalization, his examination of remedies underlines, as Gowland well knows, "the infinite, chaotic, and labyrinthine nature of a subject beyond the reach of understanding."[20] Particularism in cures as well symptoms hardly rescues Burton's method from doubt and confusion but it certainly does not prompt him to abandon formal categories to turn experimenter, clinician, or empiric.[21] After

---

[17] Galen, "On Medical Experience," in *Three Treatises on the Nature of Science*, trans. Richard Walzer and Michael Frede (Indianapolis: Hackett, 1985), 89.

[18] Aristotle, too, in *On Rhetoric: A Theory of Civic Discourse*, trans. George A. Kennedy (New York: Oxford University Press, 2007), 1356b30–33, recognizes medicine's pragmatic struggle to manage infinite possibilities.

[19] Gowland, *The Worlds of Renaissance Melancholy*, 83.

[20] Gowland, *The Worlds of Renaissance Melancholy*, 112. In his commentary on the category of the symptom, Burton is not demonstrating "a Galenic sensitivity to the particularity of every patient's case," as Tilmouth, "Burton's 'Turning Picture,'" 534, recently claims for Burton's method elsewhere in *The Anatomy*.

[21] Quacks were often associated with "empirics," because they did not take formal medical training. Burton makes the same cultural association: "there be many Mountebankes, Quackslavers, Empericks, in every street almost, and in every village, that take upon them this name [physitian], make this noble and profitable Art to be evil spoken of and contemned, by reason of these base and illiterate Artificers" (2:11).

starting from ostensibly Galenic assumptions, he has found himself in a dogmatist nightmare, where logic has failed to confine the innumerable, and diagnostic action appears indefinite. He bears witness seemingly reluctantly to the Babel event erupting in medical discourse, despite his efforts at supplying the means of containment.

Burton's admission of chaos may, in part, vocalize the common Renaissance challenge of submitting nosology to a methodical order. Ian Maclean has drawn attention to the organizational difficulties that beset sixteenth-century semiology, which drew upon "bewilderingly diverse doctrine" "scattered throughout the Hippocratic and Galenic corpus."[22] Burton's admission of chaos may also, in part, express frustration with debates in Renaissance Galenism. Nancy Siraisi has shown how Leonhart Fuchs and Giovanni Argenerio were "alert to the philosophical objections, logical contradictions, and inconsistencies in the Galenic account" of disease and symptoms and how Jean Fernel's clinical experience "stressed the practical difficulty and uncertainty of diagnosing internal disease."[23] Yet the confusion bred by Burton trying to delimit melancholy's various symptoms does not merely stem from the logical knots and hermeneutic quandaries confronted by the medical writer and compiler. In Burton's treatise, the Babel event typifies the sufferer's actual experience with melancholy. Melancholy not only produces symptoms in language but more tellingly produces voices, tongues, and languages as symptoms. Not only might it generate babbling noises on the verge of linguistic communication, such as "laughing grinning, fleering, murmuring, talking to themselves, with strange mouthes and faces, inarticulate voices, exclamations" (1:382), not only might it generate mental states and utterances, such as "complaining, grieving, vexing, suspecting, grudging" (1:387), but it also quite literally generates languages as symptoms in and of themselves. Melancholics can be "daemonicall persons, and such as speake strange languages" (1:384); "*in their fits you shall heare them speake all manner of languages, Hebrew, Greeke, and Latine, that never were taught or knew them before*" (1:400); Apponensis "speakes of a mad woman that spake excellent good Latine" (1:400); and *Guianerius* had an otherwise illiterate patient who could write Latine verses (1:400). The symptomatic voice can range from beast to eloquent scholar: "He howles like a wolfe, barks like a dog, raves like *Ajax* and *Orestes*…or that woman in *Sprenger*, that spake many languages, and said she was possessed: That Farmer in *Prosper Calenus* that disputed and discoursed learnedly in Philosophy and Astronomy, with *Alexander Achilles* his master" (1:407). Given that melancholics "learne without a teacher" (1:410), they can "talke of Astronomy, and other unknowne sciences to them (of which they have been ever ignorant,) and can hear "many such illusions and voices, which proceede most part from a corrupt Imagination" (1:426–27). Since

---

22 Maclean, *Logic, Signs, and Nature in the Renaissance*, 279–80.

23 Nancy G. Siraisi, "Disease and Symptom as Problematic Concepts in Renaissance Medicine," in *Res et Verba in der Renaissance*, ed. Eckhard Kessler and Ian Maclean (Weisbaden: Harrassowitz in Kommission, 2002), 230 and 232.

melancholics may "speake strange languages" (1:410) and certain individuals may even "speake severall languages" (1:427), the medical inquirer, according to Burton, literally confronts a Babel-like predicament. Whether a sufferer exhibits a single symptom or books of symptoms, the disease possesses a semiotic potential that exceeds language's ability to circumscribe it. We should expect nothing less from the infinite.

After claiming that the alphabet makes fewer words than melancholy does symptoms, Burton acknowledges the methodological impasse while doggedly, if not dogmatically, continuing with his method:

> They are so confused, I say divers, intermixt with other diseases. As the species be confounded (which I have shewed) so are the symptomes. ... [W]ho can distinguish these melancholy symptomes so intermixt with others, or apply them to their severall kindes, confine them into method? Tis hard I confesse yet I have disposed of them as I could & will descend to particularize them according to their species. (1:407)

Its symptoms not only make the individual species difficult to disentangle from one another but also complicate the diagnosis of other diseases. Though acknowledging the medical mayhem created by an infinite symptomology, Burton does not pursue fully its implications for the rest of nosology. His world is too dominated by melancholy to bother with diagnosing alternative ailments. His treatise tenaciously accumulates its encyclopedic girth as though melancholy were the core of all nosology, the genus of all diseases, the only real medical problem.

With reference to classification, the confusion of *The Anatomy*'s medical categories, what Rosalie Colie calls "the interchangeability of cause, symptom, and cure," has been a major question in Burton studies.[24] Followed by Judith Gardiner and Martin Heusser, Stanley Fish finds in the treatise the same schematic collapse: "Melancholy is so pervasive that it is the cause of all effects and effect of all causes, simultaneously symptom and disease, the prominent thread not only runs through the divisions and subdivisions of the superstructure, but finally undoes them."[25] Recently, Christopher Tilmouth—a "new rationalist" if you will—has trivialized this question in scholarship, arguing that *The Anatomy* does not consume itself in contradictions but demonstrates melancholy's self-propagating nature whereby a symptom can be a cause and, "therefore, indirectly, mother of itself."[26] As much as melancholy obviously compounds its severity and intensity

---

[24] Rosalie Colie, *Paradoxica Epidemica: The Renaissance Tradition of the Paradox* (Princeton: Princeton University Press, 1966), 431. For example, Burton earlier on acknowledges the elision between etiology and diagnosis: as Hippocrates has shown, "They beget on another and tread in a ring, for Sorrow is both Cause and Symptome of this disease" (1:256)—a circularity Burton explicitly finds in fear too (1:259).

[25] Stanley Eugene Fish, *Self-Consuming Artifacts: The Experience of Seventeenth-Century Literature* (Berkeley: University of California Press, 1972), 334.

[26] Tilmouth, "Burton's 'Turning Picture,'" 538.

by fanning its own flames so to speak, Tilmouth's ingenuous effort to impose a stable medical scheme on the text willfully ignores the implications of Burton's expressed problematization of that scheme.[27] Nevertheless, I do not want to side entirely with late twentieth-century new critical or biographical scholarship, which has been much too quick in aestheticizing or personalizing the contradictions inherent in Burton's medical categories and fails to recover the conceptualization and contextualization of Burton's peculiar symptom.[28]

To recognize that *The Anatomy* interchanges its medical categories with one another is to realize that melancholy resists a ready placement within a method necessary for knowing and treating the disease. As one seventeenth-century medical writer puts it, "[s]emiology is the 'knowledge of all indications of a therapeutic method, discovered by rational doctors through their own mental resources (instrumenta), for the sake of effecting a cure.'"[29] With the blurring of significant distinctions—causes that can be symptoms and cures that can be causes—how can readers ever go about finding a suitable treatment in Burton's treatise? Martin Heusser poses the question pointedly when noting solitude's simultaneous involvement in etiology and treatment: "If the line between cause and effect is so fine that even the reader (and the author) sometimes fails to observe it, how is the melancholic supposed to be able to make the distinction?"[30] Theoretical questions of indeterminacy and ambiguity aside, which Burton does not explore, interchangeable medical categories throw into doubt the possibility of ever assembling a temporal chain of symptom, disease, and cause, from which an inquirer can determine a suitable cure.

Consequently, all four medical categories begin to resemble symptoms in Burton's text, if what we mean by symptom is, in the loosest sense possible, a sign

---

[27] Tilmouth, "Burton's 'Turning Picture,'" 541ff., uncritically separates the Galenic regimen from rhetoric as though these two discourses never interpenetrated one another. He of course locates the instability of the text on the level of style, while preserving a stable medical core. The preface then is a stylistic domain in contrast to medical domain of the text proper. The distinction is too simplistic.

[28] Ruth A. Fox, *The Tangled Chain: The Structure of Disorder in the "Anatomy of Melancholy"* (Berkeley: University of California Press, 1976), 42, reads Burton's interchangeability as equivocation—"symptom is cause is cure and all are species"—but finally centres the "tangled chain" on the disease: "The pattern of the *Anatomy of Melancholy* is one of structures which equivocate but define all equivocation in a single word: melancholy" (273). Judith Kegan Gardiner, "Elizabethan Psychology and Robert Burton," *Journal of the History of Ideas* 38 (1977): 382, who examines *The Anatomy* as a manifestation of early modern psychology, also realizes that Burton often breaks down his own categories, showing the interpenetration of cause and effect, symptom and cure. She links this interchangeability to the interchangeability of the author and the reader and finally to Burton's empathetic humanistic psychology.

[29] Quoted in Maclean, *Logic, Signs, and Nature in the Renaissance,* 281.

[30] Martin Heusser, *The Gilded Pill: A Study of the Reader-Writer Relationship in Robert Burton's Anatomy of Melancholy* (Tübingen: Stauffenburg, 1987), 48.

arising from, associated with, or accompanying a disease. For Burton, causes and cures display the same Babel-like semiosis that symptoms produce. They multiply out of pragmatic control: "It is a most difficult thing (I confesse) to be able to discerne these causes whence they are, and in such variety to say what the beginning was" (1:171). Burton even expresses a desire to include within the division of necessary causes accidental ones, blurring an important distinction (1:328): if the contingent, the random, and the accidental can cause melancholy, what cannot bring on the affliction? Thus melancholy's innumerable causes stand comparison, as he claims later on, with the infinite diversity of symptoms (1:381). Where cures are concerned, Burton finds "a vast *Chaos* of medicines, a confusion of receipts and magistrals, amongst writers, appropriated to this disease" (2:241). Such a discursive predicament resonates with the earlier passage on the "Chaos of melancholy" that surpasses the tower of Babel's confusion of tongues. His partition on cures accomplishes on a large scale what he explicitly concludes on a small scale when examining the remedial benefits of the simple purgative antimony: "'tis the whole subject of bookes, I might cite a century of Authors *pro* and *con*" (2:230). If the compiler's experience with causes and cures looks like the same Babel-event of the symptom in which all the medical categories have the potential to intermix chaotically, then melancholy cannot be properly called a disease per se. For Burton, it is only ever symptomatic—a symptom that continually exceeds itself without getting the sufferer any closer to therapy.

Burton's avowed inability to master the melancholic symptom with the Galenic method finds compelling corroboration in the symptomatic nature of his own writing. Besides confessing to suffer from melancholy, Burton exhibits its symptoms in the very process of enunciating his expansive medical topic. The scholarship on *The Anatomy* well knows that "[m]any of the symptoms of melancholy described explicitly or indirectly through records of representative cases may be observed in the author himself with an astonishing degree of concordance."[31] For instance, Burton enacts what he describes as the melancholic's habit of wandering in thoughts and deed (1:397): this symptom manifests itself generally in his meandering composition, both on the level of the sentence with its lists and ambages and on the level of the subsection, the most famous example of which is the digression of air, where he imagines himself to be a peregrine falcon

[31] Heusser, *The Gilded Pill*, 167. When explaining in the preface why a divine would concern himself with matters of physicke, Burton pinpoints the origin of his text in his actually having contracted the disease: "but at this time I was fatally driven upon the Rocke of Melancholy, and carryed away by this by-streame, which as a Rillet, is deducted from the maine Channell of my studies in which I have pleased and busied my selfe at idle houres, as a subject most necessary and commodious" (Preface:20). What Reinhard H. Friederich, "Training his Melancholy Spaniel: Persona and Structure in Robert Burton's 'Democritus Junior to the Reader,'" *Philological Quarterly* 55 (1976): 208, concludes about the preface can be applied to the three partitions too: "The whole discourse turns out to have been a madman's melancholy seizure: 'And now methinks upon a sudden I am awaked as it were out of a dream; I have had a raving fit ....'"

circuitously soaring through knowledge. Another related sign Burton describes in melancholics yet continually manifests himself is the inconstant, erratic behaviour that takes the sufferer from extreme to extreme (1:390). Our first exposure to this behaviour comes right at the beginning of the preface where Burton refuses to be known but then, in an about face, proceeds to give reasons for his pseudonym, title, and subject. Probably the most memorable example of inconstancy occurs near the end of the preface, when Burton defies the reader with brave words, only to retract them in cowardly repentance (Preface:112). His erratic speech leads to a withdrawal of what he has just said—although it is not the first time he craves pardon (Preface:16).[32] Burton's act of producing discourse, what Benveniste calls *énonciation* as distinguished from *énoncé*, the resultant utterance, comes already contaminated with symptoms as though the signifier at the moment of concretizing the Galenic category of the symptom escapes the control of the subject by showing itself to be already residually symptomatic.[33] His utterance continually lags behind his enunciation. The symptomatic always exceeds his efforts to capture it in discourse.

Burton acknowledges his residually symptomatic utterance by choosing the pseudonymous epithet, Democritus Jr, in honour of the pre-Socratic anatomist. He could have just as easily named himself after Galen, who championed the practice of dissection to advance medical knowledge and rather famously made many anatomical discoveries.[34] But Burton instead identifies with a failed anatomist who could not master the cut of dissection.[35] Democritus's wild anatomical activities—visually depicted in the frontispiece and verbally depicted in the preface—helped to convince the citizens of Abdera that he was a lunatic (Preface:33). Yet, as if that were not enough, he is renowned for another, more bizarre, incision. Burton does not let us forget that Democritus gouged out his own eyes, thereby turning himself into a self-dissecting anatomist. Why enucleate? Clearly it is a melancholy gesture. Burton proffers an explanation, when first presenting some of his namesake's biographical details: enucleation took away those distractions that prevented his mind's eye from focusing on intellectual objects (Preface: 2). However, a less noble reason appears later on in partition three: "as Tertullian reports of Democritus, that put out his eyes, because he could not looke upon a woman

---

32 But this peculiar symptom may be found well beyond the satirical preface, famous for its playfulness. In the subsection on women's melancholy, he suddenly undercuts his authority on the matter by a self-reproach: "What have I to doe with Nunnes, Maids, Virgins, Widowes?" thus resigning himself to exit the fray: "I will say no more." The very next sentence exposes his irresolution and fickleness: "And yet I must and will say something more, adde a word or two" (1:417).

33 Emile Benveniste, *Problèmes de Linguistique générale*, vol. 2 (Paris: Gallimard, 1974), 80.

34 See Temkin, *Galenism*, 30–36.

35 For a sustained discussion of the epistemology of Burton's cut and anatomical discourse, see my article "Disfiguring the Body of Knowledge: Anatomical Discourse and Robert Burton's *The Anatomy of Melancholy*," *ELH* 68.3 (2001): 593–613.

without lust, and was much troubled to see that which he might not enjoy" (3:329). The torment of an uncontrollable libido prompted him to gouge out his eyes, until we discover still later on that Burton proffers another reason: "*Democritus* put out his eyes ... because he could not abide to see wicked men prosper" (3:412). Locating the impulse of self-dissection in the intellect, then in the passions, and finally in the conscience, Burton seems to formulate the explanation according to the shifting context of his treatise: the cut is said to originate with Democritus's irrational rationality in a mad, melancholic world, then is said to originate in love melancholy, and finally is said to originate in religious melancholy. Burton fails to gain leverage on his namesake's symptom through the medical nomenclature of genus and separate "species."

The anatomical cut, far from penetrating the mystery of melancholy, provides only another radically residual symptom. As such, it parodies the early modern fashion of performing literary and textual dissections.[36] Imitating a self-blinded anatomist does not inspire confidence in the opening up of knowledge to the inquirer's probing gaze. Once more, Burton's tireless pursuit of medical rationalism substantiates an empiricist-sounding conclusion over the uncertainty of settling on truths about corporeal interiority: the seventeenth-century medical empiricism of Sydenham and Locke doubted that anatomy could improve upon the practice of physic or "assist a man in the finding out and establishing a true method."[37] For them, the physician's responsibility was "to confine his observations to the 'outer husk of things,' for God shaped his faculties to perceive only the superficies of bodies."[38] What separates Burton from Sydenham and Locke is that he does not abandon his anatomical method even as he enacts its blindness, irrationality, and failures. In his text, the anatomical cut becomes itself frustratingly symptomatic, not heuristic of aetiology and diagnosis. The Democritean symptom exceeds containment by the metadiscourse of Galenic medicine as though Burton were arriving at empiricist skepticism by taking the longest route available to him.[39]

---

[36] The early modern literature of dissection has been explored extensively by Jonathan Sawday, *The Body Emblazoned: Dissection and the Human Body in Renaissance Culture* (London and New York: Routledge, 1995) and more recently by Richard Sugg, *Murder after Death: Literature and Anatomy in Early Modern England* (Ithaca: Cornell University Press, 2007).

[37] Kenneth Dewhurst, "Locke and Sydenham on the Teaching of Anatomy," *Medical History* 2 (1958): 4.

[38] David E. Wolfe, "Sydenham and Locke on the Limits of Anatomy," *Bulletin of the History of Medicine* 35.3 (1961): 210.

[39] If Galenic knowledge entails subjugating corporeal interiority to vision, then the disabling reflexivity of the Democritean cut takes the ground out from under the anatomist. Democritus's blindness has implications for reading the preface, where Burton continually responds to the world's madness with the following refrain: "what dost thou thinke Democritus would have done, had he beene spectator of these things?" (Preface: 41). Appealing to the sight of a blind wiseman undercuts his medical authority. The Democritean cut prevents the medical gaze from defining melancholy.

Another popular architectural analogue typifies Burton's particular disorientation within symptomology. Burton claims that both those who have melancholy in disposition and those who have it in habit are overwhelmed with affliction: because melancholy in disposition is "the Character of Mortalitie" (1:136), persons who cannot implement Paul's wise counsel of enduring suffering as a good soldier will "precipitate themselves into a Labyrinth of cares, woes, miseries," it falling out "oftentimes that these *Dispositions* become *Habits*" (1:138); and idle persons who develop melancholy from habit may over-stimulate their imaginations and thus "runne earnestly on in this labarinth of anxious and solicitous melancholy meditations" (1:243).[40] Briefly put, it is a symptom of melancholy to be disoriented by melancholy symptoms. Put another way, melancholy engulfs and loses the sufferer in a symptomological maze. Is this not what has happened to Burton who has tried to collect the diverse signs of this disease into an orderly edifice? He has found himself lost in the labyrinthine symptom. The trope colours his entire outlook on existence: "what's the world it selfe? A vast Chaos, a confusion of manners, as fickle as the Ayre, domicilium insanorum, a turbulent troope full of impurities, a mart of walking Spirits, Goblins, the Theater of hypocrisie…." (Preface:50–51).[41] During a discussion of discontents and miseries in partition one, he presents a similarly nightmarish vision: "In a word, the world it selfe is a maze, a labyrinth of errors, a desert, a wilderness, a denne of thieves, cheaters, &c." (1:273).

Burton's experience of the world emerges out of his labyrinthine experience of the symptom: the world as symptom and the symptom as world vertiginously confound one another in his text. How could the *umwelt* not appear labyrinthine to a melancholic whose infinite symptoms plunge him into disorientation? When Burton first tries to delineate the species of melancholy after defining the disease, he reaches an impasse:

> In such obscurity therefore, variety and confused mixture, of Symptomes, causes: how difficult a thing is it to treat of severall kindes apart; to make any certainty or distinction among so many casualities, distractions, when seldome two men shall be like affected *per omnia*? 'Tis hard, I confesse, yet neverthelesse I will adventure through the midst of these perplexities, and led by the clue or thread of the best Writers, extricate my selfe out of a Labyrinth of doubts and errors, and so proceede to the Causes. (1:171)

---

[40] Burton says the same thing for melancholics who give themselves up to perturbations: "they precipitate and plunge themselves into a Labyrinth of cares, blinded with lust, blinded with ambition" (1:256).

[41] But he does not restrict such an outlook to the Erasmian preface, where he asserts, "we are also giddy, vertiginous and lunaticke within this sublunarie Maze" (Preface: 66) and "[many are] unawares precipitated insensibly, into an inextricable labyrinth of debts, cares, woes, want, griefe, discontent; and melancholy it selfe" (Preface: 99).

But, as we have seen earlier, his desire to resume the Galenic method as though the rational metadiscourse could rescue him from perplexity leads only to further impasses and perplexities. Later on he returns to the same predicament:

> In this Labyrinth of accidental causes, the farther I wander, the more intricate I find the passage, *multae ambages*, and new causes, as so many by-paths offer themselves to be discussed: to search out all, were an *Herculean* worke, and fitter for *Theseus:* I will follow mine intended thred; and point onely at some few of the chiefest. (1:356)

Burton here admits that he cannot map out the maze. There is no position from which to command a full view of the disease.

I want to contend that such disorientation is not one symptom among others but the overriding symptom of Burton's text. The precipitation of *The Anatomy* into labyrinthine moments is yet another rendition of what we have noted as the Babel event. These two architectural tropes for confusion complement one another, having intersected long before Burton's time: as with several other famous cities, Babylon was, as Penelope Doob notes, linked to the labyrinth during the Middle Ages, there being a tradition in which Nimrod, the builder of the Tower of Babel, had a son named Icarus.[42] The story of the tower provides an etymological explanation for Babylon's disorderly and riotous cosmopolitanism and commemorates the "making labyrinth" of that city. Language as event—sheer linguistic proliferation and disorientation—interrupts the best laid architectural plans. The builders are plunged into a semiotic labyrinth utterly alienated from one another and their common project.

In his encounter with the infinite symptom, Burton experiences the alienating effects of the "pure event of language," in which discourse does not speak the subject's identity and desires but stammers out the incomprehensible. "That is why subjectification, the production of consciousness in the event of discourse," according to Giorgio Agamben, "is often a trauma of which human beings are not easily cured." The unreliable and "fragile text of consciousness" means that there is a potential "desubjectification in every subjectification."[43] Melancholy stages for Burton the pure event of language where semiosis exceeds the speaker's or the writer's knowledge of himself. The phenomenology of this decidedly non-rhetorical experience—if conventional rhetoric assumes the instrumentality of discourse—may be described by what I call "the Babel event," to which Burton's insistence on infinite semiosis makes frequent allusion.

Burton's recognition of the Babel event, however, does not imply that he revels in chaos. Like Nimrod, he does not intend his enterprise to be undermined by a linguistic labyrinth. In the preface, he clearly figures his text through benign

---

[42] Penelope Reed Doob, *The Idea of the Labyrinth from Classical Antiquity through the Middle Ages* (Ithaca: Cornell University Press, 1990), 116–17.

[43] Giorgio Agamben, *Remnants of Auschwitz: The Witness and the Archive* (New York: Zone Books, 1999), 123.

architectural tropes, which suggest control over written space. He refers to his readers as guests (Preface:13) and himself as a Dutch Host (Preface:14) as if *The Anatomy* were a "German Inn," at which travellers could find comfortable lodgings. He argues that he did not correct the errors of the first edition since carpenters often find that it is easier to "build a new sometimes, then repaire an old house" (Preface: 19) and if readers think his castle too secular, he will make amends in another publication by erecting a religious house (Preface: 23).[44] But for all these tropes of architectural familiarity and residence, if not domesticity, Burton bears witness to his text degenerating into labyrinthine confusion. What was once a home has morphed into a heterological space, alien even to its builder. Burton has become a failed Theseus or a bemused Daedalus rather than the master of his own domain, the event of language rendering the text uninhabitable and unfamiliar. Burton places his trust again and again in the Galenic method but watches it disperse into strange tongues and infinite signs.

In an effort to understand *The Anatomy*'s conceptualization of symptoms, I have examined Burton's recurrent tropes for his semiological disorientation. These tropes suggest the powerlessness of a metalanguage to master the infinitely residual symptom. One conclusion to draw from Burton's reluctant deviations from Galenism might involve privileging the authorial. His medical vision is a unique and personal, if not quirky and misguided, approach to early modern disease. But his symptom is not just his own. The epistemological and experiential construction of *The Anatomy*'s symptom emerges from a cultural matrix larger than the sphere of Burton's autonomous subjectivity. Nothing prevents us, then, from asking the question "what are Burton's infinite, labyrinthine, and chaotic symptoms symptomatic of?"

Near the beginning of the preface, Burton announces, "I have read many Bookes, but to little purpose, for want of good method, I have confusedly tumbled over divers Authors in our Libraries, with small profit, for want of Art, Order, Memory, Judgement" (Preface:4). These capitalized metadiscourses of "Art, Order, Memory, Judgement"—and one might add "Galenism"—cannot rescue Burton from a phenomenological experience of books that can be tersely described as confusion. He continues that he is neither poor nor rich and lacks nothing for "all my treasure is in *Minerva*'s Towre" (Preface:4). As the preface unfolds, the reader discovers that Burton's roving humour has to do less with a personal lack of academic discipline than with the current state of learning. Minerva's tower is in a Nimrod-like crisis.

The current state of learning presumably explains why Burton devotes considerable energy to the preface's catalogue of madmen. The wisest men of the classical tradition were fools, and "their Bookes and elaborate Treatises were full of dotage" (Preface:29), because, ultimately, all people have a never ending capacity to produce madness: "'Tis an in-bred malady in every one of us, there

[44] Burton has an ambivalent attitude toward massive monumental projects (Preface: 81, 106), which definitely reflects upon his own encyclopedic ambition.

is *seminarium stultitiae*, a seminarie of folly, *which if it be stirred up, or get a head, will run* in infinitum, *& infinitely varies, as we our selves are severally addicted*" (Preface: 32). This passage on stupidity running to infinity should not be read as a conventional warning about the dismal state of European education. Burton studies usually handles the problem of knowledge in *The Anatomy* through invoking Erasmian paradox, famously embodied by Folly's encomium, which morally upbraids prideful wisdom for being foolish.[45] For Burton, "In infinitum" does not, however, refer to a moral shortcoming but to an ineluctable force, figured confusingly as rushing water and an expanding institutional space—the seminary of folly. What will later appear as the vexing "infinite," which Burton uses to modify the causes, symptoms, and cures of melancholy, already at this juncture signals a giddy material production of madness and the concomitant lack of control over that production. In *The Anatomy*, the "infinite" is a sign overwritten with anxieties about epistemological crisis.

The alarm is sounded on the very first page of *The Anatomy*,[46] even before Burton grapples with his bête noire "melancholy." He warns the reader about misidentifying *The Anatomy* by firmly denying that it is "some ridiculous Treatise (as I my selfe should have done) some prodigious Tenent, or Paradox of the Earths motion, of infinite Worlds *in infinito vacuo, ex fortuitâ atomorum collisione*, in an infinit wast, so caused by an accidental collision of Motes in the Sunne, all which *Democritus* held...." (Preface: 1). The first time Burton mentions the "infinite," we encounter the sign embedded within the controversy over Copernican cosmology. Developed by Epicurus yet best represented by Lucretius's *On the Nature of Things*, Democritean atomism theorizes a materialist vision of the cosmos in which the random clash of infinite atoms constitute the world and, indeed, makes possible a plurality of worlds. In the Renaissance, the revival of atomism along with astronomical challenges to the Ptolemaic system helped to promote the theory that there are contingently produced infinite worlds, not a singularly created earth as the centre around which the spheres revolve. Burton enters into the fray of this controversy later in Partition Two, predictably recording the cosmological disputations and debates, if not actually siding, as Richard G. Barlow argues, with the new astronomy.[47] That said, this controversy, one among a myriad in

[45] Michael O'Connell, *Robert Burton* (Boston: Twayne, 1986), 49, claims that "there are two books coexisting" in the text: the medical treatise and a book that "finds its ancestor in Erasmus's *Praise of Folly*." Colie, *Paradoxica Epidemica*, 458, similarly asserts, "Burton's book is, first and last, a paradox of the fundamental kind, a praise of folly."

[46] The alarm is not sounded in the 1621 edition where he has no preface but a conclusion.

[47] Barlow argues that "The Digression of Air" structures itself around the device of the Lucianic cosmic voyage—Burton sending his hawk-like imagination through the ether—in order to explore the cosmos and express his belief in the plurality of worlds. At one point, Burton sympathetically postulates,

If our world be small in respect, why may we not suppose a plurality of worlds, those infinite stares visible in the Firmament to be so many Sunnes, as the Sunne hath his dancing

*The Anatomy*, really has only a limited epistemological significance. As Burton avers, his treatise has nothing to do with the "Prodigious tenet" (Preface: 1) of infinite worlds. And yet in a treatise whose author, an inveterate reader, confesses to having "never travelled but in Mape or Card" (Preface: 4) and expresses his experiences through quoting other writers, "infinite Worlds" evocatively introduces the reader to bookish constellations.[48] Indeed, the tenet illuminates the symptom of epistemological crisis at the heart of *The Anatomy*.

Instead of literally pursuing the ramifications of the new cosmology, Burton's preface immediately voices anxieties over the multiverse of print:

> *there is no end of writing bookes*, as the Wise-men found of old, in this scribling age, especially wherein *the number of Bookes is without number* (as a worthy man saith) *Presses be oppressed* and out of an itching humor, that every man hath to shew himselfe, desirous of fame and honour (*scribimus indocti doctique*——.) he will write no matter what, and scrape together it bootes not whence. (Preface: 8)

Burton articulates the epistemological crisis with phrasing conceptually reminiscent of Democritean atomism. The production of a book does not observe any rational explanation essential to the book's content. Itching humors—abitrary impulses—motivate authors to "write no matter what, and scrape together it bootes not whence" as if books were products of "an accidentall collision of motes" (Preface: 1). Contingent circumstances shape and reshape the matter that, Burton laments, gets recycled and remixed daily into more books (Preface: 9). Consequently, learning has spawned vast labyrinthine discourses, understood as a kind of expanding spatial contingency. Scholasticism, for instance, is nothing but a "labyrinth of intricable questions, unprofitable contentions, *incredibilem delirationem*" (Preface:101). Beyond the preface, Burton echoes these sentiments on a grand scale: "What is most of our philosophy, but a Labyrinth of opinions,

---

still round him? ...Though they seem close to us, they are infinitely distant, and so *per consequens*, there are infinite habitable worlds: what hinders? Why should not an infinite cause (as God is) produce infinite effects, as *Nic. Hill Democrit. philos.* disputes. (2:52) Barlow, "Infinite Worlds: Robert Burton's Cosmic Voyage," *Journal of the History of Ideas* 34.2 (1973): 292–93, says, "[M]ost scholars base their remarks on Burton's early editions where he favours the old astronomy" but "he gradually accepted the point of view that there are infinite worlds." In his digression, for instance, he challenges the impenetrability of the spheres (296), a key concept for the fixity of the Ptolemaic system. Robert M. Browne, "Robert Burton and the New Cosmology," *Modern Language Quarterly* 13 (1952): 147, says that despite Burton's objections, "his absorption with the idea [of the new cosmology] indicates an imagination enthralled by vistas of space endlessly far-flung and of countless scattered worlds."

[48] Even when expressing his experience outside of books, he opts to ventriloquize the lines of others: "Concerning my selfe, I can peradventure affirme with *Marius* in *Salust, that which others heare or read of, I felt and practiced my selfe, they get their knowledge by Bookes, I mine by melancholizing*" (Preface:8).

idle questions, propositions, Metaphysicall tearmes"? It is in this light that we can view Burton's own methodological lapses into the labyrinthine (1:171, 356) as well as his rhetorical propensity to lose the reader in long lists and in his sprawling synoptic diagrams. *The Anatomy* can be seen to extend the discursive labyrinths that replicate and convolute out of control because of the contingency of book production.

Like the plurality of worlds, book production offers no end in sight, presenting a disturbingly materialistic vision as indicated by the punning polyptoton "presses be oppressed." The printing press is an instrument of its own oppression, which overshadows its otherwise weighty impressions on paper. The tables are turned: the press is ironically pressed down by the mass of its own production. Burton shortly returns to this pun to explain the impact that the crisis has on him:

> What a catalogue of new bookes all this yeare, all this age (I say) have our *Franc-furt* Marts, our Domesticke Marts brought out? …So that which *Gesner* much desires, if a speedie reformation be not had, by some Princes Edicts and grave Supervisors, to restraine this libertie, it will run on *in infinitum. Quis tam avidus librorum helluo*, Who can read them? As already, wee shall have a vast *Chaos* and confusion of Bookes, we are oppressed with them, our eyes ake with reading, our fingers with turning. (Preface: 10–11)

With its brute materiality, the overproduction of books fatigues the human body. In the passage, reading, devoid of any idealism, appears more like the physically demanding activities of the compositor and the corrector. Here the infinite threatens to plunge us, the hapless readers, into a "vast *Chaos* and confusion of Bookes" (Preface:11), an ordeal which ultimately explains Burton's personal predicament of "confusedly" tumbling over various authors in libraries, without "Art, Order, Memory, Judgement" (Preface: 4).

The oppressive printing press has brought about the Babel event plaguing Minerva's tower and *The Anatomy* itself. Burton cannot find resolutions to the controversies he painstakingly traces out in the various discourses of learning, especially in the medical record on melancholy, because the mass production of books, a veritable cacophony of strange tongues, does not allow writers to coordinate and order their communication. Such profusion of voices yields only an oppressive mass. Burton says that he decided not to compose a theological treatise because there are so many of them "that whole teems of Oxen cannot draw them" (Preface: 20). He observes that likewise the law is oppressively confounded by its own Babel event of controversies, wistfully approving a "Laconike brevitie" after Tertullian, who championed "certa sunt paucis, there is much certaintie in fewer words" (Preface: 73); but "hee that buyes and sells a house, must have a house full of writings, there bee so many circumstances, so many words" (Preface: 73). The public sphere of print and writing manufactures a dense chaos. Burton agrees with Gesner that Protestant-like measures taken by stern authority figures must occur if the catastrophe is to be averted. This totalitarian "reformation" starkly contrasts Burton's criticism of modern divines who peevishly reject the mathematical demonstrations of Copernican astronomy (2:53). Remarkably enough, the new astronomy has not disrupted Burton's world as much as the printing press has. The proliferation of infinite bookish constellations poses a graver threat to knowledge than does any notion of a decentered cosmos.

Burton's anxiety over such chaos tempers the popular critical judgement that he holds a conventional sceptical position vis à vis knowledge, aptly summarized by Joan Webber: "While he believes in authority, he has no belief that one authority can know everything, or that one medicine can heal all men. He is most skeptical about absolute, generalizing statements on any subject."[49] Within the context of medicine, such a judgement could be used to argue that Burton advocates medical empiricism, whose classical precedents marshalled scepticism against prevailing dogmatist models of disease.[50] If in his doubts over method Burton appears to be empiricist, he acquires his sceptical stance not through expository rigour, as does Montaigne, to whom he is often compared, but through empirically confronting the irreconcilable and clashing voices on melancholy.[51] Driven to keep up with book production by incorporating new sources into his treatise's successive editions, Burton is overwhelmed with polyphonic, dialogical confusion.[52] He is a reluctant sceptic and a failed rationalist, who arrives at conclusions sounding of uncertainty and indeterminacy only after doggedly struggling to manage typographical semiosis with Galenic categories.

Burton's treatise topples into the same crisis that throughout the preface he encounters elsewhere in his world. His experience of the infinite symptom, however, is neither the confusion arising from the organizational challenges of information overload, nor the perplexity in removing the logical inconsistencies arising from classifying the disease. Infinite semiotic proliferation gestures toward a pathological dimension to language that always exceeds the efforts of the compiler and sufferer to understand. The printing press's insane production has made words, voices, and tongues strange, foregrounding language's oppressive materiality and vertiginous contingency. During a discussion of the numerous

---

49 Joan Webber, *The Eloquent "I": Style and Self in Seventeenth-Century Prose* (Madison: University of Wisconsin Press, 1968), 86. Bud Korkowski, "Genre and Satiric Strategy in Burton's *Anatomy of Melancholy*." *Genre* 8 (1979): 83, claims that he subscribes to "fideistic scepticism." Heusser, *The Gilded Pill*, 154, emphasizes Burton's "attitude of scepticism towards the absolute" and O'Connell, *Robert Burton*, 45, claims, "What we are witnessing [in Burton's text] is the copia of Renaissance humanism becoming skepticism by its own most cherished method."

50 Bailey, *Sextus Empiricus and Pyrrhonean Scepticism*, 86–7.

51 For a comparison between Burton and Montaigne, see E. Patricia Vicari, *The View from Minerva's Tower: Learning and Imagination in* The Anatomy of Melancholy (Toronto: University of Toronto Press, 1989), 194–95.

52 After the first edition, Burton expanded and revised *The Anatomy* for publication four times. For its publishing history, see Faulkner, Kiessling, and Blair, "Textual Introduction" in Robert Burton, *The Anatomy of Melancholy*, vol. 1, ed. T.C. Faulkner, N.K. Kiessling, and R.L. Blair (Oxford: Clarendon Press, 1989), xxxvii–lx.

mental and physical recreations capable of curing melancholy, Burton proposes a salutary meditation: "By this art [algebra] you may contemplate the variation of the 23 letters, which may be so infinitely varied that the words complicated and deduced thence will not be contained within the compasse of the firmament" (2:92). Only the property of type to combine and recombine itself in infinite possibilities could make visible this image of language as being centred on neither meaning nor subjectivity, on neither the human will nor the human body, but as being endlessly varied according to its own principle of random computation, its sheer materiality ultimately overflowing all worldly boundaries. The printing press reveals language to have an incomprehensible life of its own—to be an idiotic Babel machine, whose dead letters are absolutely other to communication.

*The Anatomy*'s own semiotic construction matches that which Burton laments the symptoms to be: a cacophony of clashing voices and tongues that make melancholy virtually incommunicable. Burton's phenomenology of language thus situates the symptom in a realm outside rhetoric, taken here to mean the practice and discourse of persuasion foundational to Renaissance humanism, education, and learning. As inherited from classical times, rhetoric assumes that the voice, either spoken or read, functions as a dialogical instrument for maintaining and building up the polis. As Stephen Pender observes in a discussion on medical reasoning's debt to rhetorical inquiry, "[t]he health of the body, the soul, and the polity are inextricably linked; one of their ligatures is the 'therapeutic word.'"[53] In contrast, Burton's tropes of linguistic disorientation spell out the breakdown of efficacious, healthy communication within the public sphere. The Tower of Babel represents voices as degenerating into civic chaos, and the labyrinth figures textuality as an alienating and bewildering architectural space. Ultimately, melancholy cannot be talked about with "a therapeutic word." For Burton the infinite symptom is symptomatic of the strange and unmanageable excesses and materialities of language in the age of print production.

[53] Stephen Pender, "Between Medicine and Rhetoric," *Early Science and Medicine* 10.1 (2005): 44.

# Chapter 10
# Medicine's Political Rhetoric: The Case of Bertini's *La medicina difesa*

Nancy S. Struever

This paper focuses on Anton Francesco Bertini's *La medicina difesa dalle calumnie degli uomini volgari, e dalle opposizioni de dotti* (1699). This tract is entirely political, since it is devoted to the negotiation, or renegotiation of the status of a discipline, its place among other disciplines; Bertini deals with the archetypically political construct of authority, that functions in medicine as the prestige that justifies the doctor's income, but, as well, as an essential factor in cure, the confidence in cure. Because the tract is political, it is highly rhetorical. In the preface he states the current predicament that has imposed his oratorical duty of defense: never, he claims, has medicine accomplished more, and, while it ought to be praised for its many beautiful *ritrovamenti*, never has it been so reviled.[1] Here he claims his rhetorical persona is that of a simple *dialogista*; when he states that he will speak in "*un modo de dire ordinario e piano*", he specifies not only his audience, but his ambition, the renegotiation of public opinion, the liberation of medicine from calumny; he wishes to rehabilitate, "*ripulire*", the doctor's reputation (233–34). What needed to be addressed were the public perceptions of a career, rather than the specific theories or therapies of the discipline. Chaim Perelman has argued that the primary rhetorical task is to create "adhesion of spirits" to the shared values of the community, and thus, he claims, the primary rhetorical genre is epideictic. This would define the *Difesa* as a quintessentially rhetorical enterprise, for the text of the dialogue is divided between the two epideictic genres of praise and blame. Bertini has his three protagonists, Diego, Francesco, and Vincislao, who represent national as well as theoretical identities, consider in the first book the *topoi* of blame; then Bertini assembles their responses in a second book of the *topoi* of praise, a book that is a display of tactics both of rebuttal and justification.

---

[1] *La medicina difesa /Dalle calumnie degli uomini volgari, e /Dalle opposizioni de dotti, /divisa/ in due dialoghi, e consacrata/ all'alto merito dell'/Em. Rever. Sig. Cardiinale /Jacopo Antonio Morigia ... Lucca: per i Marescandoli,* 1699. His defense, *Lo specchio, che non adula... Apologetica respondente ... Leida:* apresso Giordano, 1707, is in good part directed to attacks on his philological and rhetorical competence. The preface of the *Difesa* describes the occasion: "Non essendo mai stata la Medicina tanto colitvata da' suoi Professori, quanto nel Secolo presente, ne giammai in alcun tempo ridotta in tanto avvilamento, come oggigiorno... ," n.p.

Crucial to an account of Bertini's text is a phenomenological observation: Bertini's arguments draw heavily upon a common experience, a shared perception of a gap between medical theory and medical practice. This is, to be sure, a perennial context of traditional claims and counter claims about medicine. It is, as well, a shared perception that qualifies the judgments of a range of professions: law, and politics, and rhetoric as well as medicine. Most certainly it is an aporia that rhetoric and medicine share; and, both are beset by accusations of instability, relativism rooted in the "impurity" of their theoretical allegiances. But Roger French's *Medicine before Science* has pointed to some specific seventeenth-century issues; here he describes a double failure of both medical theory and practice; on the one hand, the seventeenth-century physician—whom he characterizes as the "Rational and Learned Doctor"—responds to a crisis in natural philosophy, the general discipline that supports medical theorizing.[2] Bertini observes that the traditional Aristotelian-Galenic system, with its *potenze, virtù, qualità,* cannot digest the new discoveries, new mechanical metaphors, new concepts of elements—*corpicciuoli, atomi, particelli. (*26*)* On the other hand, the major epidemics the practitioner confronts, such as the new "French disease", fail to respond to systemic therapies, elude systemic explanations. Further, French notes the continuation of earlier rivalries with other guilds: apothecaries, *speziali*, surgeons, which both challenge the theories and contest the boundaries of practice of the Rational and Learned Doctor.

That is to say, the theoretical training that establishes the physician's identity is perceived as having a difficult relation to clinical practice; this theory can be seen as old and outworn, or as too novel—that is, with no present connection to pharmacy or cures—or, as simply irrelevant to disease. The seventeenth century, with its bold new initiatives in theoretical paradigms becomes simply an outstanding historical example of the phenomenology of misperception. Thus, the discussion of medicine must take into account the general confusion about systems, distrusts of medical fashion, as well as suspicions of the ephemeral, ever-changing practices of cure. And, as well, a prominent issue in the historical accounts of medicine is the dark intrusion of socio-economic ambition in the practitioners of cure. Yet, one could argue Bertini's dominant strategy is word-play, discursive tactics to counter discursive events; the discussion is pervaded by modes of reflexivity, concern with discursive effect, "spin". Still, the word-play is not frivolous; Bertini's is a well-motivated response to early modern medical experience: to the perceived intransigence of the gap between theory and practice, a gap, moreover, that afflicts rhetoric, law, and politics as well as medicine, in all the professions of contingency. Thus we see in Bertini's text the disjunctions migrate, and the medical issues take on rhetorical, legal, and political coloring.

Still, Bertini claims he is not a panegyrist, not purely an encomiast. The project in no way can be defined as a simple praise of medical truth. The "cultivation"

---

[2] Roger French, *Medicine before Science; the Business of Medicine from the Middle Ages to the Enlightenment,* Cambridge: Cambridge University press, 2003.

of theories and practices is his topic only in so far as it does not meet with its proper positive response. Bertini does not simply recapitulate the beautiful *"ritrovamenti"*. The counter-intuitive move in Bertini's text is the seeming concession that dwelling on scientific issues is useless in the campaign for medical prestige; he does not proffer a simple narrative of the initiatives of medical research, or of the introduction of new models of the nature of medical-scientific inquiry. "Science", in our modern sense, seems beside the point; true, early errors can be corrected by later science, thus Democritus stands corrected by Galileo (199), but the great recent achievements have not been effective in preventing or silencing the revilings.

Bertini, then, deals in the rhetorical coinage of beliefs, not knowledge. The material sources of the text are the mass of *topoi*, the rubrics of common sense, available in the traditional literature: Pliny, Celsus, Galen, of course, but also Petrarch and Boccaccio. Bertini both presents and critiques the shared opinions, *endoxa,* the attitudes and dispositions of the historical communities from Classical times onward. The peculiar seventeenth-century context is a cloud of epistemological uncertainty, the pervasive attitude of skepticism on the part of the learned, and the puzzled credulity on the part of the vulgar, psychological attributes both perservering and subject to constant modification in the medical discourse. The task is not so much the explication of a medical *episteme*, but the reorientation of the audience towards the mass of medical topoi.

## The Strategies of the *Difesa*

Bertini ranges all the topics of discussion, and thus of the disconnection of theory from practice under four headings: first, medicine itself, that is, the present state of theory; second, the practitioners of medicine; third, the "practical" reception by the vulgar; and fourth, the reception by the learned enemies of medicine, the elite reception of theory. Under the first rubric, Bertini of course takes note of theoretical flux: he laments *"l'inconstanza d'opinioni"(25);* but he acknowledges that medicine transpires in the domain of the probable (43), and thus that the radical contingency of medical practice is a source of difficulty (18–19). At the same time, he responds to Celsus' critique of medicine as an *ars coniecturalis* (7), for conjecture is honorable, based on reason (145). He is certainly aware of the seventeenth-century confrontation of old and new systems. He is receptive, in general, to the new disciplinary matrices of natural philosophy, and contrasts the contemporary programs of reliance on observation and experience with the servility of the *settatori* of Aristotle (233; cf 37). But the new systems are not crucial to his argument, not capable of resolving the issues of perception of status. His historical account rehearses the traditional *topoi* of blame, but in the process he discounts them, to a certain extent, as not fresh, not appropriate. On the other hand, he recognizes that some contemporary investigative strengths may be of dubious value for contemporary practice; he is aware that there are disconnections between the *naturalisti* and the *medici*; theory may be ahead of practice (269); and here his account of the use of the microscope is exemplary of the problem of theoretical impertinence (45–50). One must note the, perhaps strategic, confusion: the division of opinions between the three dialogic protagonists both divide and muddle the theoretical issues.

His account of the *medici* as profession takes into account the Galenic aphorism that the ability to create confidence is at times essential to cure; our confidence in them is therapeutic. Still, at times he seems cognizant of an elite that gets, but does not deserve deference, and thus confronts the issue of just deserts. He rehearses Pliny's long list of fraudulent and dysfunctional practices of the doctors (Book 29; 12, 59–60) His narrations of specific practices seem "novelistic", creating hypercharacters in hyperplots. Many of the practices are discursive: inflated praise, *maldicenza*, duplicity in criticism, displays of false learning, plagiarism (59f). But the account includes issues of solidarity, "guildsmanship", and he cites the tradition's examples of a collaboration that preys upon the individual patient. Thus he remarks Petrarch's (Pliniesque) condemnation of the *turba medicorum* (57) the crowd of physicians attending the rich and powerful as either destructive of diagnosis, or simply too large a group for decorum (11) The incessant, indecorous quarrels and conflicts are necessarily destructive of confidence, and he dwells upon the contests of Ramazzini and Moneglia, a scandal of the late seventeenth century (51–2).

The tone shifts in the next section on, not just the practitioners, but the "vulgar" patients. There are errors of reception as well as production of medical discourse. The contests of the *medici* of course confused and afflicted not only the "volgo" but the educated, "*persone di senno e di capere*" (51–2). He characterizes vulgar error, however, in his phrase deploring the *"rozzezza del volgo"* (90f.); rawness, roughness stipulate receptive incapacity. The pretentiousness of medical learnedness is badly matched by the credulity, the indulgence in credulity of the ordinary patient. Just so, Ramazzini, a prolific and talented medical rhetorician, claimed that the *populares* are content to believe, rather than to know; they prefer a blind confidence to a confident judgment.

Then, Bertini's distress at the hostility to medicine of the learned is, I would argue, one of the sources of his disinterest in the defense of medicine as science (298–99). He can react to this criticism as a range of responses in good faith, to the use of skepticism, for example, as basically a considered reaction to the theoretical disarray of medicine, or to theoretical presumption, or to deficient systems, but, as well, to medical theoretical naivete. Bertini's statements on Lionardo Di Capoa are exemplary of his attitude to the learned enemies (109). Di Capoa is the Neapolitan author of *Il parere*, a medical-legal opinion that argues for a *libertas philosophandi*, freedom of medical inquiry as the best response to the endemic uncertainty in medical theory and practice. On the one hand, Bertini acknowledges Di Capoa's leadership, as physician, in the movement that contests the therapeutic value of bloodletting. (32). On the other hand, Bertini is appalled by the epistemological sophistication that Di Capoa displays in the remarkably dense historical account of medical theory and practice from the suggestions in the Homeric text on. Of course, both Bertini and Di Capoa are engaged in negotiating a place for a corporate discipline among other corporate disciplines in a period of considerable institutional and theoretic flux. But Di Capoa's desirable solidarity is one of theoretic methodology, Bertini's of professional, that is exclusive, authority. Di Capoa's skepticism has the practical goal of reform of contemporary medical institutions and research. The primary interest for Bertini pertains to the politics of cure, the necessity of maintaining the authority of the *medici* in the community of patients; thus, Di Capoa's strenuous critique, by describing only too well the gap between theory and practice, seems to undermine the authority of the doctor. It subverts as well the implicit assumption of Bertini that uncertainty in medicine should enhance, not detract, from the authority of the doctor. Again, there is a gross differentiation in motive between Bertini and Di Capoa; Di Capoa also may assemble the *topoi* of praise and blame, but these nourish his investigative ambitions, his reform program for corporate inquiry, which rejects dogmatism. But one should not attribute to Bertini's rhetorical division between the book of attack and the book of defense the aim of the formal rhetorical structure of debate *in utramque partem,* an aim to achieve a skeptic's suspension of judgment, a bracketing, *epoche.* Di Capoa's use of Montaigne, in contrast, is an effort to move the discussion to a different, higher plane. When Di Capoa notes the divergence between natural philosophical speculation and medical practice he opts for theoretical inclusiveness, eclecticism as sponsoring a diversity useful for progress, as a response to incoherence in practice. Bertini abets a rehabilitation of a corporate *political* identity, rather than a scientific posture.

## Medicine's Political Rhetoric

Rhetoric, according to Martin Heidegger's 1924 lectures on Aristotle, is not an autonomous linguistic *technē*, but functions *inside* politics. In his revisionary account of Hellenic thought, he claims the "original argument" transpired in the public discourse of the courts, the assemblies, and the oratory of the games; this was the competence of rhetoric, the original discipline; the philosophical and scientific tasks of dialectic and logic are thus late, derived. [3] One should consider Bertini's text as devoted to this originary rhetoric and its construal of community, constructions he describes as well as employs; thus he notes the doctors' political consciousness: "ciò facevano … per buona politica, volendo eglino provedere all loro riputazione" (42). Certainly, the historian of rhetoric will be struck by the lengthy, detailed treatment Bertini inserts of the Quintilianesque *declamatio: Pro matrem contra patrem,* which explores the moral implications of medical

---

[3] M. Heidegger, "*Grundbegriffe der aristotelischen philosophie*", 1924, notes by. W Bröcker, Herbert Marcuse-Archiv. 51. See the account of these lectures in P. Christopher Smith, *The Hermeneutics of Original Argument; Demonstration, Dialectic, Rhetoric.* Evanston: Northwestern University Press, 1998, esp. 21–34..

interventions (122f).[4] This tactic simply emphasizes Bertini's basic presupposition that medicine transpires in the domain shared with rhetoric, in the sphere of probability (205–206), where contingency requires that canons of decorum (202), appropriateness (145) be applied at all points. But the lamentable controversy, which concerns the mother's attack on the father's decision to allow the physician to sacrifice one brother to diagnose and cure the other, forces Bertini's reader to the awareness that the physician is embroiled in maneuvers of reception, of discursive effect, a concern with the patient as audience, and thus with the skills of persuasion, making-believe. And Bertini's organization itself points out that the physician must deal with the difficult divarication in audience between the *"rozzezza"* of the vulgar and the malice of the learned. (90f. 104f) The doctor must be cognizant as well of medical contests as disfiguring (50–51, 57–8, 232f.); he must become tactful in the use of praise and blame (249–50). Further, medical solutions themselves are of the form of rhetorical conclusions; that is, medical wisdom condenses in aphorisms, *topoi* that respond to the necessity of address to the general public. [5] And, of course, decorum itself, sensitivity to person, place, time, is part of the solution. (28f., 42, 126)

In sum, the Bertini text is of great value in exposing rhetoric as medicine's tarbaby, the indispensable liability, the discipline that shares untoward assumptions, offers questionable strategies. Reading Bertini on the guild's pronouncements, one would conclude that no other professional group has to work harder to maintain by means of discourse, not only its status and integrity, but to maintain the integrity of the discourse itself. And for the doctors, like the rhetoricians, even rhetorical success, as in the Quintilian controversy, prejudices the public: eloquence generates queries of integrity.

## Medical Rhetoric in History

Bertini's text is central, not peripheral, to the understanding of seventeenth-century medicine as cultural practice. Bertini historicizes the perennial medical experience depicted in the traditional texts; he considers the lived experience of cure, described as a manifold of affects, attitudes, beliefs, desires, temperaments—all the issues of character and passion, the rhetorical domain of argument. It contributes material to a Diltheyan project in intellectual history, an anthropology of a strand of seventeenth-century culture.[6] Dilthey claimed that all the major categories we

[4] The critical edition of this *Declamatio* is that of A. Stramiglia, *I gemelli malati: un caso di vivisezione,* in *Declalamzioni maggiori*, vol. 8.

[5] French, *Medicine before Science,* 229–30: he describes Bacon's and De Gorter's programs as essentially the revision, reclassification, and arrangement of the controlling aphorism or *topoi.*

[6] Wilhemn Dilthey, "Die Funktion der Anthropologie in der Kultur des 16. Und 17. Jahrhunderts", in *Weltanaschauung und Analyse des menschen seit Renaissance und Reformation,* in *Gesammelte Schriften*, II. Stuttgart: Teubner, 1960.

use in our rationalizations and justifications are derived from fundamental life-experiences; thus *our* historical descriptive psychology specifies the values of *their* anthropology, their speculation about beliefs, capacities, habits of action.

Bertini describes a "science" project, and I use *science* here in its modern definition, encapsulated in, or imprisoned in, a political predicament: he is concerned with a tissue of political responses to necessities of dealing medically with physical events of the life-world. Science is to one side of the argument because it acts within, is modified by, a predicament. The predicament of medicine as a practice, discipline perseveres through the strong novel changes in theoretical paradigms of medicine as science. The scientific initiatives function within the general experience of cure; systems face the radical instability of contingent events of discourse and therapy, thus novel theories produce novel theoretical consequences. This Diltheyan perspective illumines the motives of medical humanism in the sixteenth and seventeenth centuries, for example; humanists are not philosophers, Dilthey claims; their interest is not in metaphysics, logic, epistemology; they are, rather, psychologues and anthropologues. In so far as Bertini's rehearsal of classical-renaissance texts is humanistic, it is an effort marked by his humanist competence as psychologue, anthropologue, his capacity to appeal to emotions and desires, to change, affirm, or negate beliefs; his skill is in the depiction of medical experience.

My argument has been that the perceived gap between theory and practice in medicine is, in effect, unbridgeable. Theory can be refined, or discarded, or replaced; practice can be reformed, and institutionally reoriented, but the disconnection itself remains the topic of endless, and endlessly mutating debate. I would suggest the usefulness of the account of endless debate of W.B. Gallie's and Eugene Garver's development of the notion of essentially contested concepts and arguments. Gallie has claimed the perspicacity of the notion of essentially contested concepts for the history of thought, its usefulness for the characterisation of a vital genre of argument.[7] These are the concepts "the proper use of which inevitably invokes endless disputes about their proper use on the part of users".[8] But further, Gallie claims a "civilising function" for the distinction.

Recognition of a given concept as essentially contested implies recognition of rival uses of it (such as oneself repudiates) as not only logically possible and humanly likely, but as of permanent critical value to one's own use or interpretation of the concept in question; whereas to regard any rival as anathema, perverse, bestial, or lunatic means, in many cases, to submit oneself to the chronic human peril of underestimating or of completely ignoring, the value of one's opponents' positions. One desirable consequence of the required recognition in any proper

---

[7] See E. Garver, "Essentially Contested Concepts; The Ethics and Tactics of Argument", *Philosophy and Rhetoric*, 23 (1990), 251–70, here 251; henceforth cited by page number.

[8] Garver, "Rhetoric and Essentially Contested Arguments", *Philosophy and Rhetoric*, 11 (1978), 156–72; here 164. Henceforth cited by page number.

instance of essential contestedness might therefore be a marked raising in the quality of arguments in the disputes of the contested parties. And this would mean prima facie, a justification of the continued competition for support and acknowledgment between competing parties. (cited on 258).

Garver modifies Gallie's thesis by asserting contest precedes contest; as a theorist of rhetoric, he employs Aristotle's account in the *Rhetoric* of the formal structures of argument to claim that one does not start with substantive, hard-edged essentially contested concepts, but rather, the partisans of the argument determine the degree of contestability; it is a range of argumentative experiences that produces essential contest. The concepts are both parts of essentially contested arguments and are composed of essentially contested arguments, both the material for, and the products of arguments. His example of an essentially contested concept is "religion", with Judaism and Christianity as simply opposed versions of a single concept: they compete for the title (257). Just so, perhaps, Galenic and Hippocratic systems are competing versions of theory- for-practice. Garver goes on to assert that it is the radical particularity of rhetorical argument—its embeddedness in life-experience—that both insures the lack of theoretical closure, the certainty of the universal conclusions of dialectic, and promotes rhetorical strategies for particular practical ends.

Thus at the very core of rhetorical experience as well as medical experience is the aporia of theory-practice. Garver's motive is to show that "it is unreasonable and undesirable to demand that practical uses of theory possess more closure than essentially contested concepts will be found, after all, to possess" (252). The use of the construct is to separate theoretical from practical consequences; it is a more sophisticated, more intellectually advanced understanding of one's opponents and arguments. Bertini, I would argue, not only engages in an essential contest, but has a certain self-conscious, rhetorically self-conscious, relish about doing so. Certainly there is something *pro forma* about, not simply his listing of the traditional critiques, but of the traditional rebuttals of these critiques; the attacks are not so much refuted as acknowledged, the moral issues are not dismissed, but reviewed, reassessed. The aim, according to Garver, of essential contest is not to shut off debate, to demolish the opponent, but to amplify the argument in such a manner as to refine and specify new attributes of the essential concept. There is an odd generosity about Bertini's review of the failings, intellectual inconsistencies, practical vagaries in medicine. Accepting the radical contingency of practice is, in a way, a positive gesture, a proclamation of the difficulty and obscurity of the field itself, as both persevering exercise and enduring challenge. Just so, of course, in political speculation difficulties and challenges enhance rather than detract from the status of political agents and actions. Gallie, with Garver's help, makes us understand how the *Difesa* cannot function as an exercise in pure theory, because there cannot be a purely theoretical defense of a practice.

For the intellectual historian, then, Bertini's narrative of contest is of intrinsic interest; it suggests a continuity of predicament enclosing French's opposition of pre-scientific and scientific medicine which argues discontinuity. In considering medicine as a cultural practice, the primary essentially contested concept **is** the essentially contested argument concerning theory/practice as a duality, the difficult relationship that sponsors interminable, intractable debate. While modern "scientific" medicine offers an armamorium of weapons of defense against traditional attacks, weapons both procedural and discursive, the relation between theory and practice continues to trouble, engendering endless debates, producing, for example, an infinity of committees and commissions on medical ethics, and on the definition of the tasks of bioethics in general.

First, the most difficult problems arise from what one could call *metaphysical* differences, from arguments over systemic, fundamental notions of life and the status of living creatures within the practice as well as theory of medicine. In short, every issue can become, on some moral or political level, an issue of life or death. This stipulates gross difficulty in defining goals; not even a minor procedure can be protected from heavy-handed philosophical and theological appropriations and critique. According to Gallie and Garver, the assumptions in the contest are absolutely basic, truly contradictory, and intractable; both sides may command deep allegiances. Yet, the currency of medical contest is never pure idea; we are are dealing primarily with experiences: beliefs as energized knowledge, dispositions, habits of action. These beliefs are, at times, organized into narratives and become myths. If the Hippocratic interest in case histories is a medical taste for exemplary but idiosyncratic events, this places the discussion, as particularized, in the rhetorical domain; in the histories and doctor's *consilia* much depends on the effect of telling. What rhetoric deals with extremely well is the experiences and perceptions of cure and effect, and the putative inexhaustibility of experience makes the exercise valuable to medicine, even as it complicates and prolongs the contest. [9]

Second, there is, in medicine as discipline, a tendency to *bad theory*. Bertini's *Difesa* most certainly collects bad as well as good theory, and seems, for the most part, aware that the durability of the contest and its concepts has a source in the situation where medical practice and its discourse, with its strong, enduring professional obligations and constraints works against clarity and inventiveness in theory selection and formation. [10] The paths of theoretical and institutional developments often diverge; mathematical certainties may be unhelpful in therapy;

[9] It should be noted that Bertini, does not, like the seventeenth-century French physician, Marin Cureau de la Chambre, avail himself of rhetorical theory, the psychology that underwrites technique and effect; De La Chambre, of course, claimed that there were two essential elements to understanding humankind: the intellectual capacity of animals, and the character of the passions. The psychology behind Classical rhetorical theory posits an Aristotelian interactive continuum of faculties and actions—an inter-species as well as intra-species continuum, thus supports psychosomatic medical therapies; see my "Rhétorique et philosophie naturelle au XVIIe siècle; Le cas de Marin Cureau de La Chambre", in *Ethos et pathos: Le statut du sujet rhétorique*, ed. F. Cornilliat and R. Lockwood, Paris: Champion, 2000, 133–52.

[10] French, *Medicine before Science:* "...the university-trained doctor used his rationality and learning in the interests of professional success", 251; this has also a motive of self-promotion, 252.

or, "pure" physical theory is difficult to translate into tactful practice. But, can an element of contest be rooted in the resistance of the profession to flexible, perspicacious theory? Is there a conservatism built into professional defensiveness that fights against innovative theory? Bertini's text illumines the seventeenth-century dispositions and attitudes motivating medical modifications of theoretical language; practice requires appropriate, decorous theory, yet professionalism perceives a need for the holistic justifications of systemic theory. Thus medical practice itself insures endless contest; while it is the goal of medical research to seek certainty, truth, the doctors, like lawyers and politicians, do not have the luxury of exclusive concern with certainty; they must act.[11] As a result, the only profession encumbered with more pieties than theology is medicine; this Tartuffism sponsors almost continuous efforts of self-delusion.[12] "Professional", then, should not be easily or simply equated with "practical". Professionalism's ambivalence qualifies practical achievement in cure. The kind of theoretical elegance that prospers in texts, and supports status, is difficult to institutionalize. Certainly, public reception and learned critique are at odds, constantly, but also, as we note in modern times, no sooner does a new therapy, full of theoretical promise, appear, than a strenuous debate as to its delivery, its cost, its very access arises. Much of the discourse muddies the waters, confuses the issues by exploiting extraneous thematizations for professional advancement; the "status" "dignity" of medicine which is the topic of Bertini can sponsor an improper mutation of investigative concern.

Third, the issues as intractable, essentially contested, are reinforced in their obduracy by *politics*; the medical practitioner at every turn is beset by political demands. The individual doctor had to be a rhetorician, dealing in probabilities, concerned with audience, adept in negotiation; thus Bertini attributes to the doctor the motive of acting *"per buona politica".(42).* Fumaroli would argue, perhaps, that Bertini's text, like Moliére's *La malade imaginaire,* engages the practice of the "diplomacy of the spirit", the negotiations of new status in new societies.[13] And again we note perseverance: even the choice of silence, the eschewal of communicative skills of the modern trained medical professional is a moral/political choice, an attempt to signal that the doctor is above rhetoric. The modern invocations of the prestige of science can simply function as another rhetorical strategy. And, what are the constraints on the invocations that prevent them from being damaging to cure?

---

[11] This is a point made not only by French but by R. Jonsen and S. Toulmin in their *The Abuse of Casuistry.* Toulmin and Jonsen connect clinical medical practice with religious casuistry in the seventeenth century; in both cases, theoretical speculation must always be embedded in a practice.

[12] See French, *Medicine before Science,* 233f, on the weird pseudo-religious efforts in the eighteenth century on the part of Hoffmann, Stahl, and Rosetti.

[13] M. Fumaroli, *La diplomatie de l'esprit de Montaigne a La Fontaine*. Paris: Hermann, 1994. He sees *La malade imaginaire* as exemplary of the diplomacy of the spirit, the literary negotiations of that socialization of both the discipline or profession and of the public reception, embodying *"cette attention à autrui qui rendent sociable la vie sociale",* xv–xvi.

The need for decorous, appropriate cure imposes temporicity. There is a temporal dimension to these political careers in the confrontations of contingency, the unending challenges to produce the appropriate response; and "political" qualifies their contesting careers as producing victories and defeats, but not closure; all truly political issues must be grasped as open-ended, by their nature recalcitrant to closure. Thus Bertini's politics: in a sense, *La difesa* is an early modern political essay of intrinsic interest. On the one hand, Bertini deals with the central political problem of authority, a fundamental issue in all political theory and practice, all governmental definition, all legal process, but of peculiar interest to the seventeenth-century political discussion. But authority is an ancient medical issue. Edelstein has argued that Hellenic philosophers do not so much appropriate medical science and its methods for their inquiry, but, rather, they envy and try to appropriate the power of the doctor over the patient, seek to duplicate this authority in their relation to their disciples. The possession of a personal dominance even in, or even because of, the context of uncertainty, and in spite of any disjunctions between theory and practice, is what is enviable; they find remarkable authority persists through the imperfections, failures of performance.[14]

Still, Bertini's experience, and the medical experience of authority Edelstein describes is *anti-* political. If politics is defined rhetorically as the discursive negotiation of differences over matters of public utility, then doctor/patient rhetoric, in so far as the doctor's position is non-negotiable, and represents not a "political" but an autocratic regime. The range of issues, and the modes of dealing with the issues of Bertini's account, has the effect, at times perhaps unintended, of revealing the incoherence of the beliefs and activities that Bertini found in need of defense, and at a critical juncture when traditional theory and practice faced major revisionary moments.

## Medicine and Rhetoric

In the seventeenth century, Bertini historicized the medical experience, the phenomenology of doctor-patient interaction reported in the topoi of the tradition, and thus connected the seventeenth-century quarrels to the past. French, in his contrast of pre-scientific and scientific modes, emphazies disconnection in describing the seventeenth-century innovations in medical science as radically innovative; he seems to claim that modernity, at least modern medicine, escapes the phenomenological predicament, and thus escapes the endless debate of essentially contested concepts, and achieves closure. He notes that the early modern initiatives in the pathology of epidemics places medicine on the path to "science" through general remedies; solving a specific problem of response to a pathogen does offer certainty. Yet, the context of multiple and unintended consequences endures. And, people still die; a strong constraint on medical rhetoric.

14 L. Edelstein, *Ancient Medicine*, Baltimore: Johns Hopkins University Press, 1967.

Just so, a *New York Times Magazine* article carries the banner headline "Half of What Doctors Say Is Wrong" (note the use of "say", not "know", the emphasis on effecting discourse.) The article, in essence, simply reiterates the obduracy of the medical predicament Bertini described, for the *Difesa* is simply a prolonged exercise in the description of obduracy.[15] Bertini's detailed, compendious consideration of medical rhetoric not only saves the medical phenomena, but illustrates a peculiar reciprocity of medical and rhetorical experience. It points as well to a special, and originary, crux that invests the relation of medicine to rhetoric. B. Cassin, in her "Bonnes et mauvaises rhétoriques: De Platon à Perelman", confronts the judgments of rhetoric, and tries to counter the Platonic philosophical definition of rhetoric that, by reducing rhetoric either to sophistic (*Gorgias*) or to philosophy (*Phaedrus*), erases rhetoric as such.[16] The *Gorgias* example which argues that rhetoric is sophistic is a medical one. Gorgias, Plato's protagonist, narrates how the orator was able to persuade a patient to a cure where the doctor could not. Obviously, this asserts, on the one hand, that practice, cure, can not segregate the medical discursive art from medical science. But for Cassin, the use of the Gorgian example is as illustration of the basic character of rhetoric: rhetoric belongs in the problematic of effect, not intention. The account of medical experience is diagnostic of rhetorical capacity. For, and this is the topic of a brilliant article by Cassin on Quintilian's *Institutio oratoria* XII, 3, 12, "*philosophia enim simulari potest, eloquentia non potest*", dissimulation of authority—of doctor's systemic allegiances—is easy, dissimulation of the experiences of eloquence's audience—of patienthood—not; in Classical theory, only effect is *index sui*, not capable of *pseudos.*[17] Cassin then goes on to query Perelman's version of the dictum that effect defines, where he claims that, if the auditor's experience decides effect, the proper auditor for rhetoric to address is the Kantian universal auditor, the elite as rationalist. But this, according to Cassin, simply makes rhetoric the "ventriloquist" of philosophy; we are back to the *Phaedrus;* Cassin prefers a resolute pragmatism, an eschewal of intention, or philosophical ambition, for specific effect on specific, historical, audiences.

If we return to Bertini's *Difesa*, we can admire the pragmatic sophistication of his focus on medical rhetorical discourse. In his compilation of theoretical and practical difficulties in the reception of medicine—and this treatment is both "Classic", established, and anxiously contemporaneous—the auditors are

[15] We observe in modern discourse heavy entanglements of medical and political factors: attempts to clothe Senator Frist and Governor Dean in the garb of their medical authority; politicians seeking medical issues—abortion, prescription drugs, tobacco use, for political excitement.

[16] B Cassin, "Bonnes et mauvaises Rhétoriques: De Platon à Perelman", in *Figures et conflits rhétoriques*, ed. M. Meyer and A. Lempereur. Brussels: Editions de l'Université de Bruxelles, 1990, 17–37. "Si bien qu'à partir de Platon, le diagnostic complet devient, selon la sévère équation deux égale zéro: il n'y a pas une, mais deux rhétoriques, c'est à dire pas de rhétorique du tout, puisqu'au lieu de la rhétorique on rencontre ou bien la sophistique, ou bien la philosophie", 17.

[17] "Bonne et mauvaises Rhétoriques", 34; see "Philosophia enim simulari potest, eloquentia non potest, ou: le masque et l'effet," *Rhetorica* 13 (1995): 105–124.

necessarily both vulgar and elite, and even the elite is not equivalent to the pure Kantian universal auditor. Bertini describes a rhetoric of justification functioning inside medical politics, an atmosphere of revilings. Thus, where the Gorgian example illumines rhetoric's focus on effect, not intention, Bertini's rhetorical analysis of effect diagnoses bad politics, faulty intention, both an authoritarian *ethos,* and passionate bad faith in reception. True, as Cassin agrees, rhetoric is not political science; she repeats the Aristotelian claim that when it leaves the commonplaces for the specific places of politics, it leaves rhetoric for politics. But surely in Bertini we see his rhetorical acuteness in discriminating when the medical person's appeal to authority as source of cure becomes a bad appeal, charlatanry, the source of the "revilings" of the audience. Bertini discriminates good and bad performance within the context of the endless contest.

From another perspective, Gerald Bruns' article, "The Hermeneutical Anarchist", glosses Cassin's pragmatism; here he argues that it is the "provisionality" of rhetorical argument that is the source of its strength, is key to the quality of rhetoric.[18] Provisionality is the source of pragmatic strength. It is as well, I would claim, the argumentative interest that qualifies the medical axiom: "Do no harm". That is, consider specific effects, not system, not authority, and not, surprisingly, intention. Bruns as well glosses Garver's claim for the usefulness of essential contest as diagnostic; it supports Garver's argument that lack of theoretic closure may protect practice. Together, Cassin's problematic of effect, Bruns' premise of provisionality in argument, and Gallie and Garver's essential contest, describe a rhetorical hermeneutic that can not only save the medical phenomena, but may save medicine itself. The shared parameters of the medical and rhetorical domains underwrite shared investigative tactics. The hermeneutic explains the very peculiar weight of the maxim "do no harm": utilizing the rhetorical habits of inquiry protects practice from the combination of theoretic certainty and heroic intention, an intentionalist fallacy—from the coalescence of an aspiration for theoretic isolation, purity and invocations of moral reductionism in practice. Finally, Bruns goes on to argue that provisionality is a primary characteristic of modernity, or, at least, of modernity in art: "… this experience of possibility is what modernism is". [19] This suggests that Bertini's devotion to the durability, perseverance of the endless, essential contest is, not so much in opposition to French's assignment of modernity to the seventeenth-century medical science, as an illumination of a different definition of modernity and thus a different continuity. The rhetorical hermeneutic of predicament endures as "emancipatory", to use Bruns' term.

---

[18] Gerald Bruns, "The Hermeneutical Anarchist", in *Gadamer's Century: Essays in Honor of Hans-Georg Gadamer*, ed. J. Malpas, U. Arnswald, J. Kertscher, Cambridge; MA., MIT Press, 2002, 45–76.

[19] "The Hermeneutical Anarchist", 64: "Indeed it is not too much to see an internal link between hermeneutical experience and modernism itself, given that any experience of the modernist work at all presupposes the kind of reversal of consciousness "that characterizes the emancipatory character of hermeneutical experience", 63.

# Afterword
# The Place of Medicine in a General Account of Early Modern Intellectual History

Nancy S. Struever

What is most useful to situate the medical developments in early modern inquiry is not, it seems, Roger French's narrative of a simple progress from pre-science to science, as a disciplinary solidification of a specific investigative enterprise; rather, the French account subsists as a central, but narrow explanation of particular moments in the history of medicine. In general, it has not been helpful to consider early modern medicine as either pre-science, as anticipatory, or as anti-science, of a distressing theological bent; rather, it takes place in an encompassing inquiry practice that operates without the assurance, certitudes of science with its successive ordering paradigms.

It is perhaps more useful to employ Richard Rorty's figure, defining the history of thought as an enduring "general conversation," complicated, capacious, embracing disparities in theory, at times expansive of possibilities, at times constrictive. It is a conversation that is, over all, quite disheveled in nature, as responsive, always, to questions posed not simply in disciplinary arguments, but questions aimed from the general environment, requiring an externalist as well as internalist historical narrative. Thus, for example, we have David North's and Blair Worden's accounts of seventeenth century political theory and practice; North's focus is on a pervasive pessimism that required not Roman republican but Augustan texts to promote political speculation, and clarify political events, or Worden's dismissive claim that the republican accomplishments of the period, of both revolution and restoration, were small. Or, consider work in the history of science that argues that the Kuhnian domain of the Newtonian paradigm derives a great deal of energy from retrograde alchemical, mystical motives as well as straightforward experiential ones. Scientific triumphalism has some strange allies.

Then, medicine, beleaguered by extra-medical motives and demands, was and is a peculiar inquiry domain with its particular constraints that modify both traditional and innovative "modern" initiatives. Schmitters describes the Spinozan and Cartesian constructions of novel dualisms of mind/soul and body as both less generous in accounting for pertinent factors in medicine and more powerful in controlling the beliefs and habits of action in medical inquiry. They proffer an overpowering naturalism, acting simply as an obdurate necessitarianism. Schmitters, in claiming "vulnerability" as basic condition of possibility of cure, describes a "naturalistic" metaphysics as troublesome as the supernatural it replaces; to counter vulnerability Descartes proposes we attempt a "felt autonomy", and suggests, for example that Princess Elizabeth read Seneca for cure: a solipsism she rejects. Spinoza offers as response the creation of a super-identity, the body politic, but generated in a politics seemingly without words, without rhetoric.

Gross questions the commonplace—theology is necessarily anti-science—in his account of Melanchthon's Lutheran corrections of the Aristotelian theory of the passions, corrections that ground the "human sciences" as "meta-practical," and furnish a psychological basis for rhetorical/medical interventions. A rich German development intricates the ethical with the physical in a "physics of persuasion," and requires the transfer of techniques from rhetoric to medicine, to theology, to politics: to spiritual cure.

Solomon deploys two rather baffling tactics for a collection on rhetoric and medicine: she does not use Aristotle's *Rhetoric* on the passions in presenting the Aristotelian tradition, and she "demedicalizes" both the modern scholarship and the early modern accounts of the passions. She argues strongly for the prevalence, if not predominance of orthodox, traditional (Stoic) scenarios of rational control of the will, the appetites, the passions as both possible and necessary: reason as cure.

Williams argues the expansiveness of possibilities: claiming a symmetry between the structure of melancholy as disease and the structure of Burton's book as a treatment of melancholy as topic, he describes an infinite semiotic proliferation, a proliferation that tells us more, perhaps, about general early modern investigative habits than about specific medical work. Both the Babel and labyrinth tropes describe not so much an epistemological crisis as an epistemological frolic. Williams does not use the technical term "eclecticism," but this is, certainly, eclecticism rampant, resisting schools, colonising ranges of investigations.

Pender considers epistemological issues, resonances, if one can use such a fancy adjective to describe medical claims to knowing. Or, rather, Pender cites medical recognitions of the limits of knowing, specifying the probable as domain and uncertainty as parameter: medicine as "endless guesswork," conjecture. Yet, at the same time Pender provocatively suggests the sense of uncertainty as liberating. He notes that Cabanis, like John Cotta before him, proposes rhetoric as model for an inquiry practice of experiment, for cautious openness to "practical certitudes"; and, he argues Cabanis' "physiological monism" insures the moral relevance of medical interventions, the propriety, decorum of medical rhetoric.

To be sure, this collection focuses not so much on rhetorical and medical interventions, as on the general context for theorizing and intervening. Carlino makes a case for humanism as positive environment for medical inquiry by describing the intimate and very specific connections of Vesalius with northern Italian humanistic sodalities. He argues for a rather straightforward humanistic commitment, claiming that Vesalius saw his work as continuance as well as critique of classical anatomical investigations. But, as a general rule the peculiar and exasperating conformations of medicine as discipline modifies medical appropriations of general intellectual historical moments. In my paper on Bertini's *La medicina difesa* I have argued that a basic, persistent factor in the history of medicine is the gap between theory and practice, a gap perhaps unbridgeable and, as unbridgeable, modifying, dominating medical inquiry. There is a tension between an ambition for systemic, holistic theory (and its prestige), and the primary medical duty of decorous response to clinical circumstances. And certainly, medical inquiry, as part of the general intellectual historical conversation is at times inventive, expansive of possibilities, quite inclusive of different modalities—strict rationalist orthodoxy, Aristotelian psychological continua, eclectic tastes for contingency, or physical necessitarianism—but still resistant to the solidification of paradigm formation: medical initiatives could be as well "post-science" as pre-science.

In contrast, perhaps, the relations between rhetorical and medical moments are quite straightforward. As the present collection argues, it is not simply the case that medical and rhetorical activities are frequently intricated, but, as well, rhetorical investigations and motives illumine medical ones, often bringing out hidden or repressed dispositions. To focus on rhetoric sharpens the focus on medicine, on its issues and strategies, on its repetitive difficulties, minor or greater successes in its daily engagements.

Thus, both are rather shaky disciplines, both definable as what Ian Hacking called the "low sciences" of early modernity. They are disciplines certainly engrossed with the radically contingent, committed to dealing with phenomena not readily reduced to rigorous order; yet, certainly the historian must recognize that the strengths of an explanatory monoculture are countered by its weaknesses in confronting the irreducible diversity of a society's medical / political phenomena. They share a practical interest in a topic exemplary of those that subvert rigor, the passions—an interest expressed in formulations that are wide-ranging, declamatory, but often refined: passions as sources of error, health, power, virtue, illness. They share, or should share—partly through a recognition of troubling, irrepressibly obdurate factors such as the passions—epistemological modesty.

Consider Giglioni's strategic reversal: instead of the usual rhetorician's account of medicine, he offers a *medicus*'s view of rhetoric. We can count on Cardano for preferring investigations of dysfunction. His sense of the pathologies of rhetoric is acute. Here epistemological modesty—a sense of the incapacity for proper communication of proper knowledge—compounds almost equal parts of cynicism and moralism; the inadequacies in inquiry are delivered in delusions, self-delusions of expression. But Cardano's program is a civil one: "cognitive solipsism and moral self-sufficiency"—as in Stoic philosophy—are of neither theoretical nor practical value. Medicine and rhetoric serve a community; self-sufficiency, autonomy (of the inquirer) is not a desirable goal. Further, Cardano claims rhetoric as an allied inquiry, a *scientia animi*, with the capacity to diagnose dispositions, intentions that impinge on our welfare. Its canon of decorum—appropriateness—recognizes tactics proper to time, place, person.

From the classical definition of rhetoric as mastery of the possible means of persuasion, we derive thick accounts of the historical use of persuasive techniques; here are disclosed similarities in the technical initiatives of medicine and politics that run from the truly ingenious to the acutely embarrassing; embarrassing medical rhetorical uses were, of course, taken account of by classical critics. The texts of antiquity of course deal with the techniques deployed by the physicians to instill confidence in cure, central to therapeutic success. But the goal of securing the patient's confidence in cure is seamlessly connected with gaining society's belief in the status, prestige of the profession. The rhetorical techniques surface again in the civic-economic preemptions in Bath of medical therapies, exploiting modes of cure for civic-developmental ends. Moss describes medicine's complicity with, impatronisation by, civic spin. Here the emphasis is less on the persuasive use of rhetoric in building a patient's confidence than on a civic mission of persuading a general audience, a public, into patienthood, to feel the need for cure. Simple medical interventions, water therapy, become imbricated with the strategies of puffery, of an economic environment where medicine subsists as a local industry: early modernity as precociously modern.

The vogue of medicine is another factor. Just so, Sugg describes the excitement with which art and literature in general took up the medical news of the period. "Anatomising" as verb came to describe the best efforts of inquiry in general. Anatomy had strong connotations of invasiveness, violence, prurience, but also precision, rigor, skill. The pervasiveness of the usage illumines the reach of medical fashions. Here, certainly, the pervasiveness, stylishness is not the result of our modern retrospective historical judgments, but of a local, contemporaneous enthusiasm, for which rhetoric functions as evidence.

Finally, and counter-intuitively, metaphysical commitments, allegiance to very basic beliefs is exceptionally strong in medicinal justifications, exaggerated in rhetorical tactics of definition. Medical polemics engage a given society's presuppositions, and quite strongly and often. The complications of medical problematic are, in short, political and rhetorical ones. The sociality that defines a society's medical problems challenges, troubles their solutions.

# Bibliography

## Selected Primary Sources


Adamson, Henry. *The Muses Threnodie*. Edinburgh, 1638.

Aquinas, St. Thomas. *The Summa Theologica of Saint Thomas Aquinas*. 2 vols. Translated by Fathers of the English Dominican Province. Chicago: Encyclopedia of Britannica, 1952

Aristotle. *The Basic Works of Aristotle*, edited by Richard McKeon. New York: Random House, 1941.

———. *The Complete Works of Aristotle*, edited by J. Barnes. 2 vols. Princeton: Princeton University Press, 1984.

Augustine. *City of God*, translated by Henry Bettenson. New York: Penguin Books, 1984.

Bacon, Francis. *Advancement of Learning*. 1605. Edited by Brian Vickers. Oxford: Oxford University Press, 1996.

Bacon, Francis. *The Works of Francis Bacon*, edited by James Spedding et al. 14 vols. London: Longman, 1857–1874.

Baglivi, Giorgio. *The Practice of Physick*. Second Edition. London, 1723.

Barbaro, Daniele. *I dieci libri dell'Architettura di M. Vitruvio tradutti e commentate*. Venitia: Francesco Marcolini, 1556.

———. *In tres libros Rhetoricorum Aristotelis Commentaria*. Lyon: Sebastianus, 1544

Barrough, Philip. *The Methode of Phisicke*. London, 1583.

Baynes, Paul. *The Diocesans Tryall*. Amsterdam, 1621.

Bertini, Anton Francesco. *La medicina difesa dalle calumnie degli uomini volgari, e dale opposizioni de dotti*. Firenze, 1699.

Billingsley, H., trans. Preface to *Euclid, The Elements of Geometrie*. London, 1570.

Boyle, Robert. *The Works of Robert Boyle*. Edited by Michael Hunter and Edward B. Davis. London: Chatto and Pickering, 1999.

Bright, Timothie. *A Treatise of Melancholie*. London, 1586.

Bruele, Gualtherus. *Praxis Medicinæ, Or, the Physicians Practice*. London, 1632.

Buoni, Thomas. *Problemes of Beautie and All Humane Affections*. London, 1606.

Burton, Robert. *The Anatomy of Melancholy*, edited by Floyd Dell and Paul Jordan Smith. New York, 1927.

———. *The Anatomy of Melancholy*. Edited by T.C. Faulkner, N.K. Kiessling, and R.L. Blair. 3 vols. Oxford: Clarendon Press, 1989–1997.

Cabanis, Pierre-Jean-Georges. *An Essay on the Certainty of Medicine*, translated by R. LaRoche. Philadelphia, 1823.

———. *Du degré de certitude de la médicine*. 1798. In *Oeuvres Philosophiques de Cabanis*, edited by Claude Lehec and Jean Cazeneuve, Vol. 1. 2 vols. Paris, 1956.

Camillo, Giulio. *L'idea del theatro*. Fiorenza. Lorenzo Tormentino, 1550.

———. *L'opere di M. Giulio Camillo*. Venetia: Domenico Farri, 1579.

Cardano, Girolamo. *De ludo aleae*, edited by Massimo Tamborini. Milan: Angeli, 2006.

———.*Opera omnia*, edited by Charles Spon. 10 vols. Lyon: Jean-Antoine Huguetan and Marc-Antoine Ravaud, 1663.

Castiglione, Baldassare. *The Book of the Courtier*, translated by Sir Thomas Hoby (1561), and edited by J.H. Whitfield. London: Dent, 1974.

Celsus. *De medicina*, translated by W.G. Spencer. 3 vols. Cambridge, MA.: Harvard University Press, 1940.

Charleton, Walter. *A Natural History of the Passions*. London, 1674.

Charron, Pierre. *Of Wisdome*, translated by Samson Lennard. London, n.d. (before 1612).

Chiaramonti, Scipione [Scipio Claramontius]. *De coniectandis cuiusque moribus et atitantibus animi affectibus libri decem; Opus novi argumenti et incomparabile, cura H. Conringii recensitum*. Helmstedt: J. Müller, 1665.

Cicero. *Ad C. Herennium. De ratione dicendi (Rhetorica ad Herennium)*, translated by Harry Caplan. Cambridge, Mass.: Harvard University Press, 1989.

———. *De divinatione*. In *De senectute, De amicitia, De divinatione*, translated by W.A. Falconer, 1.14.24. Cambridge, MA.: Harvard University Press, 1923.

———. *De natura deorum*, translated by H. Rackham. Cambridge, MA.: Harvard University Press, 1933.

Cicero. *Tusculan Disputations*, translated by J.E. King. Cambridge, MA.: Harvard University Press, 2001.

Coëffeteau, F. N. *A Table of the Humane Passions*, translated by E. Grimestone. London, 1621.

Coghan, Thomas. *Epistolarum familiarium M. T. Ciceronis epitome secundum tria genera [...]*. Cambridge, 1602.

———. *The Haven of Health.* London, 1584, 1588, 1589, 1596, 1605, 1612, 1636.

———. *The Well of Wisdome, Conteining Sayinges Gathered out of the Olde Testament.* London, 1577.

Conring, Hermann. *De habitus corporum germanicorum antiqui ac novi causis dissertatio*. Helmstedt: H. Müller, 1645.

———. *De civili prudentia liber unus*. Helmstedt, H. Müller, 1662.

———. *Disputatio politica de civitate nova*. Helmstedt, H. Müller, 1662.

Cooper, Thomas. *The Mysterie of the Holy Government of our Affections.* London, 1620.

Cotta, John. *A Short Discoverie of the Unobserved Dangers of Severall Sorts of Ignorant and Unconsiderate Practisers of Physicke in England.* London, 1612.

Crooke, Helkiah. *Microcosmographia: A Description of the Body of Man.* London, 1615.

da Carpi, Berengario. *Commentaria.* Bologna, 1521.

Descartes, René. [A]. *Oeuvres philosophiques de Descartes,* edited by Ferdinand Alquié. 3 vols. Paris: Garnier Frères, 1963, 1967, 1973.

———. [AT]. *Oeuvres de Descartes,* edited by Charles Adam and Paul Tannery. 1 vols. Paris: Leopold Cerf, 1897–1913.

———. [CSM]. *The Philosophical Writings of Descartes,* translated by John Cottingham, Robert Stoothoff, Dugald Murdoch, and Anthony Kenny. 3 vols. Cambridge: Cambridge University Press, 1991.

———. *Treatise of Man.* Translated by Thomas Steele Hall. Cambridge, MA., 1972.

———. *The Passions of the Soul.* Translated by Stephen H. Voss. Indianapolis: Hackett, 1989.

Di Capoa, Lionardo. *The Uncertainty of the Art of Physic.* Translated by John Lancaster. London, 1684.

Dryander, Joannes. *Anatomia Capitis Humani.* Marburg, 1536.

———. *Anatomiae [...] corporis humani dissectionis.* Marburg, 1537.

Edguard, David. *De Indiciis et Praecognitionibus opus apprime utile medicis.* London, 1532.

Elder, W. *Pearls of Eloquence, or The School of Complements.* London, 1656.

Elster, Jon. *A School of Abuse.* 1579. In *Markets of Bawdrie: The Dramatic Criticism of Stephen Gosson,* edited by Arthur Kinney. Salzburg: Instut für Englische und Literatur, Universität Salzburg, 1974.

———. *Playes Confuted in Five Actions.* 1582. In *Markets of Bawdrie: The Dramatic Criticism of Stephen Gosson,* edited by Arthur Kinney. Salzburg: Instut für Englische und Literatur, Universität Salzburg, 1974.

Elyot, Thomas. *Castel of Helthe.* 1541. Edited by Samuel A. Tannenbaum. New York: Scholars' Facsimiles and Reprints, 1937.

Erizzo, Sebastiano, 1554, *Dell'istromento et via inventiva degli antichi,* Venetia: Plinioérotique. Toulouse: impr. Veuve J. & R. Colomiez, 1610. Paris: D. Moreau, 1623.

Fenner, William. *A Treatise of the Affections; or the Soules Pulse.* London, 1641.

Fernel, Jean. *Medicina.* Venice: Baldassarre Costantino, 1555.

Ferrand, Jacques. *Traité de l'essence et guérison de l'amour, ou De la Mélancolie*

Fletcher, Phineas. *The Purple Island, or the Isle of Man.* In *Poetical Works of Giles and Phineas Fletcher*, edited by F. S. Boas. 2 vols. Cambridge: Cambridge University Press, 1908.

Galen. *On the Passions and Errors of the Soul*, translated by Paul W. Harkins. Columbus: Ohio State University Press, 1963.

———. *Galen on the Therapeutic Method; Books I and II,* edited by R. J. Hankinson. Oxford: Clarendon Press, 1991.

Goineo, Giovanni Battista. *Defensio pro Romuli Amasei auditoribus [...].* Bologna: Bonardi, 1537.

Guidott, Thomas. *A Century of Observations [...] and an Account of the Lives and Character of the Physicians of Bathe.* London, 1675.

———. *A Collection of treatises Relating to the City and Waters of Bathe.* London, 1724.

Harvey, William. *Lectures on the Whole of Anatomy,* edited and translated by C.C.O'Malley, F.N.L. Poynter, and K.F. Russell. Berkeley and Los Angeles: University of California Press, 1961.

Heseler, Baltasar. *Andreas Vesalius first public Anatomy at Bologna, 1540,* edited by R. Eriksson. University Presspsala: Almquist & Wiksells, 1959.

Heywood, Thomas. *Apology for Actors.* London, 1612; rpt. New York: Garland Publishers, 1973.

Hobbes, Thomas. *Leviathan,* edited by C.B. Macpherson. Harmondsworth: Penguin, 1968.

———. *The English Works of Thomas Hobbes of Malmesbury*, edited by Sir William Molesworth. Aalen: Scientia, 1966.

Jorden, Edward. *A Discourse of Naturall Bathes and Minerall Waters.* London, 1631.

———. *A Briefe Discourse of a Disease Called the Suffocation of the Mother.* London, 1605.

La Chambre, Marin Cureau de. *Les charactères ces passions.* 5 vols. Paris, 1660–62.

Leonicenus, Nicolaus. *De Plinii, et plurim aliorum medicorum in medicina erroribus opus primum.* Ferrara, 1492.

Lessius, Leonard. *Hygiasticon, or The Right Course of Preserving Health.* Cambridge, 1634.

Luther, Martin. *Dr. Martin Luthers Werke: kritische Gesamtausgabe.* Weimar: Böhlau, 987 [1883].Mee, Dr. *The Character of a Compleat Physician.* London, 1680.

Melanchthon, Philip. *A Melanchthon Reader.* Edited and translated by Ralph Keen. New York: Peter Lang, 1988.

———. *Corpus reformatorum Philippi Melanthonis opera omnia,* edited by C.B. Bretschneider and H.E. Bindseil. 28 vols. Halle: C.A. Schwetschke, 1846.

———. *De rhetorica.* Wittenberg: Johannes Grunenberg, 1519.

Montaigne, Michel de. *Essays,* translated Donald M. Frame. Stanford: Stanford University Press, 1958.

Morhof, Daniel Georg. *Polyhistor literarius philosophicus.* Revised edition. Lubeck: Böckmann, 1714.

Nashe, Thomas. *The Anatomie of Absurditie.* London, 1589.

Papadopoli, Niccolò Comneno. *Historia Gymnasi Patavini.* Venetia: apud Sebastianum Coleti, 1762.

Paracelsus [Theophrast von Hohenheim]. *Sämtliche Werke,* edited by K. Goldhammer and Franz Steiner. Wiesbaden: Steiner, 1973.

Perkins, William. *The Whole Treatise of the Cases of Conscience.* London, 1606.

Placotomus, Johannes. *Oratoria de ratione discendi, ac praecipue medicinam.* Leipzig: Valentini Papae, 1552.

Primaudaye, Pierre de la. *The French Academy,* translated by T.B. London, 1586.

Protospartarius, Theophilus. *Theophili Protospartari de corporis humani fabrica libri quinque a Iunio Puolo Crasso Patavino in Latinam orationem conversi. Hippocratis preterea de purgatoriis medicamentis Libellus* [..]. Venetiis: Ottaviano Scoto, 1536.

Quintilian. *Institutio oratoria*, translated by H.E. Butler. 4 vols. Cambridge, MA., 1996.

Reynolds, Edward. *A Treatise of the Passions and Faculties of the Soul of Man.* London, 1650.

Securis, John. *A Detection and Querimonie of the Daily Enormities and Abuses Committed in Physick.* N.p., 1566.

Senault, J.F. *The Use of the Passions,* translated by Henry Earle of Monmouth. London, 1649.

Seneca. *On Anger.* In *Moral Essays*, translated by John W. Basore. 3 vols. Cambridge, MA: Harvard University Press, 1935.

Serlio, Sebastiano. *Il primo libro d'architettura* [...]. Paris: [Jean Barbé], 1545.

———. *Il secondo libro di perspettia [sic] [...].* Paris: Jean Barbé, 1545.

———. *Livre extraordinaire de Architecture [...].* Lyon: G. de Tourne, 1551.

Spinoza, Baruch. *The Complete Works,* translated by S. Shirley. Indianapolis: Hackett, 2002.

Stowe, John. *The Annales of England.* London, 1594.

Tomitano, Bernardino. *Ragionamenti della lingua toscana dove si parla del perfetto Oratore e Poeta volgari dell'eccellente medico e philosopho B.T. [...].* Venetia: Giovanni de' Farri, 1545.

Underwood, Robert. *A New Anatomie.* London, 1605.

Valla, Laurentius. *Opera.* Basil, 1540.

Varchi, Benedetto. *Opere.* Trieste: Lloyd, 1858–59.

Vaughan, William. *Directions for Health, Naturall and Artificiall.* London, 1612. Venezia: Francesco Marcolini, 1556.

Vesalius, Andreas. *De humani corporis fabrica libri septem.* Basileae: I. Oporinus, 1543.

Vettori, Pietro. *Petri Victorii commentarii in tres libros Aristotelis De arte dicendi. Positis ante singulas declarationes Graecis verbis auctoris.* Florentia: Giunta, 1548.

Wesenfeld, Arnold. *Dissertatio de natura definitionis.* Frankfurt, 1692.

———. *Passiones animi.* Frankfurt, 1713.

Wright, Thomas. *The Passions of the Minde in generall.* London, 1604; rpt. Urbana: University of Illinois Press, 1971.

Wylkinson, John. *The Ethiques of Aristotle.* London, 1547.

## Selected Secondary Sources

Agamben, Giorgio. *Remnants of Auschwitz: The Witness and the Archive.* New York: Zone, 1999.

Androeni, Annalisa. "Sangue perfetto che poi non si beve .... Le lezioni di Benedetto Varchi sul canto XXV del Purgatorio." *Rinascimento* 44 (2004): 139–223.

Angelici, Annarita. . *Sapienza, prudenza, eroica virtù. Il mediomondo di Daniele Barbaro,* Firenze: Olschki, 1999.

Arthur, T. J. "Anatomies and the Anatomy Metaphor in Renaissance England." PhD. diss., University of Wisconsin-Madison, 1978.

Atwill, Janet M. *Rhetoric Reclaimed: Aristotle and the Liberal Arts Tradition.* Ithaca: Cornell University Press, 1998.

Avesani, Rino. "La professione dell' 'Umanista' nel Cinquecento." *Italia Medievale e Umanistica* 17 (1970): 205–232.

Bailey, Alan. *Sextus Empiricus and Pyrrhonean Scepticism.* Oxford: Clarendon Press, 2002.

Barlow, Richard G. "Infinite Worlds: Robert Burton's Cosmic Voyage." *Journal of the History of Ideas 34.2* (1973): 291–302.

Baron, Hans. *The Crisis of the Early Italian Renaissance: Civic Humanism and Republican Liberty in an Age of Classicism and Tyranny.* Princeton: Princeton University Press, 1966.

Baulmin, James and Tita French Baumlin. "Psyche / Logos: Mapping the Terrains of Mind and Rhetoric." *College English* 51.3 (1989): 245–61.

Beier, Lucinda McCray. *Sufferers and Healers: The Experience of Illness in Seventeenth-Century England.* London: Routledge and Kegan Paul, 1997.

Bennett, Jonathan. "Descartes's Theory of Modality." *The Philosophical Review* 103 (1994): 639–67.

Benveniste, Emile. "La doctrine médicale des Indo-Européens." *Revue de l'histoire des religions* 65 (1945): 5–12.

———. *Problèmes de linguistique générale*. 2 vols. Paris: Gallimard, 1966, 1974.

Berwald, Olaf. *Philipp Melanchthons Sicht der Rhetorik.* Wiesbaden: Harrassowitz, 1994.

Beyssade, J-M. *La Philosophie Première de Descartes*. Paris: Flammarion, 1979.

Bolzoni, Lina. *Il teatro della memoria. Studi su Giulio Camillo*. Padova: Liviana, 1984.

———. "L'idea dell'eloquenza. Un'orazione inedita di Giulio Camillo." *Rinascimento* n.s., 23 (1983): 126–66.

Bonahue, Jr., Edward T. "'I Know the Place and the Persons': The Play of Textual Frames in Baldwin's *Beware the Cat.*" *Studies in Philology* 91:3 (1994): 283–300.

Bourgey, Louis. *Observation et expérience chez les médicins de la collection Hippocratique.* Paris, 1953.

Bouwsma, William J. "The Two Faces of Humanism: Stoicism and Augustinianism in Renaissance Thought." In *Itinerarium Italicum*: *The Profile of the Italian Renaissance in the Mirror of its European Transformations*, edited by Heiko A. Oberman and Thomas A. Brady, Jr., 3–60. Leiden: Brill, 1975.

Breymayer, Reinhard. "Bibliographie zum Thema 'Luther und die Rhetorik.'" *Linguistica Biblica* 21 / 22 (1973): 39–44.

Broughton, J. and J. Carriero, eds. *A Companion to Descartes*. Oxford: Blackwell, 2008.

Brown, Deborah. "The Rationality of Cartesian Passions." In *Emotions and Choice from Boethius to Descartes*, edited by Henrik Lagerlund and Mikko Yrjönsuuri, 259–76. Boston: Kluwer, 2002.

———. *Descartes and the Passionate Mind.* Cambridge: Cambridge University Press, 2006.

Browne, Robert M. "Robert Burton and the New Cosmology." *Modern Language Quarterly* 13 (1952): 131–48.

Bruni, Francesco. "Sperone Speroni e l'Accademia degli Infiammati." *Filologia e Letteratura* 13 (1967): 24–71.

Bruns, Gerald. "The Hermeneutical Anarchist." In *Gadamer's Century: Essays in Honor of Hans-Georg Gadamer*, edited by J. Malpas, U. Arnswald, and J. Kertscher, 45–76. Cambridge, MA.: MIT Press, 2002.

Burke, Peter. "Images as Evidence in Seventeenth-Century Europe." *Journal of the History of Ideas* 64 (2003): 273–96.

Burnyeat, M. F. "Enthymeme: Aristotle on the Logic of Persuasion." In *Aristotle's Rhetoric: Philosophical Essays*, edited by David J. Furley and Alexander Nehamas, 3–55. Princeton: Princeton University Press, 1994.

Burton, Robert. *The Anatomy of Melancholy*, edited by Thomas C. Faulkner, Nicolas K. Kiessling, Rhonda L. Blair. 3 vols. Oxford: Clarendon Press, 1994.

Bylebyl, Jerome J. "The School of Padua: Humanistic Medicine in the Sixteenth Century." In *Health, Medicine and Mortality in the Sixteenth Century*, edited by Charles Webster, 335–70. Cambridge: Cambridge University Press, 1979.

———. "The Manifest and the Hidden in the Renaissance Clinic." In *Medicine and the Five Senses*, edited by W.F. Bynum and Roy Porter, 40–60. Cambridge: Cambridge University Press, 1993.

Campana, Augusto. "The Origin of the Word Humanist." *Journal of the Warburg and Courtauld Institutes* 9 (1946): 60–73.

Capp, Bernard. *The World of John Taylor the Water-Poet 1578–1653*. Oxford: Clarendon Press, 1994.

Cardano, Girolamo. *Book of My Life*, translated by J. Stoner. New York: New York Review Books, 2002.

Carlino, Andrea. *La fabbrica del corpo*. Torino: Einaudi, 1994.

———. *Books of the Body: Anatomical Ritual and Renaissance Learning*, translated by John Tedeschi and Anne C. Tedeschi. Chicago: University of Chicago Press, 1999.

Carpo, Mario. *Alberti, Raffaello, Serlio e Camillo*. Genève: Droz, 1993.

Cartwright, Julia. *Baldassare Castiglione: The Perfect Courtier*. 2 vols. London: John Murray, 1908.

Cassin, B. "Bonnes et mauvaises Rhétoriques: De Platon à Perelman." In *Figures et conflits rhétoriques*, edited by M. Meyer and A. Lempereur, 17–37. Brussels: Editions de l'Université de Bruxelles, 1990.

Cavallo, Sandra. *Artisans of the Body in Early Modern Italy: Identities, Families and Masculinities.* Manchester: Manchester University Press, 2007.

Chamberland, Celeste. "Honor, Brotherhood, and the Corporate Ethos of London's Barber-Surgeon's Company, 1570–1640." *Journal of the History of Medicine and Allied Sciences* 64.3 (2009): 300–332.

Chambers, E.K. *The Elizabethan Stage*. 4 vols. Oxford: Clarendon Press, 1923.

Chapman, George. *Bussy D'Ambois*, edited by Maurice Evans. London: Ernest Benn, 1965.

Ciliberto, Michele. "I rapporti tra Vesalio e Varchi alla luce di documenti inediti." *Episteme* 4 (1972): 30–39.

Clark, Stuart. *Thinking with Demons: The Idea of Witchcraft in Early Modern Europe.* Oxford: Oxford University Press, 1997.

Colie, Rosalie. *Paradoxica Epidemica: The Renaissance Tradition of the Paradox*. Princeton: Princeton University Press, 1973.

Cook, Harold J. *The Decline of the Old Medical Regime in Stuart London*. Ithaca: Cornell University Press, 1986.

Conley, Thomas M. *Rhetoric in the European Tradition.* Chicago: University of Chicago Press, 1994.

Copeman, W.S.C. *Doctors and Disease in Tudor Times*. London: Dawson's of Pall Mall, 1960.

Copenhaver, Brian, "Aristotelianisms." In *The Columbia History of Western Philosophy*, edited by Richard H. Popkin, New York: Columbia University Press, 1999.

Corsano, Antonio. "La 'dialectica' di Girolamo Cardano." *Giornale Critico della Filosofia Italiana* 40 (1961): 175–80.

Crane, Mary Thomas. *Shakespeare's Brain: Reading with Cognitive Theory*. Princeton: Princeton University Press, 2001.

Crozier, Ivan Dalley. "Social Construction in a Cold Climate: A Response to David Harley, 'Rhetoric and the Social Construction of Sickness and Healing' and to Paolo Palladino's Comment on Harley." *Social History of Medicine* 13 (2000): 535–46.

Cruttwell, Patrick. "Physiology and Psychology in Shakespeare's Age." *Journal of the History of Ideas* 12 (1951): 75–89.

Cunliffe, J.W., ed. *The Complete Works of George Gascoigne*. 2 vols. Cambridge: Cambridge English Classics, 1907–1910.

Cunningham, Andrew. *The Anatomical Renaissance. The Resurrection of the Anatomical Projects of the Ancients*. Aldershot: Ashgate, 1997.

Cushing, Harvey. *A Bio-bibliography of Andreas Vesalius*. Second Edition. Hamden: Archon Books, 1962.

Damasio, Antonio R. *Descartes' Error: Emotion, Reason and the Human Brain.* New York: Putnam, 1994.

Dear, Peter. *Discipline and Experience: The Mathematical Way in the Scientific Revolution.* Chicago, 1995.

Des Chene, Dennis. *Life's Form: Late Aristotelian Conceptions of the Soul*. Ithaca: Cornell University Press, 2000.

Deswarte-Rosa, Sylvie, ed. *Sebastiano Serlio à Lyon. Architecture et imprimerie.* Vol.1. Lyon: Mémoire Active, 2004.

Dewhurst, Kenneth. "Locke and Sydenham on the Teaching of Anatomy." *Medical History* 2 (1958): 1–12.

Digby, Anne. *Making a Medical Living: Doctors and Patients in the English Market for Medicine 1720–1911.* Cambridge: Cambridge University Press, 1994.

Dilthey, Wilhelm. *Introduction to the Human Sciences: an Attempt to Lay a Foundation for the Study of Society and History*, translated by Ramon J. Betanzos. Detroit: Wayne State University Press, 1988.

Dinsmoor, William Bell. "The Literary Remains of Sebastiano Serlio." *The Art Bulletin* 24 (1942): 55–91.

Dockhorn, Klaus. *Macht und Wirkung der Rhetorik: Vier Aufsätze zur Ideengeschichte der Vormoderne.* Bad Homburg: Gehlen, 1968.

———. "Luthers Glaubensbegriff und die Rhetorik." *Linguistica Biblica* 21/22 (1973): 19–39.

Doob, Penelope Reed. *The Idea of the Labyrinth from Classical Antiquity through the Middle Ages.* Ithaca: Cornell University Press, 1990.

Duby, Georges. *Les trois ordres ou l'imaginaire du féodalisme.* Paris: Gallimard, 1978.

Dumezil, Georges. *L'idéologie tripartie des Indo-Européens.* Bruxelles: Latomus, 1958.

Eco, Umberto. *Semiotics and the Philosophy of Language.* Bloomington: Indiana University Press, 1984.

Edelstein, Ludwig. "Vesalius, the Humanist." *Bulletin of the History of Medicine* 14 (1943): 547–61.

———. *Ancient Medicine*, Baltimore: Johns Hopkins University Press, 1967.

Eden, Kathy. *Poetic and Legal Fiction in the Aristotelian Tradition.* Princeton: Princeton University Press, 1986.

Edmunds, W.M. and D.L. Miles. "The Geochemistry of Bath's Thermal Waters." In *Hot Springs of Bath,* edited by G.A. Kellaway, 143–56. Bath: Bath City Council, 1991.

Else, Gerald F. *Aristotle's Poetics: The Argument.* Cambridge, MA..: Harvard University Press, 1957.

Elster, Jon. *Alchemies of the Mind: Rationality and the Emotions.* Cambridge: Cambridge University Press, 1999.

Entralgo, Pedro Lain. *The Therapy of the Word in Classical Antiquity*, translated L.J. Rather and John M. Sharp. New Haven: Yale University Press, 1970.

Fahnestock, Jeanne. *Rhetorical Figures in Science.* Oxford: Oxford University Press, 1999.

Ferrari, G.R.F. *Listening to the Cicadas: A Study of Plato's* Phaedrus. Cambridge: Cambridge University Press, 1987.

Firpo, Massimo. *Gli affreschi di Pontormo a San Lorenzo. Eresia, politica e cultura nella Firenze di Cosimo I.* Torino: Einaudi, 1997.

Fish, Stanley Eugene. *Self-Consuming Artifacts: The Experience of Seventeenth-Century Literature.* Berkeley: University of California Press, 1972.

Foster, E. "From a Patient's Point of View: Illness and Health in the Letters of Lisolette von der Pfalz (1652–1722)." *Bulletin of the History of Medicine* 60 (1986): 297–320.

Foucault, Michel. *The Order of Things: An Archaeology of the Human Sciences*, translated by Alan Sheridan. New York: Vintage, 1970.

———. *The Birth of the Clinic: An Archaeology of Medical Perception*, translated by A.M. Sheridan Smith. New York: Vintage, 1975.

Fox, Ruth A. *The Tangled Chain: the Structure of Disorder in* The Anatomy of Melancholy. Berkeley: University of California Press, 1976.

French, Roger. "The Anatomical Tradition." In *Companion Encyclopedia of the History of Medicine*, edited by W. F. Bynum and Roy Porter, 81–101. Vol. 1. London and New York: Routledge, 1993.

———. *Medicine before Science: The Business of Medicine from the Middle Ages to the Enlightenment*. Cambridge: Cambridge University Press, 2003.

Friederich, Reinhard H. "Training his Melancholy Spaniel: Persona and Structure in Robert Burton's 'Democritus Junior to the Reader.'" *Philological Quarterly* 55 (1976): 195–210.

Fumaroli, Marc. *L'âge de l'éloquence.* Geneva: Droz, 1980.

———. *La diplomatie de l'esprit de Montaigne a La Fontaine*. Paris: Hermann, 1994.

Furdell, Elizabeth Lane. *The Royal Doctors 1485–1714: Medical Personnel at the Tudor and Stuart Courts*. Rochester: University of Rochester Press, 2001.

Gadamer, Hans-Georg. "Hermeneutics as a Theoretical and Practical Task." In *Reason in the Age of Science*, translated by Frederick G. Lawrence, 113–138; 119. Cambridge, MA.,MIT Press, 1981.

———. *Truth and Method*, translated by Joel Weinsheimer and Donald G. Marshall. 2nd, revised edition. New York: Crossroad, 1989.

———. *The Enigma of Health: The Art of Healing in a Scientific Age*, translated by John Gaiger and Nicholas Walker. Oxford: Polity Press, 1996.

Gardiner, Judith Kegan. "Elizabethan Psychology and Robert Burton." *Journal of the History of Ideas* 38 (1977): 373–88.

Garin, Eugenio. *L'Umanesimo italiano.* Rome and Bari: Laterza, 1964.

Garrett, Don. "Spinoza's Ethical Theory." In *The Cambridge Companion to Spinoza*, edited by D. Garrett, 267–314. New York: Cambridge University Press, 1996.

Garver, Eugene. "Rhetoric and Essentially Contested Arguments." *Philosophy and Rhetoric* 11 (1978): 156–72.

———. *Machiavelli and the History of Prudence.* Madison, 1987.

———. "Essentially Contested Concepts: The Ethics and Tactics of Argument." *Philosophy and Rhetoric* 23 (1990): 251–70.

———. *Aristotle's Rhetoric: An Art of Character.* Chicago, 1994.

Gatens-Robinson, Eugenie. "Clinical Judgement and the Rationality of the Human Sciences." *Journal of Medicine and Philosophy* 11 (1986): 167–78.

Gaukroger, Stephen. *Descartes' System of Natural Philosophy*. Cambridge: Cambridge University Press, 2002.

Giglioni, Guido. "Girolamo Cardano on the Passions and Their Treatment." *Bruniana & Campanelliana* 12 (2006): 25–40.

———. "Bolognan Boys are Beautiful, Tasteful, and Mostly Fine Musicians: Cardano on Male-Sex Love and Music." In *The Sciences of Homosexuality in Early Modern Europe*, edited by Kenneth Borris and George Rousseau, 201–220. London and New York: Routledge, 2008.

———. "Una nuova edizione del *De ludo aleae* di Girolamo Cardano." *Rivista di Storia della Filosofia* 25 (2008): 75–8.

Gilbert, Neil W. *Renaissance Concepts of Method.* New York: Columbia University Press, 1963.

Ginzburg, Carlo. *Myths, Emblems, Clues*, translated by John and Anne C. Tedeschi. London: Hutchinson Radius, 1990.

———. *History, Rhetoric, and Proof.* Hanover: University Press of New England, 1999.

Goldie, Peter. *The Emotions: A Philosophical Exploration.* Oxford: Oxford University Press, 2000.

Gowland, Angus. *The Worlds of Renaissance Melancholy: Robert Burton in Context.* Cambridge: Cambridge University Press, 2006.

Grabes, Herbert. *The Mutable Glass: Mirror-imagery in Titles and Texts of the Middle Ages and English Renaissance*, translated by Gordon Collier. Cambridge: Cambridge University Press, 1982.

Grafton, Anthony. *Cardano's Cosmos: The Worlds and Works of a Renaissance Astrologer.* Cambridge, MA.: Harvard University Press, 1999.

Grassi, Ernesto. *Rhetoric as Philosophy: The Humanist Tradition*, translated by John Michal Krois and Azizeh Azodi. Carbondale: Southern Illinois University Press, 1980.

Green, Lawrence D., ed. and trans. *John Rainolds's Lectures on Aristotle's Rhetoric.* Cranbury, NJ: Associated University Presses, 1986.

Grimaldi, W.M.A. *"Semeion, Tekmerion, Eikos in Aristotle's* Rhetoric.*" American Journal of Philology* 101 (1980): 383–98.

Gross, Daniel M. "Melanchthon's Rhetoric and the Practical Origins of Reformation Human Science." *History of the Human Sciences* 13.3 (2000): 5–22.

———. *The Secret History of Emotion: From Aristotle's* Rhetoric *to Modern Brain Science.* Chicago: University of Chicago Press, 2006.

Gusdorf, Georges. *Introduction aux sciences humaines; essai critique sur leurs origines et leur développement.* Paris: Les Belles Lettres, 1960.

Hall, John. *John Hall and his Patients: The Medical Practice of Shakespeare's Son-in-Law*, edited by Joan Lane. Stratford-Upon-Avon: Shakespeare Birthday Trust, 1996.

Harley, David. "Political Post-mortems and Morbid Anatomy in Seventeenth-century England." *Social History of Medicine* 7 (1994): 1–28.

———. "Rhetoric and the Social Construction of Sickness and Healing." *The Society for the Social History of Medicine* 12 (1999): 407–435.

Harris, William V. *Restraining Rage: The Ideology of Anger Control in Classical Antiquity.* Cambridge, MA.: Harvard University Press, 2001.

Hartfelder, Karl. *Philipp Melanchthon als Praeceptor Germaniae*. Nieuwkoop: B. de Graaf, 1964.

Have, Henk Ten. "Medicine and Cartesianism." *Theoretical Medicine* 8 (1987): 235–46.

Heidegger, Martin. *Being and Time*, translated by John Macquarrie and Edward Robinson. New York: Harper, 1962.

Helm, Bennett W. *Emotional Reason: Deliberation, Motivation and the Nature of Value*. Cambridge: Cambridge University Press, 2001.

Hembry, Phyllis. *The English Spa 1560–1815: A Social History*. London: Athlone Press, 1990.

Henry, John. "The Matter of Souls: Medical Theory and Theology in Seventeenth-Century England." In *The Medical Revolution of the Seventeenth Century*, edited by Roger French and Andrew Wear, 87–113. Cambridge: Cambridge University Press, 1989.

Heusser, Martin. *The Gilded Pill: A Study of the Reader-Writer Relationship in Robert Burton's* Anatomy of Melancholy. Tübingen: Stauffenburg, 1987.

Hill, Christopher. "The Medical Profession and Its Radical Critics." In his *Change and Continuity in Seventeenth-Century England*, 157–78. New Haven: Yale University Press, 1991.

Hodges, Devon L. *Renaissance Fictions of Anatomy*. Amherst: University of Massachusetts Press, 1985.

Hoffman, Paul. *Essays on Descartes*. Oxford: Oxford University Press, 2009.

Hunter, Kathryn Montgomery. *Doctors' Stories: The Narrative Structure of Medical Knowledge*. Princeton: Princeton University Press, 1991.

———. "Narrative, Literature and the Exercise of Practical Reason." *Journal of Medicine and Philosophy* 21 (1996): 303–320.

Hutchinson, D.S. "Doctrines of the Mean and the Debate Concerning Skills in Fourth-Century Medicine, Rhetoric, and Ethics." In *Method, Medicine and Metaphysics*, edited by R.J. Hankinson. *Apeiron* 21 (1988): 17–52.

Ingegno, Alfonso. *Saggio sulla filosofia di Cardano.* Florence: La Nuova Italia, 1980.

Jacyna, L.S. "Medical Science and Moral Science: The Cultural Relations of Physiology in Restoration France." *History of Science* 25 (1987): 111–146.

Jaeger, Werner. *Paideia*, translated Gilbert Highet. 3 vols. New York, 1939–44.

James, Percival Rowland. *The Baths of Bath in the Sixteenth and Early Seventeenth Centuries*. Bristol and England: Arrowsmith, 1938.

James, Susan. *Passion and Action: The Emotions in Seventeenth-Century Philosophy*. Oxford: Oxford University Press, 1997.

Jay, Martin. *Songs of Experience: Modern American and European Variations on a Universal Theme*. Berkeley: University of California Press, 2005.

Johnson, Mark. *The Body in the Mind.* Chicago: Chicago University Press, 1987.

Johnson, Ronald C. *George Gascoigne*. New York: Twayne, 1972.

Jones, Matthew L. *The Good Life in the Scientific Revolution: Descartes, Pascal, Leibniz, and the Cultivation of Virtue*. Chicago: University of Chicago Press, 2006.

Jones, Whitney R.D. *William Turner, Tudor Naturalist, Physician and Divine.* London: Routledge, 1988.

Kahn, Victoria. *Rhetoric, Prudence and Skepticism in the Renaissance.* Ithaca: Cornell University Press, 1985.

Kelley, Donald R. *Foundations of Modern Historical Scholarship: Language, Law and History in the French Renaissance.* New York: Columbia University Press, 1970.

———. Donald R. *History, Law, and the Human Sciences.* London: Variorum, 1984.

———. "Eclecticism and the History of Ideas." *Journal of the History of Ideas* 62.4 (2001): 577–92.

———. *The Descent of Ideas: The History of Intellectual History.* Aldershot: Ashgate, 2002.

Kennedy, George A. *Classical Rhetoric and Its Christian and Secular Tradition from Ancient to Modern Times.* Chapel Hill: University of North Carolina Press, 1999.

Knox, Dilwyn. "Erasmus' *De civilitate* and the Religious Origins of Civility in Protestant Europe." *Archiv für Reformationsgeschichte* 86 (1995): 107–135.

Knutilla, Simon. "Medieval Theories of the Passions of the Soul." In *Emotions and Choice from Boethius to Descartes*, edited by Henrik Lagerlund and Mikko Yrjönsuuri, 49–83. Boston: Kluwer, 2002.

Kocher, Paul H. "Lady Macbeth and the Doctor." *Shakespeare Quarterly* 5 (Autumn, 1954): 341–49.

Korkowski, Bud. "Genre and Satiric Strategy in Burton's Anatomy of Melancholy." *Genre* 8 (1979): 74–87.

Kristeller, Paul Oscar. "Humanist Learning in the Italian Renaissance." *The Centennial Review* 4 (1960): 243–66.

———. "Studies on Renaissance Humanism during the Last Twenty Years." *Studies in the Renaissance* 9 (1962): 7–30.

———. "The Humanist Movement." In *Renaissance Thought and Its Sources*, edited by M. Mooney, 21–32. New York: Columbia University Press, 1979.

———. *The Classics and Renaissance Thought.* Cambridge, MA.: Harvard University Press, 1995.

Kusukawa, Sachiko. *The Transformation of Natural Philosophy: The Case of Philip Melanchthon.* Cambridge: Cambridge University Press, 1995.

La Nave, Francesco. *Logica formale e dialettica nella filosofia di Girolamo Cardano.* Rome: Pontificia Universitas Gregoriana, 2004.

———. *Logica e metodo scientifico nelle* Contradictiones logicae *di Girolamo Cardano.* Pisa: Istituti Editoriali e Poligrafici Internazionali, 2006.

Lebuffe, Michael. "Spinoza's *Summum Bonum*." *Pacific Philosophical Quarterly* 86 (2005): 243–66.

Lehec, Claude and Jean Cazeneuve, ed. *Oeuvres Philosophiques de Cabanis.* 2 vols. Paris, 1956.

Levi, Anthony. *French Moralists: The Theory of the Passions 1585 to 1649.* Oxford: Clarendon Press, 1964.

Levin, A. "Venel, Fourcroy, Cabanis, and the Idea of Scientific Revolution: The French Political Context and the General Patterns of Conceptualisation of Scientific Change." *History of Science* 22 (1984): 303–320.

Lidz, Joel Warren. "Medicine as Metaphor." *Journal of Medicine and Philosophy* 20 (1995): 527–41.

Lin, Martin. "Memory and Personal Identity in Spinoza." *Canadian Journal of Philosophy* 35 (2005): 243–68.

Lloyd, G.E.R. *Polarity and Analogy: Two Types of Argumentation in Early Greek Thought.* Cambridge: Cambridge University Press, 1971.

Long, Pamela O. "Objects of Art / Objects of Nature. Visual Representation and the Investigation of Nature." In *Merchants and Marvels. Commerce, Science and Art in Early Modern Europe*, edited by Pamela H. Smith and Paula Findlen, 63–82. New York and London: Routledge, 2002.

Louis-Courvoisier, M. and A. Mauron. "'He Found Me Very Well; for Me, I Was Still Feeling Sick': The Strange Worlds of Physicians and Patients in the Eighteenth and Twenty-First Centuries." *Journal of Medical Ethics: Medical Humanities* 29 (2002): 9–13.

MacDonald, Michael. *Mystical Bedlam: Madness, Anxiety, and Healing in Seventeenth Century England.* Cambridge: Cambridge University Press, 1981.

Maclean, Ian. "The Interpretation of Natural Signs: Cardano's *De subtilitate* Versus Scaliger's *Exercitationes*." In *Occult and Scientific Mentalities in the Renaissance,* edited by Brian Vickers, 231–52. Cambridge: Cambridge University Press, 1984.

———. "Cardano's Eclectic Psychology and its Critique Julius Caesar Scaliger." *Vivarium* 46 (2008): 392–417.

———. *Logic, Signs, and Nature in the Renaissance: The Case of Learned Medicine.* Cambridge: Cambridge University Press, 2002.

———. "The Medical Republic of Letters before the Thirty Years War." *Intellectual History Review* 18.1 (2008): 15–30.

Marion, Jean-Luc. *Sur la Théologie Blanche de Descartes*. Paris: Presses Universitaires de France, 1981.

Matten, Mohan. "Empiricism and Ontology in Ancient Medicine." In *Method, Medicine and Metaphysics*, Ed. R. J. Hankinson. *Apeiron* 21 (1988): 99–121.

Mazzacurati, Giancarlo. "La fondazione della letteratura." In *Il rinascimento dei moderni. La crisi culturale del XVI secolo e la negazione delle origini*, edited by Giancarlo Mazzacurati, 237–58. Bologna: Il Mulino, 1985.

McClure, George W. *Sorrow and Consolation in Italian Humanism*. Princeton: Princeton University Press, 1991.

Meyer, Michel. *Philosophy and the Passions*, translated by Robert F. Barsky. University Park: University of Pennsylvania Press, 2000.

Mikkeli, Heikki. "The Cultural Programme of Alessandro Piccolomini and Sperone Speroni at the Padua Accademia egli Infiammati in the 1540s." In *Philosophy in the Sixteenth and Seventeenth Centuries. Conversations with Aristotle*, edited by Constance Blackwell and Sachiko Kusukawa, 76–85. Aldershot: Ashgate, 1999.

———. *Hygiene in the Early Modern Medical Tradition*. Helsinki: Academia Scientiarum Fennica, 1999.

Miller, Jacqueline T. "The Passion Signified: Imitation and the Construction of Emotions in Sidney and Wroth." *Criticism* 43.4 (2001): 407–421.

Morrissey, Mary. "Narrative Authority in Spiritual Life-Writing: The Example of Dionys Fitzherbert (fl. 1608–14)." *The Seventeenth Century* 15 (2000): 1–17.

Moss, Jean Dietz. *Novelties in the Heavens: Rhetoric and Science in the Copernican Controversy.* Chicago: Chicago University Press, 1993.

———. and William A. Wallace. *Rhetoric and Dialectic in the Time of Galileo.* Washington, D.C.: Catholic University of America, 2003.

Mugnai Carrara, Daniela. *La biblioteca di Nicolò Leoniceno*. Florence: Olschki, 1991.

Nance, Brian. *Turquet de Mayerne as Baroque Physician: The Art of Medical Portraiture*. Amsterdam: Rodopi, 2001.

———. "Wondrous Experience as Text: Valleriola and the *Observationes Medicinales*." In *Textual Healing: Essays on Medieval and Early Modern Medicine*, edited by Elizabeth Lane Furdell, 101–117. Leiden: Brill, 2005.

Nauert, Charles G. "Humanists, Scientists, and Pliny: Changing Approaches to Classical Authors." *American Historical Review* 84 (1979): 72–85.

Noreña, Carlos G. *Juan Luis Vives and the Emotions*. Carbondale: Southern Illinois University Press, 1989.

Nussbaum, Martha. *The Therapy of Desire: Theory and Practice in Hellenistic Ethics*. Princeton: Princeton University Press, 1994.

———. *Upheavals of Thought: The Intelligence of Thought.* Cambridge: Cambridge University Press, 2001.

Nutton, Vivian, ed. *Galen: Problems and Prospects*. London: Wellcome Institute for the History of Medicine, 1981.

———. "The Rise of Medical Humanism: Ferrara, 1464–1555." *Renaissance Studies* 11 (1997): 2–19.

———. "Introducing Renaissance Medicine to Tudor England," In *Natural Particulars: Nature and the Disciplines in Renaissance Europe*, edited by Anthony Grafton and Nancy Siraisi, 275–93. Cambridge,MA.: MIT Press, 1999.

———. *Ancient Medicine*. London and New York: Routledge, 2004.

O'Connell, Michael. *Robert Burton*. Boston: Twayne, 1986.

Ogilvie, Brian W. *The Science of Describing: Natural History in Renaissance Europe*. Chicago and London: University of Chicago Press, 2006.

O'Malley, Charles D. *Andreas Vesalius of Brussels, 1514–1564*. Berkeley: University of California Press, 1964.

Olivato, Loredana. "Dal teatro della memoria al grande teatro dell'architettura: Giulio Camillo Delminio e Sebastiano Serlio." *Bollettino del Centro Internazionale di Studi d'Architettura Andrea Palladio* 21 (1979): 233–52.

———. "Per Serlio a Venezia: documenti nuovi e documenti rivisitati." *Arte Veneta* 25 (1971): 284–91.

Ong, Walter J. *Ramus, Method, and the Decay of Dialogue*. Cambridge, MA.: Harvard University Press, 1958; repr. 1983.

Ore, Øystein. *The Gambling Scholar.* Princeton: Princeton University Press, 1953.

O'Rourke Boyle, Marjorie. "William Harvey's Soliloquy to the College of Physicians: Reprising Terence's Plot." *Medical History* 52 (2008): 365–86.

Outram, Dorinda. *The Body and the French Revolution: Sex, Class, and Political Culture*. New Haven: Yale University Press, 1989.

Pagel, Walter. *Paracelsus: an Introduction to Philosophical Medicine in the Era of the Renaissance*. Basel: S. Karger, 1958.

———. "Medical Humanism. A Historical Necessity in the Era of the Renaissance." In *Essays on the Life and Work of Thomas Linacre, c. 1460–1524*, edited by Francis Maddison, Margaret Pelling, and Charles Webster, 375–86. Oxford: Clarendon Press, 1977.

———. *From Paracelsus to Van Helmont: Studies in Renaissance Medicine and Science*, edited by Marianne Winder. London: Variorum Reprints, 1986.

Park, Katherine. "The Organic Soul." In *The Cambridge History of Renaissance Philosophy*, edited by Charles B. Schmitt, Quentin Skinner, Eckhard Kessler, and Jill Kraye, 464–84. Cambridge: Cambridge University Press, 1988.

———. "Natural Particulars: Medical Epistemology, Practice and the Literature of Healing Springs." In *Natural Particulars: Nature and the Disciplines in Renaissance Europe*, edited by Anthony Grafton and Nancy Siraisi, 347–67. Cambridge, MA.: MIT Press, 1999.

Parker, Robert Sorlien, ed. *The Diary of John Manningham of the Middle Temple 1602–1603*. New Hampshire: University Press of New England, 1976.

Paster, Gail Kern. "Unspeakable Deeds: The Comic Actor and the History of Shame." *Elizabethan Theatre* 13 (1994): 63–77.

———. "Nervous Tension." In *The Body in Parts: Fantasies of Corporeality in Early Modern Europe*, edited by David Hillman and Carla Mazzio, 108–125. New York: Routledge, 1997.

———. "The Body and Its Passions." *Shakespeare Studies* 29 (2001): 44–50.

———, Katherine Rowe, and Mary Floyd-Wilson, eds. *Reading the Early Modern Passions: Essays in the Cultural History of Emotion.* Philadelphia: University of Pennsylvania Press, 2004.

———. *Humoring the Body: Emotions and the Shakespearean Stage*. Chicago: Chicago University Press, 2004.

Patey, Douglas Lane. *Probability and Literary Form: Philosophic Theory and Literary Practice in the Augustan Age.* Cambridge: Cambridge University Press, 1984.

Pelling, Margaret. *Medical Conflicts in Early Modern London: Patronage, Physicians, and Irregular Practitioners, 1550–1640*. Oxford: Clarendon Press, 2003.

Pender, Stephen. "Essaying the Body: Donne, Affliction, and Medicine." In *John Donne's Professional Lives*, edited by David Colclough, 215–248. Cambridge: D.S. Brewer, 2002.

———. "Between Medicine and Rhetoric." *Early Science and Medicine* 10 (2005): 36–64.

———. "Examples and Experience: the Uncertainty of Medicine." *British Journal for the History of Science* 39 (2006): 1–28.

———. "Seeing, Feeling, Judging: Pain in the Early Modern Imagination." In *The Sense of Suffering: Constructions of Physical Pain in Early Modern Culture,* edited by Jan Frans van Dijkhuizen and Karl A. E. Enenkel, 477–503. Leiden: Brill, 2009.

Pigeaud, Jackie. *L'art et le vivant*. Paris: Gallimard, 1995.

Pirotti, Umberto. *Benedetto Varchi e la cultura del suo tempo*. Firenze: Olschki, 1971.

Pomata, Gianna and Nancy G. Siraisi, ed. *Historia: Empiricism and Erudition in Early Modern Europe*. Cambridge, MA.: MIT Press, 2005.

Porter, Roy. *Disease, Medicine and Society in England: 1550–1860*. London: Macmillan Press, 1987.

Pozzi, Mario, ed. *Trattatisti del Cinquecento*. Tomo I. Milano-Napoli: Ricciardi, 1978.

Rather, L. J. "Thomas Fienus' (1567–1631) Dialectical Investigation of the Imagination as Cause and Cure of Bodily Disease." *Bulletin of the History of Medicine* 41 (1967): 349–67.

Reeve, C.D.C. *Practices of Reason: Aristotle's Nichomachean Ethics*. Oxford: Oxford University Press, 1995.

Reiss, Timothy. *Knowledge, Discovery and Imagination in Early Modern Europe: The Rise of Aesthetic Rationalism*. Cambridge: Cambridge University Press, 1997.

———. *Mirages of the Self: Patterns of Personhood in Ancient and Early Modern Europe*. Stanford: Stanford University Press, 2003.

Rico, Francisco. *Le rêve de l'humanisme de Pétrarque à Erasme*. Paris: Les Belles Lettres, 2002.

Ricoeur, Paul. *The Rule of Metaphor: Multi-Disciplinary Studies of the Creation of Meaning in Language*, translated Robert Czerny. Toronto: University of Toronto Press, 1977.

Roach, Joseph. *The Player's Passion: Studies in the Science of Acting*. Newark: University of Delaware Press, 1985.

Roberts, K.B. and J.D.W. Tomlinson. *The Fabric of the Body: European Traditions of Anatomical Illustration*. Oxford: Clarendon Press, 1992.

Rorty, Amélie Oksenberg, ed. *Essays on Aristotle's Rhetoric*. Berkeley: University of California Press, 1996.

———. "Descartes on Thinking with the Body." In *The Cambridge Companion to Descartes*, edited by J. Cottingham, 371–92. Cambridge: Cambridge University Press, 1994.

Roth, Moritz. *Andreas Vesalius Bruxellensis*. Berlin: G. Reimer, 1892.

Rutherford, Donald. "Salvation as a State of Mind: the Place of *Acquiscentia* in Spinoza's *Ethics*." *British Journal for the History of Philosophy* 7 (October 1999): 447–73.

Rütten, Thomas. "Ludwig Edelstein at the Crossroad of 1933. On the Inseparability of Life, Work, and their Reverberations." *Early Science and Medicine* 11 (2006): 50–99.

Samuels, Richard S. "Benedetto Varchi, the Accademia degli Infiammati, and the Origins of the Italian Academic Movement." *Renaissance Quarterly* 29 (1976): 599–633.

Sappol, Michael. *A Traffic of Dead Bodies: Anatomy and Embodied Social Identity in Nineteenth-Century America*. Princeton: Princeton University Press, 2002.

Sawday, Jonathan. *The Body Emblazoned: Dissection and the Human Body in Renaissance Culture*. London: Routledge, 1995.

Scheible, Heinz. *Melanchthon: Eine Biographie*. Munich: C.H. Beck, 1997.

Scheurl, Christoph. *Briefbuch, ein Beitrag zur Geschichte der Reformation und ihrer Zeit*, edited by F. von Soden and J.K.F. Knaake. Aalen: O. Zeller, 1962.

Schmalz, Tad. "The Disappearance of Analogy in Descartes, Spinoza, and Regis." *Canadian Journal of Philosophy* 30 (2000): 85–113.

Schmitt, Charles B. *Cicero Scepticus*. La Hague: Martinus Nijhoff, 1972.

———. *John Case and Aristotelianism in Renaissance England*. Montreal: McGill-Queen's Press, 1983.

———. "Aristotle among the Physicians." In *The Medical Renaissance of the Sixteenth Century*, edited by A. Wear, R.K. French, and I.M. Lonie, 1–15. Cambridge: Cambridge University Press, 1985.

Schmitter, Amy. "The Wax and I: Perceptibility and Modality in the Second Meditation." *Archiv für Geschichte der Philosophie* 82 (2000): 178–201.

———. "The Passionate Intellect: Reading the (Non-)Opposition of Intellect and Emotion in Descartes." In *Persons and Passions: Essays in Honor of Annette Baier*, edited by J. Whiting, C. Williams, and J. Jenkins, 48–82. South Bend: Notre Dame University Press, 2005.

———. "On the Eternal Truths: a Commentary on Papers G. Walski, I. Agostini, and L. Devillairs." *Descartes e i Suoi Avverari: incontri Cartesiani II*, edited by G. Belgioioso, 61–70. Le Monnier Università, Lecce 2004.

———. "How to Engineer a Human Being: Passions and Functional Explanation in Descartes." *A Companion to Descartes*, edited by J. Broughton and J. Carriero, 426–44. Oxford: Blackwell, 2008.

Schneewind, J.B. *The Invention of Autonomy: A History of Modern Moral Philosophy*. Cambridge: Cambridge University Press, 1998.

Schoenfeldt, Michael. *Bodies and Selves in Early Modern England: Physiology and Inwardness in Spenser, Shakespeare, Herbert, and Milton*. Cambridge: Cambridge University Press, 1991.

Serjeantson, R. W. "Proof and Persuasion." In *The Cambridge History of Science*, 7 Vols. Vol. 3: *Early Modern Science*, edited by Katherine Park and Lorraine Daston. 132–75. Cambridge: Cambridge University Press, 2006.

Self, Lois S. "Rhetoric and *Phronesis*: the Aristotelian Ideal." *Philosophy and Rhetoric* 12 (1979): 130–145.

Shapiro, Lisa. *The Correspondence between Princess Elisabeth of Bohemia and René Descartes*. Chicago: University of Chicago Press, 2007.

Siraisi, Nancy G. *Avicenna in Renaissance Italy: the Canon and Medical Teaching in Italian Universities after 1500*. Princeton: Princeton University Press, 1972.

———. *Tadeo Alderotti and His Pupils: Two Generations of Italian Medical Learning*. Princeton: Princeton University Press, 1981.

———. *Medieval and Early Renaissance Medicine: An Introduction to Knowledge and Practice*. Chicago: University of Chicago Press, 1990.

———. "Girolamo Cardano and the Art of Medical Narrative." *Journal of the History of Ideas* 52 (1991): 581–602.

———. *The Clock and the Mirror: Girolamo Cardano and Renaissance Medicine.* Princeton: Princeton University Press, 1997.

———. "Anatomising the Past: Physicians and History in Renaissance Culture." *Renaissance Quarterly* 53 (2000): 1–30.

———. "Medicine and the Renaissance World of Learning." *Bulletin of the History of Medicine* 78 (2004): 1–36.

Skinner, Quentin. *Reason and Rhetoric in the Philosophy of Hobbes.* Cambridge: Cambridge University Press, 1996.

Smith, P. Christopher. *The Hermeneutics of Original Argument: Demonstration, Dialectic, Rhetoric.* Evanston: Northwestern University Press, 1998.

Smith, Roger. *The Norton History of the Human Sciences*. New York: Norton, 1997.

Snow, Charles P. *The Two Cultures and a Second Look.* Cambridge: Cambridge University Press, 1963.

Sorell, Thomas. *Descartes Reinvented.* Cambridge: Cambridge University Press, 2005.

Staum, Martin S. *Cabanis: Enlightenment and Medical Philosophy in the French Revolution.* Princeton: Princeton University Press, 1980.

Stolleis, Michael, ed. *Hermann Conring (1606–1681): Beiträge zu Leben und Werk*. Berlin: Duncker and Humblot, 1983.

Struever, Nancy S. *The Language of History in the Renaissance: Rhetoric and Historical Consciousness in Florentine Humanism.* Princeton: Princeton University Press, 1970.

———. "Vico, Valla, and the Logic of Humanist Inquiry." In *Giambattista Vico's Science of Humanity*, edited by Giorgio Tagliacozzo and Donald P. Verene, 173–185. Baltimore: Johns Hopkins University Press, 1976.

———. *Theory as Practice: Ethical Inquiry in the Renaissance*. Chicago: University of Chicago Press, 1992.

———. "Petrarch's *Invective contra medicum*: An Early Confrontation of Rhetoric and Medicine." *Modern Language Notes* 108 (1999): 659–79.

———. "Rhetoric and Medicine in Descartes' *Passions de l'Āme*: The Issue of Intervention." In *Renaissance-Rhetorik / Renaissance Rhetoric,* edited by Heinrich F. Plett, 196–212. Berlin: Walter de Gruyter, 1993.

———. "Rhétorique et philosophie naturelle au XVIIe siècle: Le cas de Marin Cureau de La Chambre." In *Ethos et pathos: Le statut du sujet rhétorique*, edited by F. Cornilliat and R. Lockwood, 133–52. Paris: Champion, 2000.

Sugg, Richard. *Murder after Death: Literature and Anatomy in Early Modern England*. Ithaca: Cornell University Press, 2007.

Summers, David. *The Judgment of Sense: Renaissance Naturalism and the Rise of Aesthetics*. Cambridge: Cambridge University Press, 1987.

Temkin, Owsei. *Galenism: Rise and Decline of a Medical Philosophy*. Ithaca: Cornell University Press, 1973.

———. *The Double Face of Janus and other Essays in the History of Medicine*. Baltimore: Johns Hopkins University Press, 1977.

Thorndike, Lynn. "Medicine versus Law at Florence." In his *Science and Thought in the Fifteenth Century. Studies in the History of Medicine and Surgery, Natural and Mathematical Sciences, Philosophy and Politics*, 24–58. New York: Columbia University Press, 1929.

Tilmouth, Christopher. "Burton's 'Turning Picture': Argument and Anxiety in *The Anatomy of Melancholy.*" *Review of English Studies* 56 (2005): 524–49.

Tracy, Theodor J. *Physiological Theory and the Doctrine of the Mean in Plato and Aristotle*. The Hague: Mouton, 1969.

Trimpi, Wesley. "The Ancient Hypothesis of Fiction: An Essay on the Origins of Literary Theory." *Traditio* 27 (1971):1–78.

Valente, Micaela. "Per una storia dei rapporti tra retorica e politica nel Cinquecento: Socrate e Cardano." In *Socrate in Occidente*, edited by Ettore Lojacono, 189–99. Florence: Le Monnier, 2004.

van der Eijk, Philip J. *Medicine and Philosophy in Classical Antiquity: Doctors and Philosophers on Nature, Soul, Health, and Disease*. Cambridge: Cambridge University Press, 2005.

Vasoli, Cesare. *La dialettica e la retorica dell'Umanesimo: Invenzione" e "Metodo" nella cultura del XV e XVI secolo*. Milan: Feltrinelli, 1968.

Vianello, Valerio. *Il letterato, l'accademia, il libro: contributi sulla cultura veneta del Cinquecento*. Padova: Antenore, 1988.

Vicari, Patricia E. *The View from Minerva's Tower: Learning and Imagination in* The Anatomy of Melancholy. Toronto: University of Toronto Press, 1989.

Vickers, Brian. "Rhetoric and Poetics." In *The Cambridge History of Renaissance Philosophy*, edited by Charles B. Schmitt, Quentin Skinner, Eckhard Kessler, and Jill Kraye, 715–45. Cambridge: Cambridge University Press, 1988.

Vitrac, Bernard. *Médicine et philosophie au temps d'Hippocrate*. Saint-Denis: Presses universitaires de Vincennes, 1989.

Vives, Juan Luis. *The Passions of the Soul: the third book of De Anima et Vita*. Translated Carlos G. Noreña. Lewiston, NY: Mellen Press, 1990.

Von Staden, Heinrich. "Anatomy as Rhetoric: Galen on Dissection and Persuasion." *Journal of the History of Medicine and Allied Sciences* 50 (1995): 47–66.

———. "Science as Text, Science as History: Galen on Metaphor." In *Ancient Medicine in its Socio-Cultural Context*, 2: 499–518. 2 vols. Amsterdam: Rodopi, 1995.

Walsham, Alexandra. *Charitable Hatred: Tolerance and Intolerance in England, 1500–1700*. Manchester: Manchester University Press, 2006.

Wear, Andrew. "Making Sense of Health and Environment in Early Modern England." In *Health and Healing in Early Modern England: Studies in Social and Intellectual History*, edited by Andrew Wear. Aldershot: Ashgate, 1998.

———. *Knowledge & Practice in English Medicine 1550–1680*. Cambridge: Cambridge University Press, 2000.

Wilson, Luke. "William Harvey's *Prelectiones*: The Performance of the Body in the Renaissance Theatre of Anatomy." *Representations* 17 (1987): 62–95.

Yates, Frances. *The Art of Memory*. London: Routledge and Kegan Paul, 1966.

# Index

For Product Safety Concerns and Information please contact our EU representative GPSR@taylorandfrancis.com
Taylor & Francis Verlag GmbH, Kaufingerstraße 24, 80331 München, Germany

www.ingramcontent.com/pod-product-compliance
Ingram Content Group UK Ltd.
Pitfield, Milton Keynes, MK11 3LW, UK
UKHW022012180926
475701UK00003B/329
*9781138246225*